Mosby's
Rapid
Review
Series

MEDICAL-SURGICAL
NURSING

Mosby's Rapid Review Series

MEDICAL-SURGICAL NURSING

Series Editor

Paulette D. Rollant, PhD, RN

President, Multi-Resources, Inc.
Newnan, Georgia

Deborah A. Ennis, MSN, RN, CCRN

Professor of Nursing
Harrisburg Area Community College
Harrisburg, Pennsylvania

second edition

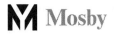

A Harcourt Health Sciences Company

St. Louis   London   Philadelphia   Sydney   Toronto

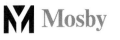

A Harcourt Health Sciences Company

Vice President, Nursing Editorial Director: Sally Schrefer
Senior Editor: Loren Wilson
Sr. Developmental Editors: Brian Dennison, Nancy L. O'Brien
Project Manager: Deborah L. Vogel
Design Manager: Bill Drone

SECOND EDITION

Mosby, Inc.
A Harcourt Health Sciences Company
11830 Westline Industrial Drive
St. Louis, Missouri 63146

Printed in the United States of America

Library of Congress Cataloging-in-Publication Data

0-323-01177-2

00 01 02 03 04 CL/MVY 9 8 7 6 5 4 3 2 1

Preface

HOW TO USE *MOSBY'S RAPID REVIEW SERIES*

Mosby's Rapid Review & Study Series is designed to help you get the most from your prep, study and review time for nursing exams. These books can be used to review essential concepts, theory, and content prior to nursing courses and challenge, certification, or licensing examinations. The rapid review series can also be used to prepare for clinical experiences and as a quick reference while in the clinical setting. *Mosby's Rapid Review Series* consists of three books:

Maternal-Child Nursing
Medical-Surgical Nursing
Nursing Pharmacology

The series is designed to highlight and prioritize important information about the specific content as indicated in each title. It is not meant to provide comprehensive, in-depth coverage of the selected area of nursing.

In the revised editions, the new features, "Fast Facts," "Warning," "Essential Odds and Ends" chapter, "WEB Resources," the updated bibliography, the glossary, and the revised questions, answers, and test tips give you the added advantage for test prep. The CD-ROM disk of 265 new higher level questions, which include management and home care content, provides an opportunity to practice for the real test.

Keep in mind that this series, in combination with other texts, should be consulted when a more comprehensive discussion of a particular topic is desired. Use these books to jog your memory, to reinforce what you know, to guide you to identify what you don't know, and to lead you to appropriate sources for more details. If you are in a formal education setting, these books are not intended as a substitute for class attendance or the completion of any required reading assignments.

Used consistently and correctly, *Mosby's Rapid Review Series* can help you to:

1. Enhance your skills to prioritize in clinical situations, especially management and home care situations, by applying the nursing process.
2. Increase your ability to easily remember essential content.

3. Increase the productivity of your review and study time to leave time for you and your family.
4. Apply new behaviors for the improvement of your test-taking skills.
5. Evaluate your strengths and weaknesses for specific content areas or testing situations.

WHAT IS UNIQUE ABOUT *MOSBY'S RAPID REVIEW SERIES?*

1. The 265-question test on an accompanying CD-ROM
2. Comprehensive rationales for each answer option
3. Test-taking tips to eliminate test-taking errors
4. Chapter format of the nursing process with prioritized content
5. Web sites and traditional bibliography for further exploration of content areas
6. Odds and Ends chapter for the unfamiliar
7. Glossary of key terms

Test questions on CD-ROM

Each book in the series is accompanied by a comprehensive exam of 265 questions. The comprehensive exam questions, like the end-of-chapter questions, include the answers, comprehensive rationales, and test-taking tips. The disk has a tutorial and a test mode. Both allow you to repeat the test as many times as you wish. The level of the questions varies from knowledge, recall, application, and analysis. In many of the questions, all the options are correct; the task of the test taker is to select the highest priority.

Comprehensive rationales

The rationales include the answers and the rationales for each option. In questions where all options are correct but they must be prioritized, rationales state why or how each option is correct and why only one option is the best answer.

Test-taking tips

These tips build your decision-making skills to set nursing priorities and for managing home care wisely. The tips help to further develop your logical thinking skills to narrow the options to two and then select the correct answer based on what you know. After working with the questions in these books or on the CD-ROM, you will more often select the correct answer on those harder questions. You will have increased confidence from new learning methods and actions to think "how can I answer this question" rather than "if I only knew. . . ." You will learn how to get the correct answer on those questions about content you don't know.

Chapter format

Each chapter contains an easy-to-follow format divided into five sections:

1. "Fast Facts" are placed at the beginning of each chapter. These items are the "must know" information in that chapter.

2. "Content Review" is organized and structured by the nursing process to help you identify what is most important. Within each chapter the highlights include:
   - All information within each heading is prioritized
   - Nursing diagnoses are prioritized
   - Goals are client-centered
   - The "Warning" feature is used throughout and focuses on critical and life-threatening issues
   - Client education is focused for the settings of hospital, clinics, and home
   - Management and home care content are included where applicable
   - You are alerted to issues regarding older adults where applicable
   - Evaluation criteria include decision-making tools about which actions to take when the client's clinical status shows improvement or deterioration
   - Tables, charts, and figures contrast, cluster, and simplify information for ease of grasp, recall, and review
3. "Review Questions" are stand-alone, four-option multiple choice questions. The test questions are of all difficulty levels and include management and home care situations for decision-making. The stems vary from being brief to lengthy to provide a realistic drill that mimics the NCLEX exam.
4. "Answers, Rationales, and Test-Taking Tips" focus on:
   - Comprehensive rationales, which are given for each option to explain why or how it is correct or incorrect. Additional information is given for less common facts or entities in the options. Other pertinent advice is also included to help your recall or review unfamiliar content or issues.
   - Test-taking tips give actions and strategies to use. For the more difficult questions, such as when options are narrowed to two; when you have no idea of a correct answer; when the content or issue is unfamiliar; or when all of the options are correct answers, specific approaches are given for each type of situation. The explanations include ways to prevent test-taking errors and ways to change your reading of the stem and options to get results— more correct answers. Specific prescriptions are given to raise your test scores.

"WEB resources" and bibliography

Web site resources for a particular condition, disorder, or topic are found throughout each book. A bibliography, including some books used in the development of the series, suggests areas for further study if more in-depth facts are needed.

Glossary

This list of key terms is provided to save you time in looking up unfamiliar terms or words.

WHAT'S IN *MOSBY'S RAPID REVIEW SERIES: MEDICAL-SURGICAL NURSING?*

This book is organized in a head-to-toe systems approach. The initial sequence of content is for the upper torso of the body: the neurological system, the cardiac system, with vascular and hematology areas, and the respiratory system. Following these chapters are the lower body systems: the gastrointestinal, the renal, the urinary, the reproductive, and the endocrine systems. The last group of chapters focuses on the body's overall safety needs with the musculoskeletal, the integumentary, and the immune systems.

This sequence will enhance your ability to recall content, especially if you have developed a review or study plan that is similar, and is also typically used to complete a physical assessment. In addition, the nursing process frames the content outline for each chapter. The outline uses consistent headings: each system's structure and function, targeted concerns, and pathological disorders, including subheadings for the nursing process: assessment, nursing diagnoses with client goals, nursing interventions, and evaluation protocol.

Each chapter is a synthesis of the many essentials needed by nurses in practice. The content is prioritized in major and minor lists. The most common elements are written to include what is essential for study and review, and to reference items in an expedient manner. The most common pathological disorders are included in each system. Acute and home care is part of each discussion.

ABOUT THE AUTHORS

The original idea, the design, and the development of the *Rapid Review Series* were by Dr. Rollant. The original co-authors were the content experts for their respective books. They provided their expertise and hard work to develop the specific content and the questions. In the first edition, Dr. Rollant expanded the rationales for the question answers and then added the test-taking tips for each question.

In this revised second edition, each book has an author who is expert in the field, and Dr. Rollant is the series editor. Dr. Rollant has directed, coordinated, and managed the consistency of the revision as well as provided additional test questions, rationales, and test-taking tips. Dr. Rollant, with the expertise of test-taking skills development, expanded the discussion in the rationales for the correct answer and the discussion of each option for the questions written by the authors.

As a team, the series editor and the authors have worked diligently to provide the best test preparation and review format available to nursing students and graduates. We wish you the best in your nursing career. We encourage you to let us know what you have found the most or least helpful and what other needs you may have for test preparation. You can contact Dr. Rollant at rollant@bellsouth.net or 22 Village Lane, Newnan, GA 30265.

ACKNOWLEDGMENTS

I express my heartfelt gratitude to those who have endured with me throughout this publication opportunity of a nursing review series: an adventure from idea to reality.

I especially want to thank the following people who were involved in the first edition of the review series:

Beverly Copland, who thought that I had the potential to complete this project and who eagerly gave me tons of strong support in the initial and ongoing book development phases.

Laurie Muench, who picked up the ball in the middle of manuscript preparation and persisted with me through the process to completion of book publication. The response "OK . . . when can I expect it?" provided silent encouragement and sometimes comic relief when my mental and physical energies ran quite low. Laurie's thoughtfulness and guidance to help me set priorities were invaluable! I am very grateful and fortunate to have worked with Laurie.

Suzi Epstein, who was full of enthusiasm and total support from the birth of the idea to the final publication of the books. Suzi's creativity and suggestions provided essential building blocks in the overall development of the series.

My *coauthors,* for their enormous efforts to produce manuscript in a short time. Their nursing expertise was helpful for the development of the unique aspects of each book.

I also want to thank the following people who were involved in this second edition of the series:

Brian Dennison, who headed up the meeting of the authors for the revisions, coordinated the manuscript schedule and provided guidance up to the production of the changes. Brian's creativity, framed with his organizational skills, allowed for the process to be quite enjoyable. Brian's patience and steadiness were of great strength to me.

Nancy O'Brien, who entered at the production phase and carried the task to completion; however, not without a lot of bumps along the way. Nancy left no stone unturned as she strongly supported my colleagues and me. I appreciate her talent, skills, and patience to enter a project midway and complete it with ease and detail.

My wonderful husband, *Dan,* for his patience, humor, support, and love. His faith in my abilities has sustained my energies and maintained my sense of self. He has been my sounding board throughout both editions of the review series and through the publication of the *Soar to Success: Do Your Best on Nursing Tests* book.

My parents, *Joseph* (deceased March 7, 2000) and *Mildred Demaske,* for their love, encouragement, and prayers.

Paulette Demaske Rollant

I would like to thank the following people for helping me through the writing and revisions of this text:

Bill, for his love and his never-ending confidence and support.

Heather and *Meghan,* for never complaining when Mom was too busy writing her book.

Mom and *Dad,* for encouraging me to go for the degree(s)—I wouldn't be where I am today without them.

Last, but not least, *Paulette,* for believing in me!

Deborah A. Ennis

Contents

INTRODUCTION
How to Use This Book
for Rapid Review
& Study

This book is designed to work for you at your convenience to save you time and energy. Read the following guidelines first. They will help save you additional time and energy for test preparation. These guidelines are divided into three areas of concern: the NCLEX-RN test plan structure, rapid study steps, and rapid review tips.

The chapters in this book are designed for short, quick intervals of review. Carry this book with you to catch those times when you are stuck and have nothing to do for that 5 to 15 minutes. Talk yourself into a brief rapid review and study period.

The directions for rapid review and study will give you the edge to:

- Maximize your individual performance on test prep and test questions
- Identify your personal priorities for test prep
- Sharpen your thinking and discrimination skills on multiple choice tests

NCLEX-RN test plan structure

The framework of *client needs* is the universal structure used on the NCLEX-RN. This framework of client needs defines the nursing actions and expected competencies across all settings for all clients. An integration of concepts and processes with nursing practice will be tested on the NCLEX-RN throughout the following four major categories of *client needs*. These categories, their subcategories, and related content, which includes, but is not limited to this list, are:

1. Safe, effective care environment
   - Management of care: advanced directives, advocacy, case management, client rights, concepts of management, confidentiality, continuity of care,

delegation, ethical practice, continuous quality improvement, incident/irregular occurrence/variance reports, informed consent, legal responsibilities, organ donation, consultation and referrals, resource management, supervision
- Safety and infection control: accident prevention, disaster planning, error prevention, handling hazardous and infectious materials, medical and surgical asepsis, standard (universal) precautions, use of restraints

2. Health promotion and maintenance
   - Growth and development through the life span: the aging process, ante/intra/postpartum and newborn stages, developmental stages and transitions, expected body image changes, family planning, family systems, human sexuality
   - Prevention and early detection of disease: disease prevention, health and wellness, health promotion programs, health screening, immunizations, lifestyle choices, techniques of physical assessment

3. Psychosocial integrity
   - Coping and adaptation: coping mechanisms, counseling techniques, grief and loss, mental health concepts, religious and spiritual influences on health, sensory/perceptual alterations, situational role changes, stress management, support systems, unexpected body image changes
   - Psychosocial adaptation: behavioral interventions, chemical dependency, child abuse/neglect, crisis intervention, domestic violence, elder abuse/neglect, psychopathology, sexual abuse, and therapeutic milieu

4. Physiological integrity
   - Basic care and comfort: assistive devices, elimination, mobility/immobility, non-pharmacologic comfort interventions, nutrition and oral hygiene, personal hygiene, rest and sleep
   - Pharmacological and parenteral therapies: administration of blood and blood products, central venous access devices, chemotherapy, expected effects, intravenous therapy, medication administration, parenteral fluids, pharmacologic actions and agents, side effects, total parenteral nutrition, untoward effects
   - Reduction of risk potential: alterations in body systems, diagnostic tests, laboratory values, pathophysiology, therapeutic procedures, potential complications after tests, procedures, surgery, and health alterations
   - Physiological adaptation: alterations in body systems, fluid and electrolyte imbalances, hemodynamics, infectious diseases, medical emergencies, pathophysiology, radiation therapy, respiratory care, unexpected response to therapies

Website: http://www.ncsbn.org/dxp.html
Other helpful sites:
National Student Nurses Association
    http://www.NSNA.org/index.htm
American Nurses Association
    http://www.ANA.org/index.htm

Rapid study steps

Step 1. Identify a study routine—What can be changed for efficiency and effectiveness?

a. What are your best days to study? First list or think about all weekly activities that are set, such as work time, your children's school obligations, or attendance at church.

b. Write these activities on the days of your personal calendar and the calendar at home – yes, the big one that everyone uses to coordinate family activities; it is usually in the kitchen on the refrigerator. Be sure to include the time needed for each activity, including travel time to and from the activity.

c. Oh! You don't use one. Maybe it is time to get one and get writing! This communicates the weekly needs to your family or support systems. It highlights the time you will be available or unavailable to them.

d. Now write in your study times. What are the best times to study? Just look at "the time left" on each day. Decide if you desire to schedule in study, relaxation, or catch-up activities at these times. Then stick to it.

e. To have designated study time written on a readily accessible calendar is a nice reminder every day to yourself that study is important to you. Be sure to cross off completed tasks! You will feel great as you cross off the completed daily or weekly study times. These actions give you a sense of accomplishment.

   1) Does the designated study time have to be blocked for at least a few hours? No. Set aside your designated study time in 15- to 30-minute increments. These times might be set when you know that others in the family will be involved in their own activities.

   2) Remember the nursing process: assessment of the immediate situation is the first step in any given client situation. Get started with the application of the nursing process to your own life. The more you use these steps in your daily life, the more skilled you become in answering those test questions based on the nursing process. Weekly, assess what time you have and what content is weak and needs attention.

Step 2. Launch a rapid textbook study routine for each given class

a. Scan the table of contents in your textbook, noting assigned required reading

   i. Put a check mark in front of the content for 10 items with which you are comfortably strong.

   ii. Circle 10 content areas with which you are shaky or which you dislike.

   iii. Prioritize the shaky content, then the comfortable content.

      1. Put numbers from 1 to 10 in front of your shaky content, and then in front of the comfortable content. Number 1 should be weakest content area and number 10 should be the strongest area within each category of shaky or comfortable content.

b. When you are feeling a high-energy day, go to the number 1 chapter of the shaky content area and read.

c. When you are having a low-energy day, go to the number 1 chapter of the comfort content area and read.

d. Continue to work your way through all 10 areas of each category. Once you have completed all areas, start again with this process for the remainder of the content.

Step 3. Resort to rapid chapter reading

a. Read the summary at the end of the chapter or the introduction if no summary is provided
b. Read the major and minor headings in the chapter in an attempt to put together a picture of the importance and the sequence of the content
   i. If you are at this point and it is before class, make a brief list of what you don't understand. Use this list as the basis of the questions that you ask during class.
   ii. If you are doing this after you have attended the class, more in-depth reading of the selected subject matter may be needed
c. Next, read each chapter. Start by first reading the sections of the unfamiliar subject matter. Use this process to read the paragraphs: Read the first and the last sentence of each paragraph. Then, if you need to read the entire paragraph, do so. Recall from English class that paragraphs are formed with the key sentences at the first and last position. Apply this "process of writing" to your "process of reading."
d. Continue to use this process for assigned readings, such as journal articles as well as for your enjoyment in reading books, newspapers or magazines

Step 4. Achieve actions for accurate and retentive rapid study

a. Develop a system of study that meets the needs of your schedule.
   i. Select time when you are least tired or stressed, both mentally and physically
   ii. Limit your study time to a maximum of 90 minutes. This time frame results in the most effective, efficient retention of content.
b. If possible, relax and take a nap after the study period to cement the information into your long-term memory. Some research reveals that sleeping for 2 to 3 hours after studying results in a 70% to 80% retention rate of content in long-term memory. In contrast only a 30% to 40% retention rate is achieved when you are active after the study session.
c. Breathe deeply and slowly three times at the onset and at the end of your study time. S-L-O-W, deep breathing with concentration on the air going in and out is one of the best ways get relaxed, both physically and mentally.
d. Use one other relaxation technique at the half way mark of your study session
e. If your time is limited, use 10- to 15 minute intervals to study small pieces of the content. For example, you may want to review the different aspects of hypertension in one study session.

Step 5. Select a theme for the day

a. When you plan at the beginning of the semester, use the approach of selecting a theme or topic for the day. For example, if there is enough time between your test and when you begin to study, review something every Monday on sodium from the book. Then, at work, find clients with sodium imbalances, review their charts, and discuss their situations with colleagues or with the clients' physicians. Continue with themes for each day such as:

  3) Tuesdays: potassium.
  4) Wednesdays: calcium.
  5) Thursdays: magnesium.
  6) Fridays: acidosis situations.
  7) Saturdays: alkalosis situations.
  8) Sundays: fun days. Don't forget to keep one day to relax and have fun. This allows your mind to work; your mind will automatically reorganize the retained content for better recall.

b. Weekly themes also might be of help. Do one system per week, such as pulmonary, endocrine, and so forth. Think of a way to associate the theme with meaning. For example, during the first week study the pulmonary system since this is the first system with BCLS. Then during the second week, study the cardiovascular system.

Step 6. Set up a study place

a. Designate a place to sit and study. Have all of your schoolbooks, references, computer, and so forth, at this location for ease of access.

b. A designated study place eliminates the "set up" time if all of your stuff is centralized and not scattered throughout the house. You can get more done in less time.

c. On days you aren't motivated to study, simply sit at this location for a minimum of 5 minutes. Within that time frame, tell yourself you might "flip through" a book. Before you know it, you will be into a productive study session.

Rapid review tips

1. Are there a few basic essential actions I can use for recall? Yes! Yes! Yes!
   a. Use yellow or lime green notebook paper or index cards. These colors enhance recall in long-term memory.
   b. Underline single words instead of phrases. The mind becomes more alert and attentive.
   c. Use a lime green or yellow highlighter
   d. PRINT with CAPS when you make notes. Recall is enhanced. Avoid cursive writing of notes.
   e. Talk out loud to whomever will listen—even talk to your pets—cat, dog or fish.
   f. Review for 15 to 30 minutes before you go to sleep.
   g. Repeat items at least 3 times.
2. How can I use this review book for a rapid review before my class?
   a. Complete the review questions at the end of each chapter for a specified content area.
   b. Review the answers, rationales, and test-taking tips.

c. Review content for the missed areas.

d. Refer to your textbook, which has more details, if you still do not understand the information.

3. How should I use my notes from class?

a. Read over your notes from class—every day! Yes, every day! Three repetitions enhance recall: You hear the instructor. You take notes. You reread your notes.

b. Every day before going to sleep, take 10 minutes for a quick read-over of your class notes.

c. Read over the notes for each class in the same sequence as the classes were attended that day.

4. What is an easy way to know key terms or content?

a. Card them.

b. Use a 3- x 5-inch index card to write the terms or condition on one side and the definitions of the key terms or the content information on the opposite side.

c. Use the nursing process format to outline critical content.

d. Look at the term and state your definition out loud.

e. Uncover the definition and read the given definition out loud.

f. Speaking the content as well as seeing the content will enhance your retention. If you have a few related terms that you can't remember, make a story out of the terms.

g. Carry the card with you for a few days to review this content again. Suggestion: put these cards on your sun visor in the car and review them at the stoplight or if stopped in traffic.

5. How can I prepare for the end of the semester comprehensive exam?

a. Complete the comprehensive exam on the CD-ROM. Use it in the test mode.

b. Review which questions were missed. Be sure to read the rationales and test-taking tips.

c. Note if the test item was missed because of a lack of content knowledge or because you simply misread the question or some of the options.

d. If a content problem is identified, list the specific content missed. Then cluster these under umbrellas of similar content. Use index cards for this activity.

   i. Prioritize these clusters, with number 1 being the least familiar content.

   ii. Review additional content as indicated by the questions that you missed.

   iii. Review the most familiar content last, or on low-energy days. Review the weakest content first, or on high-energy days.

e. If your problem was identified as misreading, make a list of where the misreading occurred—in the question? In an option? If in an option, which one? Is there a pattern to the misread options? Was the misread option a series of items or a two-part option? Did you misread the second part of the option? Identify the pattern of errors you made in reading. Most test takers have 3 to 5 consistent errors that they repeat over and over again.

Think of actions that you can take to eliminate or minimize these types of testing errors.

6. Should I repeat the same practice test questions?
   a. Yes. However, do practice questions at different times of the day than when the comprehensive test was initially done. Repeat the comprehensive exam on the CD-ROM in the test mode, and then in the tutorial mode, and then again in the test mode.
   b. Note whether the test item was missed because of a lack of content knowledge or because of simply misreading the question or some of the options.
   c. Note that even though the questions are repeated, you should evaluate how your reading of the questions and options differed.
   d. Do you have a pattern in perception and consistent ability to identify key words, terms, age, and developmental needs?
   e. Did the fatigue factor or tenseness influence your thinking skills? And what did you do or could you have done to minimize these factors to improve your abilities?
   f. Did anticipatory thinking of the correct answer enhance or hinder your selection of the correct answer?
   g. Doing the same test questions over can be helpful to reinforce content, fine tune test skills, and establish better reading habits

7. How do I evaluate my performance for testing?
   a. For any practice test questions, read all of the rationales and test-taking tips. Do this for the questions you got correct and those that you missed. The rationales and test-taking tips often contain pearls of wisdom on how to remember or get a better understanding of the content.
   b. Remember to do a relaxation exercise before you begin your questions, during the examination, and as you review the results. Do at least one mental and one physical relaxation exercise at least every 30 minutes or every 30 questions.
   c. When you miss a question ask yourself:
      i. Did I not know the content?
      ii. Did I misread the question or options?
   d. If you miss questions because of a knowledge deficit:
      i. Make a list on a 3- x 5-inch card for 3 to 4 days.
      ii. Group or cluster the content according to the steps in the nursing process, the content area, or a system.
      iii. Look up that content.
      iv. Do not look up content after every practice test. A better approach is to cluster the content and look it all up every 3 to 4 days. With this approach you will have better retention in long-term memory and the best recall at a later time.
   e. If you misread the question or the option(s):
      i. Try to identify new ways to approach reading questions and their options.
      ii. Try to identify what key words, time frames, ages, and developmental stages that you may have overlooked.

8. How can I improve my test scores?
   a. Practice, practice, and practice doing questions.
   b. Practice, practice, and practice doing relaxation before you begin the practice exam, after every 10 to 20 questions, and then at the end of the examination to refresh your thinking and diminish your tenseness or tiredness.
   c. Look for a pattern or cluster of wrong answers.
       i. Where did you miss questions?
      ii. Are there clusters of missed questions? If so, did this happen after what type of question? One related to the nursing process? One that asks for a priority and where all of the options are correct? One that had terms of "all but the following?" One that asked for the most or the least important item? One that had information you had never seen?
     iii. Did you miss clusters of questions at the beginning of the test?
          1. If so, you have a tension or anxiety problem.
          2. Simply do at least one mental and one physical relaxation exercise before the test and at question 25 to control your thinking.
      iv. Did you miss clusters of questions at the middle or the end of the test?
          1. If so, you have a fatigue or tiredness problem.
          2. First be alert to the event of "feeling tired" or fatigued.
          3. When you feel this way, get up and leave the room for 2 to 4 minutes. While you are out of the room, MOVE and be active. Touch your toes 10 times. Swing your arms from side to side. Mentally tell yourself: "I know something. I'll figure it out."
          4. Return to the test in a more sharp, attentive state.
9. What is most essential to preparation for the NCLEX? What are the most essential actions to prepare for "the big test"?
   a. Be sure to do a practice exam with the exact number of questions as the NCLEX or your "big test."
   b. Write down on a note card when you were the most tired, anxious, or nervous during this examination. List the question number you were at when you were feeling this way.
   c. Do relaxation exercises at these tense or fatigued times during the exam. Note which actions helped the most.
   d. Avoid the thought "I am tired and just want to get done with the test."
   e. Your success is directly correlated to your degree of effort to review content as well as to deal with any tension and fatigue during the review and exam processes.

Summary

We would be pleased if you use this book as a major tool to supplement your textbooks, clinical, and classroom activities. We hope that after you have used this book you will have learned to take actions to:

- Maximize your individual performance in study, review, and testing situations.
- Identify personal actions to help you set priorities for test preparation.
- Sharpen your thinking and reading skills during tests.

We hope that this book makes it easy, enjoyable, and effective to study and review at convenient times. The short, condensed, and prioritized chapter content may spark new ways to develop your skills in critical thinking and recall of content.

It is feedback from students, graduates, and practitioners in nursing that prompted the development and publication of this rapid review series. We welcome your comments. Please contact Dr. Rollant at rollant@bellsouth.net or 22 Village Lane, Newnan, GA 30265. We wish you a successful career in the nursing profession and hope that *Mosby's Rapid Review Series* has made that success a little easier to obtain!

The material on rapid study steps and rapid review tips was taken from Rollant PD: Soar to Success: Do Your Best on Nursing Tests, St. Louis, 1999, Mosby.

1

The Neurosensory System

FAST FACTS

1. Information is transmitted continuously:
   - From the periphery of the body via the spinal cord to the brain, which processes and responds to this motor and sensory information
   - From the brain via the spinal cord and out to the periphery so that muscles and organs respond to brain signals
2. Motor information is transmitted via the descending tracts in the anterior portion of the spinal cord. **Think**. . . Anterior portion: **A**way from the brain
3. Sensory information is transmitted via the ascending tracts in the posterior portion of the spinal cord. **Think**. . . **P**osterior portion: **P**oint up to the brain
4. Nervous systems:
   - Central: brain and spinal cord
   - Peripheral: cranial and spinal cord
   - Autonomic: parasympathetic and sympathetic
     - Parasympathetic: cholinergic or normal bodily functions; craniosacral
     - Sympathetic: adrenergic functions or stress response when very happy, sad, or fearful; thoracolumbar
5. Neurologic stimuli coordinate the heart and lung: a happy medium exists between the sympathetic and parasympathetic systems
   - The sympathetic system increases the heart rate, and the parasympathetic system decreases the heart rate
   - The sympathetic and parasympathetic systems work together to create a normal range for heart and respiratory rates
6. Important concerns for procedures to evaluate neurologic functioning:
   - A baseline neurologic examination is required *before* these examinations
   - Food and fluids generally are not restricted before neurologic examinations
   - The exception is the electroencephalogram (EEG): avoid drugs with stimulants such as ephedrine, and avoid foods with stimulants, such as caffeine and cocoa products

- Clients usually must lie very still for neurologic examinations and may receive sedatives to help them do so
- Clients should take their usual dose of anticonvulsant medication before an EEG unless otherwise ordered

7. Clients must be positioned for a lumbar puncture:
   - Adults, adolescents, and children: lateral decubiti or side-lying, fetal position. Instruct clients to clasp the hands on the knees to maintain this position. In certain situations a sitting position is used
   - Infants: sitting and leaning forward with support—a frog-like position

8. After neurologic tests the priority is to monitor the neurologic status, second only to airway; breathing; and circulation

9. After a lumbar puncture or spinal tap into the subarachnoid space, the following nursing actions can help prevent a headache:
   - Encouraging fluid intake
   - Keeping the client flat for 6 to 12 hours, with the head on a flat pillow
   - Medicating the client with nonnarcotic analgesics for headaches that do occur
   - These headaches normally do not last longer than 3 days after the procedure
   - If headaches persist for more than 3 days, the physician needs to be notified. A *blood patch* is usually done, which is the injection of a small amount of the client's blood into the spinal column

CONTENT REVIEW

I. The neurosensory system: definition: the neurosensory system receives and transmits information from all areas of the body and from external stimuli to control bodily functions

II. Structure and function
A. Central nervous system
  1. Protective structures
     a. Skull
     b. Meninges: membranes covering brain and spinal cord
        (1) Dura mater
        (2) Arachnoid
        (3) Pia mater
  2. Cerebrum: 80% of the bulk of the brain; right and left hemispheres, each with four lobes, connected by the corpus callosum
     a. Frontal lobes
        (1) Personality
        (2) Learning, problem solving
        (3) Moral behavior
        (4) Motor activity

(5) Broca's area: speech (on dominant side)

(6) Parietal lobes

(7) Interprets sensory information: sense of the body's position, touch

b. Temporal lobes

(1) Hearing

(2) Taste

(3) Smell

(4) Wernicke's area: comprehension of written and spoken language

c. Occipital lobes: receive and interpret visual stimuli

3. Cerebellum: two lateral hemispheres separated by the vermis (wormlike middle lobe of the cerebellum)

a. Coordinating movement

b. Equilibrium

c. Muscle tone

d. **Proprioception**

4. Brainstem

a. Midbrain: relays information about muscle movement to other areas of the brain; cranial nerves III and IV originate here

b. Pons: relays information to brain centers and lower spinal areas; cranial nerves V, VI, VII, and VIII originate here

c. Medulla oblongata: **Reflex** center for involuntary functions (breathing, sneezing, swallowing, coughing, salivation, and vomiting); cranial nerves IX, X, XI, and XII originate here

5. Cerebral ventricular system: four interconnecting ventricles that produce and circulate cerebrospinal fluid (CSF)

6. Diencephalon

a. Thalamus: relays information from the spinal cord and cerebral cortex

b. Hypothalamus

(1) Regulates body temperature

(2) Is responsible for hunger and thirst

(3) Generates autonomic nervous system responses

(4) Controls pituitary gland hormonal secretions

c. Epithalamus: contains the pineal gland believed to be important in physical growth and sexual development

B. Spinal cord

1. Protective structure: 33 spinal vertebrae, divided into five regions: cervical, thoracic, lumbar, sacral, and coccygeal

a. Thirty-one segments with a pair of spinal nerves from each segment

(1) Cervical (8): supplies neck, upper extremities, diaphragm, and intercostal muscles

(2) Thoracic (12): supplies thoracic and abdominal areas

       (3) Lumbar (5): supplies lower extremities

       (4) Sacral (5): supplies lower extremities along with urinary and bowel control

       (5) Coccygeal (1): supplies perineum

   b. Anterior portion of the cord: descending motor tracts

   c. Posterior portion of the cord: ascending sensory tracts

   d. Lateral columns: preganglionic fibers for the autonomic nervous system

C. Peripheral nervous system

   1. Cranial nerves: 12 pairs that arise from the brain

   2. Spinal nerves: 31 pairs that arise from the spinal cord

D. Autonomic nervous system

   1. Parasympathetic (craniosacral): controls normal bodily functions

   2. Sympathetic (thoracolumbar): controls stress response

E. Eye: produces vision when light is transmitted through the cornea and lens, to the retina, then to the optic nerve, and finally to the occipital lobe of the brain

   1. Exterior structures

     a. Cornea: clear fibrous covering of the eye

     b. Sclera: outer layer of the eye

     c. Eye muscles (6): allow movement of the eye

     d. Lacrimal glands: secrete tears to lubricate eyes; drains into the lacrimal ducts

   2. Interior structures

     a. Iris: muscle responsible for dilation and constriction of pupil; adds color to the eye

     b. Lens: focuses images on retina

     c. Aqueous humor: refraction medium for light; gel found in the anterior chamber

     d. Vitreous humor: refraction medium for light; gel found in the posterior chamber

     e. Chorioid: black, second layer of the eye

     f. Retina: inner, photosensitive layer of the eye

F. Ear: responsible for hearing and balance

   1. External structures

     a. Pinna: flap of cartilage that collects sound waves and transmits them into the canal

     b. Auditory meatus (external ear canal): conducts sound waves toward the tympanic membrane; ceruminous glands in the canal produce cerumen (wax) to protect the canal from small particles

     c. Tympanic membrane: pearl gray membrane found at the end of the auditory meatus; conducts sound waves to the middle ear

   2. Middle ear

     a. Ossicles: the malleus, incus, and stapes are the three small bones that vibrate and transmit sound to inner ear

b. Eustachian tube: connection between inner ear and nasopharynx; equalizes pressure between the middle ear and atmospheric pressure
3. Inner ear
   a. Cochlea: spiral tube containing the receptors for sound
   b. Controls balance

III. Targeted concerns
   A. **Pharmacology: priority drug classifications**
      1. Osmotic diuretics: increase osmotic pressure in the vascular space
         a. Expected effects: diuresis; decreases increased intracranial pressure (ICP)
         b. Commonly given drugs
            (1) Mannitol (Osmitrol)
            (2) Urea (Ureaphil)
         c. Nursing considerations
            (1) Mannitol easily crystallizes: Before infusing into the client, warm the mannitol in warm water, not the microwave, then cool to body temperature
            (2) Use in-line filter to administer mannitol to prevent infusion of crystals into the venous system
            (3) Monitor blood pressure (BP) and pulse hourly for blood volume changes
               (a) Increased BP: indicative of fluid overload, which is transient
               (b) Decreased BP: indicative of dehydration
               (c) Tachycardia can be indicative of fluid overload or dehydration
            (4) Evaluate for signs of dehydration: decreased central venous pressure (CVP), dry mucous membranes, poor skin turgor
      2. Anticholinesterase drugs: prevent destruction of acetylcholine by inhibiting acetylcholinesterase
         a. Expected effect: decrease the symptoms of myasthenia gravis (MG)
         b. Commonly given drugs
            (1) Edrophonium chloride (Tensilon): for diagnostic tests of MG only
            (2) Pyridostigmine bromide (Mestinon)
            (3) Neostigmine bromide (Prostigmine bromide)
         c. Nursing considerations
            (1) Have parenteral atropine available in the advent of cholinergic crisis when dosage is too high
            (2) Give 30 minutes before meals
      3. Anticonvulsants: increase cerebral cortex threshold to reduce its response to stimuli
         a. Expected effect: depresses seizure activity
         b. Commonly given drugs

       (1) Phenobarbital (Luminal)

       (2) Phenytoin (Dilantin)

       (3) Carbamazepine (Tegretol)

       (4) Valproic acid (Depakene)

   c. Nursing considerations

       (1) Blood levels, renal, and liver studies must be monitored at specific intervals identified by the physician for long-term use

       (2) Dilantin intravenous (IV) push must be given slowly, only into a normal saline line

       (3) Depakene must be given with food to avoid gastrointestinal (GI) distress

4. Antidyskinetic drugs: increase the release of dopamine in the brain

   a. Expected effect: reduces the effects of Parkinson's disease

   b. Commonly given drugs

       (1) Levodopa (Larodopa)

       (2) Carbidopa/Levodopa (Sinemet)

       (3) Amantadine (Symmetrel)

   c. Nursing considerations

       (1) The dosage of Symmetrel may have to be adjusted by the physician if its effectiveness decreases (i.e., if tremors recur)

       (2) Postural hypotension may be a problem

       (3) Clients must be cautioned to avoid alcohol while taking medication

5. Cycloplegic or mydriatic ophthalmic agents: cause paralysis of the ciliary muscles of the eye

   a. Expected effect: dilates the pupil

   b. Commonly given drugs

       (1) Atropine sulfate

       (2) Scopolamine hydrobromide

   c. Nursing considerations

       (1) Inform clients they will be photophobic for the length of time the drugs are effective; advise physician if photophobia lasts longer than 1 week

       (2) Inform clients they will be unable to focus on near objects for as long as 24 hours

6. Miotic ophthalmic agents: cause contraction of the sphincter muscle of the iris; vasodilate vessels where the intraocular fluid leaves the eye

   a. Expected effect: pupillary constriction; treats glaucoma

   b. Commonly given drugs

       (1) Pilocarpine hydrochloride (Pilocar)

       (2) Carbachol (Carbacel)

       (3) Physostigmine salicylate (Eserine)

   c. Nursing considerations

        (1) Instruct clients on the correct method for instillation with eyedropper: tilt head back, pull down lower lid, place drop in cup of lower lid

        (2) Instruct clients not to touch the tip of the eyedropper to the eye

        (3) Advise clients they should be evaluated periodically for changes in intraocular pressure

  7. Ophthalmic agents that are beta-blockers: lower intraocular pressure by decreasing aqueous humor formation

    a. Expected effect: treats glaucoma

    b. Commonly given drugs

        (1) Timolol maleate (Timoptic)

        (2) Betaxolol hydrochloride (Betoptic)

    c. Nursing considerations

        (1) Some agents in this group are contraindicated in clients with chronic obstructive pulmonary disease (COPD), also called chronic airflow limitation (CAL)

        (2) Same precautions as in the previous group

  8. Carbonic anhydrase inhibitors: inhibit the enzyme necessary for the formation of aqueous humor

    a. Expected effect: decreases intraocular pressure; weak diuretic

    b. Commonly given drugs

        (1) Acetazolamide (Diamox)

        (2) Ethoxzolamide (Cardase)

    c. Nursing considerations

        (1) Assess for hypokalemia

        (2) Give with food

        (3) Avoid intramuscular injections because of the extreme pain caused by injection of the medication

  9. Anti-infective ophthalmic agents: prevent bacterial cell wall synthesis

    a. Expected effect: attacks bacterial infection of the eye

    b. Commonly given drugs

        (1) Bacitracin (Baciguent Antibiotic Ointment)

        (2) Neomycin sulfate (Myciguent)

        (3) Sulfacetamide sodium (Bleph-10)

    c. Nursing considerations

        (1) Remove exudate from the eye before instilling medication to enhance action

        (2) Instruct clients on correct instillation: apply from inner to outer canthus as lower lid is pulled down or everted

B. Procedures

  1. Lumbar puncture (spinal tap): collects and evaluates CSF; measures pressure around spinal cord

  2. X-ray films of the skull, vertebral column: evaluate for abnormalities

    3. Computed Tomogram (CT) scan: evaluates for bony and soft tissue abnormalities using cutaway views of the area

    4. Magnetic Resonance Image (MRI) scan: evaluates for bony and soft tissue abnormalities using a magnetic force

    5. Positron emission tomography scan (PET scan): scans brain for structure and function using radioactive substance

    6. Cerebral arteriogram: visualizes the arteries that feed the brain by use of radiopaque dye and x-ray films

    7. Electroencephalogram (EEG): evaluates the electrical activity of the brain

    8. Electromyography (EMG): records nerve conduction in skeletal muscle

    9. Evoked potentials: records brain activity in response to stimuli such as visual, auditory, or somatosensory stimuli

    10. Snellen's test (eye chart): evaluates visual acuity

    11. Ophthalmoscopic examination: evaluates the inner structures of the eye

    12. Tonometry: tonometer measures intraocular pressure

    13. Audiogram: evaluates hearing

C. Psychosocial concerns

    1. Anger: common in clients with limiting degenerative neurosensory disorders

    2. Denial: common in clients with degenerative changes owing to neurosensory disorders

    3. Anxiety: common in clients unable to discern changes that occur owing to a neurosensory disorder

    4. Immobility: very common in clients with neurologic impairment

    5. Lifestyle changes: common in clients with neurosensory impairment owing to decreased mobility

D. Health history: question sequence

    1. What symptoms are you having that made it necessary for you to seek assistance?

    2. When did your symptoms begin, and how have they progressed?

    3. What medical problems are you presently being treated for?

    4. What medical problems have you been treated for in the past?

    5. Is there a history of neurologic or sensory disorders in your family?

    6. Have you ever been hospitalized or had surgery? What for and when?

    7. What prescription and over-the-counter medications are you presently taking?

    8. Have you found it necessary to make changes in your daily routine?

    9. What is your occupation?

    10. Are there any toxic substances that you have been exposed to at your workplace or in your home?

TABLE 1-1	Cranial Nerve Evaluation Procedures

Cranial Nerve	How to Assess
I Olfactory	Identify common smells
II Optic	Observe eye abnormalities, test vision
III Oculomotor	Test pupillary size and reaction
IV Trochlear	Client's eyes follow object in all directions
V Trigeminal	Clamp jaws, open jaws widely and back and forth; feels touch to face; sterile wisp of cotton to cornea causes blink
VI Abducens	Move eyes back and forth
VII Facial	Smile, frown, raise forehead and eyebrows, taste of different types of foods
VIII Acoustic	Auditory acuity
IX Glossopharyngeal	Uvula, palate rise symmetrically when Client says "Ah"
X Vagus	Cough, speak
XI Spinal accessory	Elevate shoulders, turn head to one side and the other, back and forward
XII Hypoglossal	Stick out tongue, move side to side

11. Have you ever blacked out? If yes, how often and how long were you unconscious?
12. Do you feel, see, or hear anything unusual before you black out?
13. Would you ever consider yourself moody?
14. Do you ever have difficulty walking?
15. Do you ever feel strange sensations in your arms and legs, or anywhere else in your body?

E. **Physical examination: appropriate sequence**
1. Airway, breathing, and circulation (ABCs): vital signs
2. Pupillary response
3. Level of consciousness, orientation, mood, affect, memory, intellect, and speech
4. Inspection of head, neck and spine, eyes, ears, and nose
5. Skull and spine palpation
6. Inspection of muscle size, tone, and strength in all major muscle groups
7. Inspection of gait
8. Evaluation of the ability to feel touch and pain
9. Evaluation of Reflexes
10. Evaluation of cranial nerves (Table 1-1)

IV. Pathophysiologic disorders
A. **Cerebral vascular accident (CVA)**
1. Definition: sudden disruption of blood supply to the brain, leading to ischemia and eventual necrosis in part of the brain

2. Pathophysiology
   a. Ischemic: decreased blood flow to the brain tissue causes infarcted areas that will become edematous as a result of the infarct; if the infarcted areas are large enough the cerebral edema may increase to the point of displacing the brain and forcing it through the foramen magnum, causing death from brain stem herniation
   b. Hemorrhagic: neurons are damaged at the site of the hemorrhage; increased ICP is a result of tissue edema from the injury and from the space-occupying blood that has spilled into the brain area and is displacing the brain; this type of CVA also can result in brain displacement through the foramen magnum, causing death from brain stem herniation
3. Etiology
   a. Ischemic: thrombosis, embolism, and decreased blood flow from arteriosclerotic or severe hypotensive changes
   b. Hemorrhagic: intracerebral hemorrhage usually from vessel damage as a result of long-term hypertension; subarachnoid hemorrhage from a rupture of an intracranial aneurysm
4. Incidence: third leading cause of death in the United States
5. Assessment
   a. Ask the following questions
      (1) Do you ever have periods of time when you feel weak?
      (2) Do you ever have difficulty speaking?
      (3) Have you ever had a period of time when your vision was impaired?
   b. Four stages of clinical manifestation
      (1) Transient ischemic attack (TIA)
         (a) Warning of impending CVA
         (b) Weakness
         (c) Aphasia: impaired language function
            (i) Expressive: (motor) words cannot be formed or spoken
            (ii) Receptive: (sensory) language cannot be understood
         (d) Drop attack: drop to the floor for no apparent reason
         (e) Symptoms gone sometimes after minutes or within 24 hours
      (2) Reversible ischemic neurologic deficit (RIND)
         (a) Similar to TIA but symptoms last longer than 24 hours
         (b) Risk of CVA is greatly enhanced at this stage
      (3) Stroke in evolution
         (a) Increasing neurologic deficits over a period of days
         (b) Clinical worsening, decreasing level of consciousness

(4) Stroke
    (a) Right- or left-sided weakness (hemiparesis) or paralysis (hemiplegia); deficit is on opposite side of infarct
    (b) Aphasia (receptive most common in left lesions)
    (c) Left neglect: seen in right lesions; physical neglect of left side of the body

c. Abnormal diagnostic tests
    (1) CT scan: identifies cause of CVA, placement in brain, and possible shift in brain contents
    (2) MRI: identifies cause of CVA, placement in brain, and possible shift in brain contents
    (3) Arteriography: identifies site of aneurysms, stenosis, vessel abnormalities, or diminished circulation

6. Expected medical interventions
    a. Thrombolytic therapy may be utilized in the face of an ischemic CVA
    b. Oral anticoagulants given to prevent further intra-arterial clot formation; this is contraindicated in hemorrhagic CVA
    c. Aspirin, ticlopidine (Ticlid), or clopidogrel (Plavix) administration to decrease clot formation especially for long term care
    d. Measures to maintain BP at acceptable levels; drug therapy to increase or decrease BP as needed
    e. Anticonvulsants to prevent seizures related to cerebral edema
    f. Mannitol to decrease cerebral edema
    g. Corticosteroids (dexamethasone) to decrease cerebral edema
    h. Amicar, an antifibrinolytic agent, used to prevent rebleeding in the case of an aneurysm

7. Nursing diagnoses
    a. Ineffective airway clearance related to decreased neurologic status
    b. Altered physical mobility related to effects of hemiparesis or hemiplegia secondary to CVA
    c. Impaired verbal communication related to altered cerebral function
    d. Risk for injury related to altered mobility, seizures, or both

8. Client goals
    a. Airway will remain clear as evidenced by clear upper airway sounds and respiratory rate of 16 to 20 breaths per minute
    b. Mobility will improve when clients begin to help turn themselves in bed and complete half of their range of motion exercises
    c. Client will verbalize one new word per week
    d. Client will not be injured during hospitalization

9. Nursing interventions
   a. Acute care
      (1) Take measures to reduce increased ICP
          (a) Head of bed elevated 15 to 30 degrees
          (b) Keep head and neck in alignment; avoid neck flexion
          (c) Advise client to:
              (i) Avoid Valsalva's maneuver; administer stool softeners
              (ii) Avoid bending, coughing, sneezing, and vomiting
              (iii) Avoid isometric energy expenditure (i.e., pushing up in bed)
          (d) Maintain quiet, darkened environment
          (e) Prohibit television and radio if they stimulate client
          (f) Encourage bed rest
          (g) Limit visitors
          (h) Prohibit giving rectal medications and taking temperature rectally due to risk of stimulation of Valsalva's maneuver
      (2) Assess client for increases in ICP
          (a) Decreasing level of consciousness
          (b) Headache
          (c) Projectile vomiting
          (d) Elevated systolic BP with a stable diastolic pressure: results in a widened pulse pressure
          (e) Bradycardia
          (f) Pupils, unequal and become fixed and dilated
          (g) Hyperthermia
          (h) Slow, deep irregular respiratory pattern
      (3) Prevent complications of immobility
          (a) Range of motion exercises to prevent contractures and frozen joints
          (b) Prevent skin breakdown by turning client to unaffected side and back every 2 hours
          (c) Pad side rails to prevent injuries owing to seizures, and so forth
          (d) Monitor bowel and bladder elimination
          (e) Administer tube feedings safely
              (i) High Fowler's position or head of bed up at least 30 degrees
              (ii) Evaluate tube position in stomach
              (iii) Feed slowly; feedings should be at room temperature with blue coloring added
              (iv) Check residual every 4 hours to evaluate for full stomach and potential for regurgitation
      (4) Maintain communication with client
          (a) Use touch and gestures to assist communication

      (b) Ask questions that can be answered by yes and no

      (c) Use communication aids such as pictures or word cards

      (d) Maintain an accepting environment

      (e) Assist with initiation of speech therapy when client is stable

      (f) Be patient

  b. Home care regarding client and family education

    (1) Many clients will start their rehabilitative phase in a rehabilitation center, and prepare for home care from that level

    (2) Goals of rehabilitation

      (a) Motor improvement

      (b) Speech improvement

      (c) Cognitive improvement

      (d) Social and mental readjustment to new limitations

      (e) Return of autonomy, especially in activities of daily living

      (f) Restoration of social activity and interpersonal relationships

10. Evaluation protocol

  a. How do I know that my interventions were effective?

    (1) No assessment findings associated with increased ICP

    (2) No complications of immobility

    (3) Nutritional needs met safely

    (4) Communication needs met with minimal frustration for the client

  b. What criteria will I use to change my interventions?

    (1) Client exhibits assessment findings associated with increased ICP

    (2) Client exhibits one or more complications of immobility (e.g., pressure sores and contractures)

    (3) Client is losing weight, indicating inadequate nutrition or intolerance of feedings; complications of tube feedings are apparent

    (4) Client is unable to make needs known and is becoming frustrated

  c. How will I know that my client teaching has been effective?

    (1) Mobility is improved

    (2) Speech is improved

    (3) Client is gaining independence related to feeding and hygiene

    (4) Client is performing one or more assisted daily living activities per week

    (5) Client is renewing interpersonal relationship with significant other

11. Older adult alert
   a. Because older clients are at higher risk for the complications of immobility, take extra care regarding prevention and early identification of problems
   b. The older adult population is most affected by CVAs
   c. When planning care for older clients after a CVA, consider other medical problems that the client may have

B. Brain tumors
   1. Definition: abnormal growth in the cranial cavity, which may be benign or malignant; a malignancy may be a primary tumor or a metastatic lesion
   2. Pathophysiology: all brain tumors can be life-threatening; early diagnosis gives a more promising outcome; the tumor occupies space, thus creating pressure on brain tissue; edema will follow; eventually herniation of the brain down into the foramen magnum will cause death
   3. Etiology: many metastatic lesions originate from the lung or breast; no known cause of primary brain tumors; primary tumors do not metastasize
   4. Incidence: equal among men and women; metastatic lesions are more common than are primary lesions
   5. Assessment
      a. Ask the following questions
         (1) Have you noticed weakness in any one area of your body?
         (2) Do you ever feel pins and needles or numbness in any area of your body?
         (3) Do you ever have difficulty speaking?
         (4) Do you ever have difficulty walking?
         (5) Do you experience headaches, dizziness, or seizures?
      b. Clinical manifestations
         (1) Weakness of an area of the body or half of the body (right or left)
         (2) Paresthesia
         (3) Difficulty speaking
         (4) Gait, personality, or vision changes
         (5) Headaches
         (6) Dizziness
         (7) Seizures
      c. Abnormal diagnostic tests
         (1) Skull x-ray films: identifies lesion
         (2) Chest x-ray films: may identify primary site
         (3) CT scan: identifies tumors, ventricular changes, and shifts in brain mass
         (4) MRI: identifies tumors, ventricular changes, and shifts in brain mass

      (5) EEG: identifies slowing of electrical activity in areas of the brain affected by the tumor

      (6) Cerebral angiogram: identifies tumor vascularity

6. Expected medical interventions
   a. Type of intervention depends on tumor type and location
   b. Chemotherapy: intrathecal (in CSF)
   c. Radiation therapy
   d. Intracranial surgery to remove or debulk tumor
7. Nursing diagnoses
   a. Anxiety related to unknown outcome of illness
   b. Pain related to pressure exerted on surrounding structures by the tumor
   c. Risk for injury related to weakness or seizure activity secondary to cerebral edema
   d. Self-care deficit; bathing and hygiene difficulty related to impaired mobility
8. Client goals
   a. Client will state that anxiety is decreased
   b. Client will state that pain is relieved or improved on a scale from 0 to 10; goal is from 0 to 2
   c. Client will not be injured during hospitalization
   d. Client will begin to bathe self, each day bathing one more body area
9. Nursing interventions
   a. Acute care: postoperative care
      (1) Measures to decrease ICP (see Cerebral Vascular Accident, Acute Care, p. 12)
      (2) Monitoring ICP: always compare postoperative vital signs and neurologic signs with preoperative signs (see Cerebral Vascular Accident, Acute Care)
      (3) Assess input and output carefully; clients usually are kept slightly dehydrated to prevent cerebral edema
      (4) Assess head dressing for drainage and bleeding
      (5) Assess for any drainage from the nose or ears; if drainage identified, do not pack ears or nose if drainage identified: may increase ICP

> **⚠ Warning!**
>
> Assess all drainage from nose or ears for glucose, which if present indicates cerebrospinal fluid.

   (6) Use scrupulous aseptic technique when caring for the incision and changing the dressing (if ordered by physician) because risk for infection or meningitis is very great

   (7) Pad side rails to prevent injury as a result of seizure activity

      b. Home care regarding client and family education
- (1) Note changes of infection
- (2) Note changes if tumor increases in size or recurs
- (3) Increasing mobility in the home
- (4) Increasing independence in the home

10. Evaluation protocol
    a. How do I know that my interventions were effective?
- (1) Client exhibits no findings associated with increased ICP
- (2) Vital signs are within 10% of baseline for the client
- (3) Intake is approximately 10% less than output, keeping the client in a minimally dehydrated state
- (4) No bleeding from incision noted
- (5) No evidence of CSF leak
- (6) No evidence of infection
- (7) No seizure activity or injury

    b. What criteria do I use to change my interventions?
- (1) Increased ICP
- (2) Vital signs are not within 10% of baseline for the client
- (3) Intake is greater than output, indicating fluid overload
- (4) Bleeding noted from incision
- (5) CSF leak noted
- (6) Increased temperature and increased leukocyte count, which are indicative of postoperative infection
- (7) Seizure activity noted

    c. How will I know that my client teaching has been effective?
- (1) Client and family are able to state signs and symptoms of infection
- (2) Client and family are able to state signs and symptoms of increasing tumor size
- (3) Client's mobility increases each day
- (4) Client becomes more independent each day

11. Older adult alert: as a normal course of aging, the older client may exhibit slower reflexes. Careful preoperative evaluation must be done to establish a baseline for these clients before surgery. Comparison of the postoperative status to the baseline will alert the nurse to appropriate changes in the postoperative period.

C. Head injury

1. Definition: trauma or injury to the skull, brain, or both, as a result of an impact to the head
2. Pathophysiology
    a. Concussion: no changes in brain tissue; brain shaken causing a brief change in neurologic status
    b. Contusion: bruise of brain itself; caused by blow to the head
    c. Skull fracture: break in the skull; may be a linear, nondisplaced, or displaced fracture

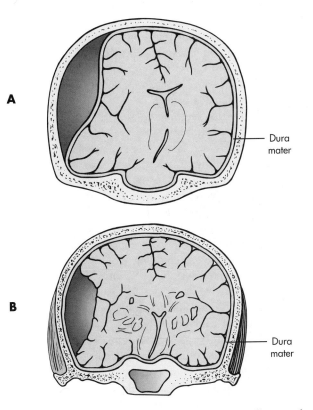

A

Dura
mater

B

Dura
mater

Figure 1-1   A, Epidural hematoma in the temporal fossa, usually a result of laceration of the middle meningeal artery. **B,** Subdural hematoma, usually a result of laceration of the subdural veins. (From Price SA, Wilson LM: *Pathophysiology: clinical concepts of disease processes,* ed 5, St. Louis, 1997, Mosby.)

    d. Hematomas (Figure 1-1)
       (1) Epidural: injury resulting in damage to an artery with blood collecting rapidly above the dura; death will occur if not treated quickly
       (2) Subdural: injury resulting in damage to a vein with blood collecting below the dura; may be slow forming, and assessment factors may not appear for weeks; classified as acute, subacute, or chronic; differentiated by the length of time for hematoma formation
       (3) Intracerebral: associated with a cerebral laceration and edema of surrounding tissue; may be seen after a contusion
  3. Etiology: trauma from motor vehicle accidents, falls, and assaults
  4. Incidence: teenagers and young adults comprise the most frequently affected age group; over 2 million injuries occur per year

5. Assessment
   a. Ask the following questions
      (1) Do you have a headache?
      (2) Did you lose consciousness after your injury?
      (3) What is your name? Do you know where you are? What is today's date?
      (4) Do you feel nauseous?
   b. Clinical manifestations may include any or all of these
      (1) Decreased level of consciousness
      (2) Posturing: usually in response to stimulation (usually bilateral but can be unilateral) (Figure 1-2)
         (a) Decorticate: indicates cortical damage
         (b) Decerebrate: indicates severe hemispheric damage
      (3) Headache
      (4) Pupil changes: size, equality, and reaction
      (5) Nausea and vomiting
      (6) Elevated systolic BP with widened pulse pressure
      (7) Bradycardia
      (8) Slow, irregular respiratory pattern
   c. Abnormal laboratory findings
      (1) Electrolytes: hypernatremia or hyponatremia related to pressure on the hypothalamus and altered production and release of antidiuretic hormone (ADH)
      (2) Serum alcohol level elevated: high percentage of injuries are alcohol related
   d. Abnormal diagnostic tests
      (1) Skull x-ray film: fractures
      (2) Cervical x-ray film: fracture or displacement; high incidence of cervical injuries are associated with cranial injury
      (3) CT scan: hematoma, shift of brain contents
      (4) MRI: hematoma, shift of brain contents
      (5) EEG: abnormal waves; used to help identify brain death
      (6) Positron emission tomography (PET) scan: brain tissue normal but metabolically hypoactive
6. Expected medical interventions
   a. Surgery: repair vascular injuries, repair skull abnormalities, drain hematomas, debride wounds, and suture lacerations
   b. Drug therapy
      (1) Mannitol: to decrease cerebral edema
      (2) Anticonvulsants: to prevent seizure activity
      (3) Corticosteroids: to prevent or decrease cerebral edema
      (4) Antibiotics: to prevent meningitis
   c. Mechanical ventilation if respiratory effort impaired; maintain slight respiratory alkalosis (partial pressure of carbon dioxide at 25 to 30 mm.Hg.) to help decrease cerebral edema for a maximum of 48 hours or if ICP is increasing; refer to physician protocol

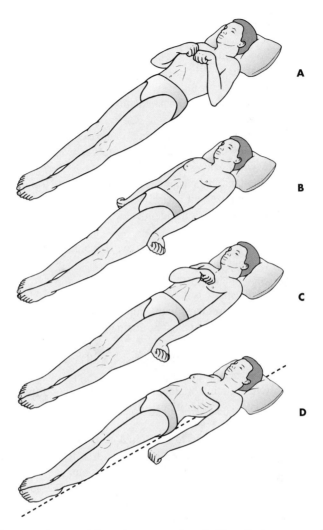

Figure 1-2 Decorticate and decerebrate posturing. **A,** Decorticate response. Flexion of arms, wrists, and fingers with adduction in upper extremities. Extension, internal rotation, and plantar flexion in lower extremities. **B,** Decerebrate response. All four extremities in rigid extension, with hyperpronation of forearms and plantar extension of feet. **C,** Decorticate response on right side of body and decerebrate response on left side of body. **D,** Opisthotonic posturing. (From Thelan LA, Urden LD, Lough ME, Stacy KM: *Critical care nursing: diagnosis and management,* ed 3, St. Louis, 1998, Mosby.)

      d. Monitoring of ICP: to identify and treat as an emergency increases in ICP of over 20

      e. Nutritional support: tube feeding or total parenteral nutrition until client is able to eat

   7. Nursing diagnoses

      a. Ineffective airway clearance related to decreased neurologic status

      b. Pain related to injured cerebral tissue

       c. Impaired verbal communication related to decreased neurologic status

       d. Fluid volume excess or deficit related to altered ADH production and release

  8. Client goals

       a. Client will maintain patent airway as evidenced by clear upper airway sounds

       b. Client will state head pain is decreased or relieved

       c. Client will communicate with staff appropriately either verbally or by writing notes to indicate needs

       d. Client will balance intake and output; daily weight is stable within 1 kg of the client's baseline

  9. Nursing interventions: identical to the care required for the client with a brain tumor or CVA

 10. Evaluation protocol: identical to the evaluation protocol for the client with a brain tumor or CVA

 11. Older adult alert

       a. A fall usually is the cause of head injuries in older clients. The fall may be associated with another neurologic impairment such as a CVA. The client must be evaluated carefully for all possible injuries

       b. Older clients are at higher risk for all complications associated with a head injury

       c. Rehabilitation of older clients may be more difficult owing to the presence of other illnesses or of decreased endurance

D. Spinal cord injury (SCI)

  1. Definition: damage to the spinal cord as a result of fractured or displaced vertebrae, resulting in a loss of sensation and motor function below the level of the cord damage

  2. Pathophysiology: any movement in the vertebrae can cause compression, tearing, or transection of the cord; common areas affected are the cervical or lumbar vertebrae

  3. Etiology: trauma, such as motor vehicular accidents, falls, diving accidents, tumors, congenital defects, and infectious or degenerative diseases

  4. Incidence: over 10,000 per year; usually seen in young adults

  5. Assessment

       a. Ask the following questions

          (1) Are you having any difficulty breathing?

          (2) Can you feel me touching you here? Touch several areas below the level of injury

          (3) Can you wiggle your toes? Your fingers?

       b. Clinical manifestations

          (1) Loss of movement below the level of injury

          (2) Loss of sensation below the level of injury

(3) Decreased or absent bowel and bladder function

(4) Loss of perspiration below the level of injury

(5) All autonomic functions are uncertain below the level of injury

(6) Pain

(7) Fever

(8) Spinal shock

    (a) Total loss of sensory, motor, and autonomic function below the level of injury (e.g., urine retention)

    (b) Hypotension

    (c) Bradycardia

    (d) Duration of several days to several months

c. Abnormal laboratory findings

    (1) Serum chemistry: hypoglycemia or hyperglycemia, electrolyte imbalance

    (2) CBC: decreased hematocrit and hemaglobin

d. Abnormal diagnostic tests

    (1) Spinal x-rays: vertebral fracture or displacement

    (2) CT scan: spinal cord edema and injury

    (3) MRI: spinal cord edema and injury

6. Expected medical interventions

a. Immobilization of entire spine requires use of Gardner-Wells tongs or Halo ring traction and a specialized bed, such as a Stryker frame or rotational bed, for turning and care (Figure 1-3)

b. Surgery to remove bone fragments and, in some instances, to place bone graft to bring stability to the vertebral column

c. Corticosteroids: high dose is now recommended

d. Support of respiratory function with the use of mechanical ventilation if necessary

e. Support fluid volume as necessary

7. Nursing diagnoses

a. Altered cardiac output related to loss of vascular tone secondary to spinal cord injury

b. Ineffective breathing pattern related to interrupted spinal cord impulses

c. Impaired physical mobility related to loss of muscle control below the level of spinal cord injury

8. Client goals

a. Client will demonstrate an appropriate cardiac output as evidenced by BP within 10% of baseline

b. Client will demonstrate an effective breathing pattern as evidenced by respiratory rate and depth within 10% of baseline

c. Client will demonstrate appropriate muscle tone in all appropriate muscle groups

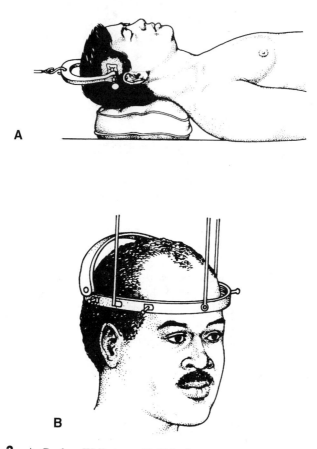

Figure 1-3 **A,** Gardner-Wells tongs. **B,** Halo ring. (**A** and **B** from Beare PG and Myers JL: *Principles and practice of adult health nursing,* ed 3., St. Louis, 1998, Mosby. **C** from Barker E. *Neuroscience nursing,* St. Louis, 1994, Mosby.)

9. Nursing interventions
    a. Acute care
        (1) Respiratory function is maintained either through the use of mechanical ventilation or through coughing and deep breathing every 2 hours
        (2) Cardiovascular status is assessed and maintained with the use of fluid and vasopressor therapy as per physician's orders
        (3) Vertebral immobility and skeletal traction with appropriate alignment is maintained as per physician's orders
        (4) Joint mobility is maintained through the advent of passive or active range of motion exercises, or both
        (5) Wrist contractures are prevented through the use of splints
        (6) Foot drop is prevented through the use of high-top sneakers or splints

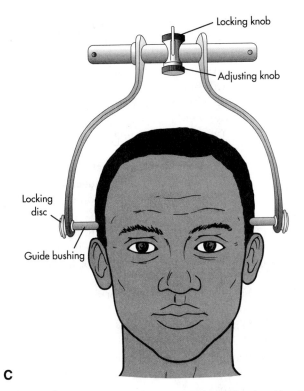

Locking knob

Adjusting knob

Locking disc

Guide bushing

C

Figure 1-3, cont'd C, Vinke tongs for cervical immobilization. (**A** and **B** from Beare PG and Myers JL: *Principles and practice of adult health nursing,* ed 3., St. Louis, 1998, Mosby. **C** from Barker E. Neuroscience Nursing, St. Louis, 1994, Mosby.)

    (7) Evaluate for pulmonary infections

    (8) Bladder function is maintained through the use of continuous or intermittent bladder drainage

    (9) Monitor for urinary tract infection: persistent low-grade fever, cloudy or smelly urine

  (10) Begin bowel training program once bowel function has resumed; daily timed Bisacodyl suppository

  (11) Prevent skin breakdown through the use of turning regime and meticulous hygiene

  (12) Meet nutritional needs as per physician's orders via tube feeding, enteral nutrition, or parenteral nutrition

  (13) Assist with psychological impact of injury

 b. Home care regarding client and family education: rehabilitative phase

    (1) Autonomic dysreflexia: any client with lesion at T6 or above is at risk

      (a) Result of noxious stimuli below the level of the injury causing organ **reflex** activity

(b) Bowel or bladder distention is the most common cause
(c) Distention causes exaggerated stimulation of sympathetic nervous system
  (i) Rapid increase in BP: risk of cerebral hemorrhage
  (ii) Bradycardia
  (iii) Severe headache
  (iv) Flushing
  (v) Profuse sweating
(d) Treatment
  (i) Remove cause: usually constipation with impaction or distended bladder
  (ii) Decrease BP with short-acting antihypertensive agent
  (iii) Elevate head of bed to help decrease BP
(2) Self-intermittent catheterization if client is able
(3) Monitoring respiratory status for findings associated with infection
(4) Monitoring urinary tract for findings associated with infection
(5) Skin care, a long-standing need
(6) Maintaining mobility
(7) Maintaining joint function and contracture prevention with active-passive range of motion exercises
10. Evaluation protocol
  a. How do I know that my interventions were effective?

> ⚠️ **Warning!**
>
> An important nursing intervention for autonomic dysreflexia is to prevent constipation and ensure regular bladder catheterization. Prevention is the key to ensure that this life-threatening complication does not occur.

(1) Appropriate respiratory status: rate is 16 to 20 breaths per minute with appropriate depth and arterial blood gas levels within 10% of client baseline
(2) BP and pulse rate within 10% of client baseline
(3) Appropriate skeletal alignment with no further cord damage
(4) Appropriate joint functions
(5) No contractures
(6) No foot drop
(7) No pulmonary or genitourinary infections
(8) Acceptable attainment of bowel training
(9) No skin breakdown
(10) Minimal or no weight loss (less than 5 kg)
(11) Psychological adjustment to impairment

    b. What criteria will I use to change my interventions?
- (1) BP, heart rate (HR), respiratory rate (RR), or depth of respiration is greater than 10% of client baseline
- (2) New neurologic instability
- (3) Joint immobility
- (4) Foot drop
- (5) Pulmonary or genitourinary infection
- (6) Fecal incontinence or constipation
- (7) Skin breakdown
- (8) Weight loss of over 5 kg
- (9) Emotional liability and inability to discuss body changes

    c. How will I know that my client teaching has been effective?
- (1) Client and family are able to state the cause, signs, symptoms, and treatment of autonomic dysreflexia
- (2) Client and family are able to demonstrate appropriate intermittent catheterization technique
- (3) Client and family are able to state findings associated with respiratory and genitourinary infections that should be brought to the attention of the physician
- (4) Client and family are able to demonstrate correct skin care technique
- (5) Client and family are able to demonstrate correct range-of-motion exercises and methods to maintain joint function

11. Older adult alert
    a. The nurse must be very aware of the complications associated with the spinal cord injured client and remember the older adult client is a higher risk for these complications
    b. The older adult client suffering from congestive heart failure or chronic lung disease may not be able to lay flat
    c. The older adult client is easily disoriented. One method to hinder disorientation is to prevent sensory deprivation by ensuring that the client is wearing glasses and a hearing aid, if needed, to maintain appropriate sensory input.

E. Chronic degenerative neurologic diseases: Parkinson's syndrome, multiple sclerosis, amyotrophic lateral sclerosis, and myasthenia gravis. For the definition, etiology, incidence, pathophysiology, assessment, and expected medical intervention, see Table 1-2

1. Nursing diagnoses
    a. Self-care deficit, bathing, and hygiene related to physical mobility impairment and weakness
    b. Body image disturbance related to changes in bodily function and inability to perform functions independently
    c. Impaired home maintenance management related to weakness and immobility
    d. Ineffective coping by the client and family members related to deteriorating health status

TABLE 1-2 Comparison of Chronic Degenerative Neurologic Diseases

	Parkinsonism	Multiple Sclerosis (MS)	Amyotrophic Lateral Sclerosis (ALS)	Myasthenia Gravis
Onset age	50-60 years	20-40 years	40-70 years	20-50 years
Sex	Male > female	Female > male	Male > female	Female > male
Etiology	Unknown	Unknown; virus/autoimmune origin suspected	Unknown; virus/autoimmune origin suspected	Unknown; autoimmune origin suspected; occurs in cool climates
Area affected	Substantia nigra cells in basal ganglia	Disseminated demyelinated plaques in white matter of brain and spinal cord	Motor neurons in brain and spinal cord	Myoneural junction of voluntary muscle
Pathophysiology	Impaired coordinated muscle movement and autonomic dysfunction because of deficiency of dopamine	Impaired nerve impulse conduction because of destruction of myelin	Impaired nerve impulse conduction because of degeneration of motor neurons	Impaired transmission of nerve impulse to skeletal muscle possibly because of acetylcholine deficiency

Findings	Rigidity Slow movements Nonintentional tremor Autonomic dysfunction	Depends on site of plaque: • Visual problems • Spastic weakness/paralysis • Poor coordination • Paresthesias • Speech defects • Intentional tremor • Bowel/bladder dysfunction • Emotional disorders • Exacerbations and remissions	Twitching Muscle weakness, progressing to atrophy and paralysis of upper and lower extremities Usually fatal 2-15 years after onset
Treatment	Supportive medication	Symptomatic	Symptomatic
Medication	Levodopa Carbidopa/levodopa (Sinemet)	Muscle relaxants Anti-inflammatories (steroids) during exacerbation	Antibiotics for respiratory and urinary tract infections

Profound or progressive muscle weakness and fatigue
Can progress to respiratory failure (myasthenic crisis)

Supportive medication
Surgery sometimes: thymectomy

Anticholinesterase:
Diagnosis—Edrophonium chloride (Tensilon)
Maintenance—Pyridostigmine bromide (Mestinon)
Anti-inflammatories (steroids) during acute phase

From AJN/Mosby: *AJN/Mosby Nursing boards review*, ed 9, St Louis, 1994, Mosby.

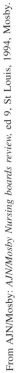

2. Client goals
   a. Client will continue to perform and assist in several aspects of the activities of daily living as long as possible
   b. Client will state comfort with changes occurring in the body
   c. Client will indicate that home maintenance is managed by other family members or resources as necessary
   d. Client will attain acceptable coping skills
3. Nursing interventions
   a. Maintain independence
      (1) Help client identify optimal activity level
      (2) Teach client to balance rest and activity
      (3) Encourage client use of devices to assist with function
   b. Prevent complications
      (1) Assist client in diet selections: planning that will prevent constipation and maintain nutritional status
      (2) Help client and family be alert to skin care needs, risk and prevention of skin breakdown
      (3) Encourage range of motion exercises and deep breathing exercises for the prevention of joint and muscle disuse and pulmonary infections
      (4) Implement the use of self-catheterization if necessary to prevent genitourinary infection
   c. Provide appropriate care and guidelines in all settings
      (1) Determining when hospitalization is necessary and when a long-term care facility may be necessary
      (2) Obtaining help in the home with care and instruction
      (3) Obtaining physical therapy and vocational therapy as needed
   d. Provide education and emotional support for client and family: assist them in making contact with appropriate support groups and agencies that offer resources for education or care assistance
4. Evaluation protocol
   a. How will I know that my interventions and teaching were effective?
      (1) Client and family are able to demonstrate independence and the ability to cope with new situations
      (2) Client and family are able to identify situations that require physician intervention or hospitalization
      (3) Client and family are able to indicate how to obtain help from community agencies and other resources
      (4) Client and family know how to prevent some of the more common complications of the disease process
5. Older adult alert
   a. The older adult client must be aggressively evaluated for complications of the disorders more often than the younger adult

F. Glaucoma

1. Definition: disorder characterized by an increase in intraocular pressure, resulting in blindness if untreated. Primary open-angle glaucoma, the most common form, has slow onset with few symptoms; closed-angle glaucoma has acute onset with severe eye pain.

2. Pathophysiology

   a. Open-angle glaucoma: resistance to flow of aqueous humor out of the posterior chamber as a result of thickened collecting channels or Schlemm's canal (normal drainage canal)

   b. Closed-angle glaucoma: iris is abnormally situated and prevents drainage through the normal drainage canal

3. Etiology

   a. Heredity

   b. Eye trauma

   c. Diabetes

   d. Eye surgery

4. Incidence: leading cause of blindness; higher incidence in the African-American population

5. Assessment

   a. Ask the following questions

      (1) Have you noticed that you have been losing the ability to see objects to your sides?

      (2) Have you noticed you have been bumping into objects lately?

      (3) Have you experienced halos around lights or blurring of vision?

      (4) Have you experienced eye pain?

   b. Clinical manifestations

      (1) Chronic open-angle glaucoma

         (a) Loss of peripheral vision

         (b) Eventual loss of central vision

      (2) Acute closed-angle glaucoma

         (a) Findings in the early stage suggest symptoms often occur in the evening and are intermittent

            (i) Blurred vision

            (ii) Halos around lights

            (iii) Frontal headache

            (iv) Eye pain

         (b) Findings in the acute stage

            (i) Severe eye pain

            (ii) Photophobia

            (iii) Increased lacrimation

   c. Abnormal diagnostic tests: intraocular pressure measured and is higher than 20 mm Hg

6. Expected medical interventions
    a. Miotic ophthalmic drops to decrease formation of the aqueous humor by the ciliary body or to constrict the pupil, or both
    b. Surgery (iridectomy) or laser (iridotomy) therapy are indicated when medical treatments are ineffective; however, the severity of blindness may guide treatment and outcome
7. Nursing diagnoses
    a. Anxiety related to vision changes and possible loss of vision
    b. Pain related to increased intraocular pressure
    c. Sensory-perceptual alteration: loss of peripheral vision related to damage to intraocular structures
8. Client goals
    a. Client will state anxiety is decreased
    b. Client will state pain or other findings are decreased or relieved
    c. Client will indicate accommodations have been made for loss of peripheral vision
9. Nursing interventions
    a. Acute care
        (1) Bed rest to help relieve pain
        (2) Quiet environment, dimmed lighting
        (3) Analgesics and antiemetics as needed
        (4) Allow sleeping on back and not on operative side
        (5) Avoid straining at stool
        (6) If eyesight is impaired
            (a) Direct all speaking to client
            (b) Avoid nonverbal communication
    b. Home care regarding client education
        (1) How to instill eye drops correctly
        (2) How to prevent further eye damage; damage is irreversible
        (3) Need for lifelong medical treatment
        (4) Need for routine eye examinations
        (5) Need for avoiding activities requiring upper body strength to prevent increased intraocular pressure
        (6) Need for instructions on how to alter diet to decrease sodium intake
10. Evaluation protocol
    a. How will I know that my interventions were effective?
        (1) Pain is relieved
        (2) Communication with client is acceptable
    b. What criteria will I use to change my interventions?
        (1) Pain continues
        (2) Communication is frustrating for the client
    c. How will I know that my client teaching has been effective?
        (1) Client is able to demonstrate correct eyedrop instillation

   (2) Client is able to state instillation of eye drops is a must for remainder of life

   (3) Client is able to state that routine examinations must be done at least yearly

   (4) Client is able to indicate activities that should not be performed to prevent increased IOP

   (5) Client is able to observe changes after eliminating salt from diet

  11. Older adult alert

   a. Glaucoma must be considered when assessing an older adult client with visual disturbances

G. Cataracts

 1. Definition: opacity of the crystalline lens of the eye

 2. Pathophysiology: the thickness and denseness of the lens increases with age as a result of the formation of new fiber cells in the lens; also a result of molecular deterioration caused by the absorption of ultraviolet radiation

 3. Etiology: breakdown of the metabolic process of the lens, or trauma

 4. Incidence: found commonly in populations over 55 years of age

 5. Assessment

  a. Ask the following questions

   (1) Do you have difficulty seeing?

   (2) Have you just recently noticed difficulty seeing or has this been a gradual change?

   (3) Do you have any pain in your eye?

  b. Clinical manifestations

   (1) Blurred vision

   (2) Gradual loss of vision

   (3) Painless changes in vision

  c. Abnormal diagnostic test: ophthalmoscopic examination indicating presence of cataracts

 6. Expected medical interventions

  a. Surgical removal of the lens, usually on an outpatient basis

  b. Intraocular lens placement after surgery

  c. Contact lenses may be prescribed after surgery, or glasses to replace natural lens

 7. Nursing diagnoses

  a. Sensory-perceptual alterations related to changes in visual acuity

  b. Risk for injury related to change in visual acuity

 8. Client goals

  a. Client will indicate having made acceptable adjustments for decreased vision

  b. Client will be free of injury

9. Nursing interventions
   a. Acute care: postoperative in recovery area for 2 to 3 hours before discharge to home
      (1) Deep breaths, no coughing (increases intraocular pressure)
      (2) Keep head of bed elevated 30 to 45 degrees
      (3) Turn client only to unaffected side to prevent an increase in intraocular pressure in affected eye
      (4) Check for bleeding under the eye shield and dressing
      (5) Treat nausea immediately to prevent vomiting, which causes increased intraocular pressure
      (6) Report severe eye pain immediately to physician; could be acute glaucoma
   b. Home care regarding client education
      (1) Do not remove eye shield or dressing until instructed to do so by physician; afterward the eye is protected with glasses or a shaded lens during the day and with an eye shield at night
      (2) Instill eye medications as ordered
      (3) Visits to physician may be for within 4 to 5 days if outpatient surgery is performed
      (4) Avoid activities that would cause straining, bending, or lifting until the initial postoperative visit to the physician
      (5) Prevent coughing and sneezing until seen by the physician postoperatively
      (6) Do not squeeze the eyelids; do not shut, rub, or place pressure on eyes until seen by the physician postoperatively
      (7) Cataract glasses
         (a) Magnify objects by one third
         (b) Vision clear only in the center of the lens
      (8) Contact lenses are more expensive but they will be make vision clearer than cataract glasses
10. Evaluation protocol
   a. How will I know that my interventions were effective?
      (1) Client is deep breathing but not coughing
      (2) Client is turning only to the unaffected side
      (3) No bleeding noted
      (4) Nausea was treated and vomiting averted
      (5) No severe pain noted
   b. What criteria will I use to change my interventions?
      (1) Client is coughing or vomiting
      (2) Client is turning to affected side
      (3) Bleeding noted on the dressing
      (4) Client admits to pain becoming more severe
   c. How will I know that my client teaching has been effective?
      (1) Client is able to state activities to be avoided

(2) Client is able to state appropriate home care for dressings, need for follow-up visit to physician

(3) Client is able to state how the cataract glasses or contact lenses will affect vision

(4) Client is able to demonstrate instillation of ordered eye medication

11. Older adult alert

a. As a common disorder in this population, cataracts must be considered when assessing older adults with visual disturbances

b. Older clients may not be able to provide self-care after surgery owing to eye shield and impaired vision; clients may require assistance for an extended period of time

H. Retinal detachment

1. Definition: fluid collecting between the neural and pigment layers of the retina

2. Pathophysiology: vitreous humor seeps through an opening in the retina and separates the retina from the pigment epithelium and choroid

3. Etiology: recent or previous trauma, retinal degeneration, and recent cataract surgery

4. Incidence: more common after aged 50 but can occur as a result of trauma at any age

5. Assessment

a. Ask the following questions

(1) Did you notice a flash of light or sparks in front of your eyes?

(2) Do you ever see small specks, spots, or clumps floating in front of your eyes?

(3) Did you experience loss of part of your vision?

b. Clinical manifestations

(1) Flashes: described as flashes of light or sparks in front of eyes; more common when entering a dark room

(2) Floaters: described as specks, spots, or clumps before the eyes

(3) Curtain effect: described as a shade being pulled over part of the visual field

(4) Blurred vision that becomes worse

(5) Loss of visual field

(6) On ophthalmoscopic examination the retina hangs like a torn curtain

6. Expected medical interventions

a. Cryotherapy or laser photocoagulation to seal any breaks in the retina

b. Scleral buckling: suturing a compatible material on the sclera at the site of the break

7. Nursing diagnoses: same as for the client with cataracts
8. Client goals: same as for the client with cataracts
9. Nursing interventions
   a. Acute care
      (1) Preoperative
         (a) Bilateral patching may be ordered to decrease eye movement
         (b) Mydriatics and antibiotic eye medications may be used
      (2) Postoperative: same as the client having cataract surgery
   b. Home care: same as the client having cataract surgery
10. Older adult alert: same as the client having cataract surgery

I. Deafness
1. Definition: complete or partial loss of hearing
2. Pathophysiology
   a. Conductive hearing loss: sounds cannot be conducted through the outer and middle ear; can be improved by hearing aid because the inner ear structures are intact
   b. Sensorineural hearing loss: impaired sensory or neural components of hearing in the inner ear; will not benefit from a hearing aid
3. Etiology: infection, ototoxic substances, trauma, noise, and the aging process
4. Incidence: most common disability in the United States; over 25 million Americans suffer from deafness
5. Assessment
   a. Ask the following questions
      (1) Do you have difficulty understanding words?
      (2) Do you have a ringing in your ears?
   b. Clinical manifestations
      (1) Progressive loss of hearing
      (2) Eventual loss of the ability to understand the spoken word
      (3) Tinnitus
      (4) Distorted or abnormal sounds
   c. Abnormal diagnostic tests: audiometric test: decreased hearing acuity, bilateral or unilateral
6. Expected medical interventions
   a. Hearing aid if found to be effective
   b. Cochlear implant
7. Nursing diagnoses
   a. Sensory: perceptual alterations: auditory related to trauma, infection, ototoxic substances, noise, and the aging process
   b. Risk for injury related to decreased auditory acuity
8. Client goals
   a. Client will state adjustments in lifestyle made to accommodate for changes in hearing
   b. Client will be injury free

9. Nursing interventions regarding client education
   a. How to care for and clean the hearing aid device
   b. Keep the device free of earwax
   c. Prevent the device from getting wet
   d. Check the battery of the device
   e. Keep the device out of extreme heat
10. Evaluation protocol
    a. How will I know that my client teaching has been effective?
       (1) Client will demonstrate correct method for placing device
       (2) Client will demonstrate how to test the battery
       (3) Client will demonstrate correct cleaning method
       (4) Client will state in what type of environment device should be stored
11. Older adult alert
    Being a common disorder, hearing assessment is an important part of the routine assessment of older adult

WEB Resources

http://www.eyenet.org/public/glaucoma/glaucoma.html
   Glaucoma

http://www.nmss.org/
   The National Multiple Sclerosis Society

http://www.spinalinjury.net/
   Spinal cord injury: Spinal cord injury resource center

http://www.amhrt.org/catalog/Stroke_catpage30.html
   Stroke with information about cerebrovascular accidents

REVIEW QUESTIONS

1. The client experienced neurologic changes from a transient ischemic attack. Family members exhibit an understanding of this condition if they discuss with the nurse that associated deficits from this pathology will be gone within what timeframe?
    1. Several hours
    2. Several days
    3. Longer than 24 hours
    4. Over 2 to 3 months

2. In reviewing a client's plan of care, the home care nurse has identified interventions that relate to the client's hemiparesis after the event of an embolic stroke. The nurse would expect to see what documentation by the support staff who had cared for this client within the past month?
    1. The use of a walker for mobility in the home
    2. Full passive range of motion
    3. Full active and passive range of motion
    4. The use of picture aids for communication

3. The nurse is assigned to four clients with various causes of increased ICP. The nurse would prioritize their ongoing assessments to include which sequence of actions?
    1. Level of consciousness, respiratory pattern, blood pressure, pupillary reaction
    2. Pupillary reaction, level of consciousness, respiratory pattern, blood pressure
    3. Blood pressure, level of consciousness, respiratory pattern, pupillary reaction
    4. Respiratory pattern, blood pressure, level of consciousness, pupillary reaction

4. When caring for the client with head trauma, a priority of care would be to prevent transient increases in ICP. A nursing intervention aimed at this action would be to
    1. Administer Ativan (ordered as required) as soon as nausea occurs
    2. Maintain the client in a flat position with proper head and neck alignment
    3. Have the television and radio continuously playing between visits from the family
    4. Perform rectal temperatures with a probe for accuracy

5. The caretaker of a client who has had a recent head injury reports these findings. Which statement requires advisement for the caretaker to call 911 or to bring the person to the emergency room?
    1. Feelings that the heart is beating out of their chest
    2. Complaints of feeling "swimmy headed" when sitting up from a lying position

  3. Vomiting that "shoots across the room"
  4. A very slow, deep breathing pattern

6. The home care nurse visits a client who had a spinal cord injury. Which of these findings indicates that the family is using proper action for the prevention of chronic plantar flexion position of the client's feet?
  1. Mid-calf boots
  2. Rubber-soled dress shoes
  3. High-top shoes
  4. Range-of-motion exercises to the lower extremities every 4 hours

7. Findings of expected complications for a client with a post-3-year spinal cord injury above the T6 level are
  1. A sudden onset of a severe increase in BP, a decreased HR, severe headache
  2. A sudden onset of a mild increase in BP, an increased HR, diaphoresis
  3. A subtle onset of an increased BP, decreased HR, agitation
  4. A subtle onset of a decreased BP, then an increased BP, then a decreased HR with dry, hot skin

8. A client who had undergone cataract surgery on the right eye two weeks ago calls the nurse to report a persistent feeling of sand being in that eye. What is the best response of the nurse?
  1. "Have you been putting in your eye drops as ordered?"
  2. "Do you have any drainage from this eye?"
  3. "This is an expected feeling after your type of surgery. It may persist for a few more weeks."
  4. "This may indicate a need to increase the frequency of your eye drops. After I speak with your doctor, I will call you back with further instructions."

9. Client teaching has been effective if when instilling eye drops the client
  1. Keeps the neck in alignment and drops the drop onto semi-open eyes
  2. Extends the neck and holds the upper lid open and allows the drop to drop onto the eye
  3. Flexes the neck and pulls down on the lower lid and drops the drop onto the eye
  4. Hyper extends the neck and pulls down the lower lid and drops the drop into the lower lid

10. Client teaching, in the holding area before surgery, for a client with a retinal detachment must include
  1. How to instill eye drops into both eyes
  2. That both eyes will continue to be patched postoperatively to prevent eye movement in the affected eye
  3. That eyeglasses with dark lens are needed before and after surgery to minimize photophobia
  4. How deep breathing, coughing and turning will be done after surgery

ANSWERS, RATIONALES, AND TEST-TAKING TIPS

Rationales	Test-Taking Tips

1. Correct answer: 1

Clients who experience a transient ischemic attack (TIA) should have resolution of findings within several minutes or within a maximum of 24 hours. Options 2 and 3 are answers for the condition of reversible ischemic neurologic deficit (RIND). Neurologic deficits from RIND typically resolve within 2 to 3 days, and can last for up to 3 to 4 weeks. Findings in an evolving stroke or CVA typically are permanent. In some clients, however, improvement may occur to varying degrees over longer periods of time such as 1 to 2 years, with minimal improvement over 2 to 3 months.

As you read the options eliminate what you know is incorrect. Options 2 and 3 are similar: the timeframe of "days" being the common element. Therefore, these two options can be eliminated. Options 1 and 4 remain. The key word in the information is "transient." This clue leads you to look for the option that is the least amount of time. Common sense plus the clue word "transient," guides you to eliminate option 4. Select option 1.

2. Correct answer: 3

The client with hemiparesis, or weakness on one side of the body, needs exercise for both sides of the body. These specific exercises are called range-of-motion exercises. They are aimed at maintaining or improving joint or muscle function, or both. However, the types of exercises differ. Active range-of-motion exercises are done on the unaffected side. Passive range-of-motion exercises are done on the side affected with the hemiparesis. Options 1 and 4 are also appropriate actions for clients who have had a stroke.

Once you read the question and the options, you might have the tendency to think the question is about the condition of a stroke. This is an error since the question is asking about hemiparesis, a specific problem rather than the general condition of a stroke. Avoid the temptation to let options such as 1 and 4 change your perception of what the question is. To select the correct option you must focus on the specific problem hemiparesis and the client's strengths, the unaffected side of the body. The unaffected side requires maintenance of the joint and muscle function. If you only focused on

However, these options are not the best answers because the question asks about specific information on the condition hemiparesis. In option 2, passive range-of-motion exercises would be indicated if a client had bilateral extremity weakness or paralysis.

"hemiparesis" your approach is too narrow and did not include the total physiologic muscle and joint needs of this client: the weak and the strong parts of the body.

3. Correct answer: 4

The client with a given clinical condition such as "increased intracranial pressure" must be assessed with the sequence of the basic life-support guidelines: airway, breathing, and circulation, the ABCs. These actions: respiratory pattern and blood pressure evaluations, are then followed by evaluations in the level of consciousness and pupillary reaction, which are the first criteria to change in any given clinical condition. In the other options, the sequence is incorrect for the given situation. Option 1 would be a proper sequence if a client had collapsed from an unknown cause. Think of basic life support in general situations in which the first step is to shake and shout: establish consciousness, then ABCs.

When clients have a given clinical condition: not a suspected or rule-out clinical condition, the ABCs set the priority for a sequence of actions. Then, the stated major dysfunction becomes the next focus. If you misread the given condition as "potential for ICP changes" or "for an increase in ICP," you likely chose options 1 or 2. You have answered *a* question and not *the* question. The question is asking about "ongoing assessments" for a specific, known clinical condition.

4. Correct answer: 1

Nausea may stimulate the gag reflex, which results in a transient increase in ICP. Therefore, timely administration of antiemetics, such as Ativan, is an appropriate action. Option 2 is an incorrect position for clients

Read the question carefully: the content being tested is about ICP. The question about the content is how to prevent transient increases in ICP. Eliminate the options you know are wrong: options 2 and 3. Be cautious not to change the question after you have narrowed

Rationales	Test-Taking Tips

after head trauma. The client's head must be elevated at least 15 to 30 degrees at all times: a low Fowler's position. The second part of this option 2 is correct. The head and neck alignment is important to maintain the drainage of CSF into the jugular veins. In option 3, stimulation by the television or radio is to be avoided since stimulation of any type may further increase ICP. Taking of temperatures rectally, option 4, is to be avoided. Rectal stimulation tends to increase ICP from a vagal or Valsalva "bearing-down" type of response by the body. Auxiliary temperatures are sufficient to monitor the temperature of clients at risk for increased ICP. However, rectal probes may be used on occasion. Remember that rectal probes are left in, thus avoiding the frequent stimulation of putting the probe in and taking it out.

options to a and d and reread option 4. It is true: rectal temperatures are usually the most accurate. However, accuracy of temperatures is not the focus. Avoid not choosing option 1 if you cannot recall what the medication is. The question is not about a medication. The clue is to associate "nausea" with "transient increases in ICP," which is the focus of the question. Avoid the assumption that head trauma clients cannot communicate if nausea occurs. No information is given in the stem to support such data. If you selected option 2, you may have made the error to put more emphasis on the second part of this option, which is correct, than the first part of it, which is incorrect. To avoid this error, after you have selected a two-part option as the correct answer, reverse your reading process. Read the second part of the option first and the first part of the option second. Practice this action until it becomes an automatic routine.

5. Correct answer: 3

Option 3 describes the situation of "projectile" vomiting, which is a classic finding with increased ICP. Increased ICP manifestations are a slow, deep, irregular respiratory pattern; bradycardia; projectile vomiting; and hypertension with a widened pulse pressure: the systolic increases and the diastolic stays about the same. Option 1, usually documented as palpitations, is a finding in clients who typically have valvular heart disease such as a

All of the options are correct for being a concern to the nurse. The clue that leads you to the best option is given in the information before the question: the client had a head injury. Therefore, as you read the given options with the focus of the neurologic system you will have a better chance to select the best option. Ask yourself which option is most associated with neurologic conditions. You might even go one step further to think of risks for increased ICP since the client has a history of a head injury. If you

prolapsed mitral valve or other cardiac malfunctions from ischemia, trauma, or untoward medication effects to the conduction system. Option 2 is a description for postural or orthostatic hypotension, which is a consistent indicator of a volume deficit in the vascular space or a temporary response to spinal or epidural therapies. Option 4 is a correct answer. However, it is not the best answer. Option 4 states neither the regularity nor the rate of the breathing pattern. Increased ICP has the findings of an *irregular* respiratory pattern. The rate of breathing varies with the degree of pressure exerted and the area affected within the cranium.

would have no idea of the correct answer, another approach would be to give each option a theme: option 1 is cardiac; option 2 is vascular volume; option 3 *is neurologic rather than gastrointestinal since the vomiting is "projectile";* and option 4 is pulmonary. An educated guess is to match the topic in the question: neurologic: with the theme in the option. Select option 3. Recall that there is one situation for "projectile vomiting" without a neurologic origin. It is during infancy with the diagnosis of pyloric stenosis.

6. Correct answer: 3

High-top shoes provide the best prevention of foot drop or plantar flexion for clients with diminished muscle tone and joint function of the lower extremity and foot. Usually, high-topped sneakers are recommended because they are less expensive than leather shoes. In option 1, midcalf boots would prevent drop foot, but they are not the best answer. With a midcalf boot more skin area is exposed to potential rubbing and pressure, with an increased risk for skin breakdown. Dress shoes do not prevent drop foot since they usually do not go above the ankle. The type of sole has nothing to do with the selection of this answer. In option 4, range-of-motion exercises for

Note that this is a more difficult question since three of the options could be the correct answer: options 1, 3, and 4. Actions for the selection of the best answer might include the use of the time element, frequency, or to close your eyes and picture the given options. With respect to frequency, options 1 and 3 are continuous therapy and option 4 is intermittent therapy. Therefore, options 1 and 3 are the better answers in this given situation. To decide between these options, think of anatomy: the ankle is the joint involved with foot drop. The item that serves the purpose with minimal skin contact would be the best choice: option 3. Avoid the temptation of getting stuck on the terminology "chronic plantar flexion." Remember to go with what you know: the client had a

Rationales	Test-Taking Tips

the lower extremities is a correct action, but not the best answer. Range-of-motion exercises keep the joint functional and support muscle tone at the time of the exercise. However, in-between the times of the exercises the foot has the tendency to plantar flex.

7. Correct answer: 1

The complication of clients with this type of injury is autonomic dysreflexia or hyperreflexia, of which can occur up until their death. Autonomic dysreflexia manifestations are a rapid onset of severe hypertension with BPs over 200/100, bradycardia, flushing, profuse sweating, and severe headache. These findings usually occur as the result of a noxious stimulus below the level of injury. The most common cause, estimated to be 95% of the time, is bowel or bladder distention, which results from constipation, or urine retention from a failure to do self-catheterization as instructed every 2 to 4 hours. The findings in option 2 are incorrect except for diaphoresis. All of the findings in options 3 and 4 are incorrect since the onset is sudden not subtle and slow.

spinal cord injury and the question is about position of the feet. If you need to, simply figure it out with a focus on what you know and not to focus on the unknown terminology.

This is a more difficult question because the name of the complication is not given. By reading the question and options, the clue of changes in BP and HR should jog your memory to the situation of a dysreflexia because the spinal cord is involved. Associate that an autonomic or sympathetic dysreflexia is a "hyper" situation that occurs quickly. Recall that the sympathetic system is used in times of emergency and not for day-to-day bodily functions. Narrow the options to 1 and 2, which have sudden onsets, and then read the findings of each option. Agitation, a change in level of consciousness that is commonly associated with head injuries, has nothing to do with a spinal cord injury, especially in the rehabilitation phase. Or you could think of days of high stress or sympathetic stimulation when most people end up with headaches. Now, if you have no idea of the correct answer, go with what you know about the options. Reread the options to note that option 1 has two key clues: a sudden onset that typically indicates complications and the word "severe," which usually indicates a need for immediate action because a complication may have occurred. Select option 1.

8. Correct answer: 3

Option 3 is a true statement. The responses in option 1 and 2 might be correct if the question was different; for example: "What is the best initial response to gather further information or to do further assessment?" The first sentence in option 4 is not correct. The second actions, to notify the physician and get back to the client, are appropriate actions.

The timeframe of 2 weeks postoperative is an important factor. If the client was not inserting drops as ordered, or if the client had drainage from the eye, other findings such as mild to severe pain or fever would have caused the client to notify the nurse before the 2 weeks. Another clue is that the finding is described by the client as "persistent," which indicates that the feeling did not change with or without the eye medication. Finally, expected complaints for 4 to 6 weeks after cataract surgery are frequent tearing from the eye and the "scratchy" feeling of sand in the eye.

9. Correct answer: 4

The correct method for a client to instill eye drops is to hyperextend the neck and the pull down on the lower lid, and place the drop on the cup formed by the lower lid, the conjunctival sac. Options 1, 2, and 3 are incorrect actions to instill eye drops.

Recall that the surface of the eye is very sensitive and this eliminates options 2 and 3, which have the eyedrop placed "onto the eye." For questions such as this one, where positions are being tested, you can act out the positions as you read the options. As you get into the given positions, it will become obvious which of the options is the correct answer. If you are unsure of what positions of the neck are: flexed, extended, and hyperextended: go back to the pictures in your basic nursing text to get them cemented into your mind. Remember that a picture is worth a thousand words.

10. Correct answer: 2

Clients must be taught preoperatively the rationale for bilateral patching: when one eye moves, the other will move as well. Thus, to restrict eye movements both eyes must be

Recall tip: retinal detachment: two words for the condition means two patches on the eyes. Cataract is one word: use one patch on the affected eye postoperative. Other approaches can be used to eliminate the three

Rationales	Test-Taking Tips
patched. In option 1, teaching of eyedrop installation is not a priority at this time. This will be taught postoperatively and usually to another family member. In option 3 most clients have photophobia after eye surgery. However, the one part of the option about the dark glasses worn in the initial preoperative period is incorrect content. Option 4 is an incorrect action. The usual postoperative techniques are not done after eye surgery. These types of exercises mimic straining and would increase intraocular pressure which then puts pressure on the surgical site in the eye.	wrong options. Use common sense to eliminate option 1. A client with any deficit eye function will not be able to see nor give a return demonstration for eyedrop installation. Associate mydriatric eye drops make the pupil larger as it relaxes it. Remember when you had your eyes dilated at the eye doctor to have the pressure and retina checked. Therefore, light enters the eye freely and results in photophobia. Mydriatric eye drops are commonly given to relax the eye after eye surgery or eye trauma. After the surgery dark glasses are worn as needed indoors and outdoors for a week or two. The usual postoperative exercises: deep breathing, coughing, and turning, are Valsalva maneuvers to be avoided postoperatively in clients who have had cranial surgery, eye surgery, or head trauma.

2

The Cardiac System

FAST FACTS

1. Weight gain or loss in a cardiac client most often is related to fluid weight gain or loss. An increase in weight of more than 2 lb/wk is the most accurate indicator of fluid weight gain: 1 kg equals 2.2 lb, which equals 1 L of fluid.
2. Tachycardia and hypotension, which are assessment factors for cardiac decompensation, occur when the body systems are unable to compensate for a cardiac disease.
3. An increased HR is the first indication of decreased cardiac output (CO), and is followed by a decreased BP.
4. Anxiety may be seen in cardiac clients as a result of fear of dying, lifestyle adjustments, and a need to depend on medications for minimum functioning.
5. Cardiac output = HR × stroke volume (SV): (1) for CO, think BP; (2) for SV, think intravascular fluid volume loss or gain; (3) when fluid volume decreases (a decreased **preload**), the HR increases to maintain CO or BP at near normal values; and (4) decompensation eventually occurs as the HR increases to over 120 to 130 beats per minute as a result of less time for ventricular filling, and thus a significant decrease in CO or the volume pumped will occur. The BP drops.
6. The heart and lungs work together, increasing or decreasing heart and breathing rates in a given situation: (1) bradycardia with bradypnea and (2) tachycardia with tachypnea.
7. The HR increases with any pathologic problem except neuropathology. The HR decreases with (1) spinal shock, (2) increased ICP, (3) autonomic dysreflexia, and (4) vasovagal reflex.

CONTENT REVIEW

I. The cardiac system
Definition—the cardiac system is responsible for pumping:
   1. Oxygenated blood (arterial) to the cells for cellular nutrition, oxygenation, and to pick up waste product such as CO_2

2. Deoxygenated blood (venous) back to the pulmonary system to get rid of wastes and replenish oxygen

II. **Structure and function**

A. **The heart is a muscular organ about the size of an adult fist and is positioned directly on the diaphragm, between the lungs**
   1. Layers of the heart and coverings
      a. Pericardium—double-thickness membrane that covers the heart and the roots of the great vessels
      b. Epicardium—outermost covering
      c. Myocardium—muscle layer itself
      d. Endocardium—innermost covering
   2. Heart chambers
      a. Right atrium—receives venous blood from the systemic and cardiac circulation
      b. Left atrium—receives arterial blood from the lungs
      c. Right ventricle—receives blood from the right atrium; pumps to the pulmonic circulation
      d. Left ventricle—receives blood from the left atrium; pumps out to the systemic circulation
   3. Valves—maintain a forward flow of blood through the heart
      a. Tricuspid—between the right atrium and ventricle and attached to papillary muscles
      b. Pulmonic—between the right ventricle and the lungs at the base of the pulmonary artery
      c. Mitral—between the left atrium and ventricle and attached to papillary muscles
      d. Aortic—between the left ventricle and aorta
   4. **Conduction** system
      a. General sequence
         (1) Specialized cardiac cells initiate an electrical impulse
         (2) The electrical impulse is transmitted throughout the heart
         (3) Chambers of the heart are stimulated to contract in a coordinated pattern
      b. Impulse sequence
         (1) Impulse originates in sinoatrial node (SA)
         (2) Impulse fans out across both atria; followed by atrial contraction
         (3) Recollects at the atrioventricular (AV) node
         (4) Travels through the bundle of His—at the top of the septum
         (5) Moves into the Purkinje fibers in the ventricles; followed by ventricular contraction
      c. Depolarization—ion exchange in conduction cells (sodium-potassium pump)
         (1) Potassium leaves cells
         (2) Sodium enters cells

(3) Calcium enters cells through slow calcium channels; calcium is released in large quantities
 d. Repolarization—ions return to normal balance
  (1) Potassium returns to cells
  (2) Sodium leaves cells
 e. Polarized state is the resting state

III. **Targeted concerns**
A. **Pharmacology—priority drug classifications**
 1. Cardiac glycosides—increase the force of myocardial contraction
  a. Expected effects—increase in CO with increased urine output in some cases; slowing of the rate of impulse initiation from the SA node and thus the movement through the AV node to decrease the HR
  b. Commonly given drugs
   (1) Digoxin (Lanoxin)
   (2) Digitoxin
  c. Nursing considerations
   (1) Hold drug for HR less than 60 beats per minute or greater than 120 beats per minute; notify physician within 2 to 3 hours
   (2) Assess for hypokalemia; most common finding is cramps in lower leg; low potassium potentiates the action of digitalis drugs and increases the risk for digoxin toxicity
   (3) Assess for digoxin toxicity, level greater than 2.5 ng/ml digoxin; most common initial findings are anorexia, nausea, and vomiting; later findings may be yellow vision, green halos around objects, and dysrhythmias
 2. Beta-adrenergic blocking agents—block sympathetic stimulation (epinephrine) to beta-receptor sites in the body
  a. Expected effects
   (1) Decreased myocardial **contractility;** decreased oxygen need of the myocardium, which prevents angina pectoris
   (2) Decreased HR
   (3) Decreased BP
   (4) Mild decrease in anxiety
  b. Commonly given drugs
   (1) Propanolol hydrochloride* (Inderal)
   (2) Metoprolol tartrate* (Lopressor)
  c. Nursing considerations
   (1) Hold drug for HR less than 50 beats per minute; notify physician within 2 to 3 hours
   (2) Caution against abrupt withdrawal—result may be severe angina pectoris

---

*The generic names of all beta-blockers end in "lol." Think of the word lull—makes the heart sleepy and slow.

(3) Assess for orthostatic hypotension—decrease in systolic BP greater than 20 mm Hg when changing from a lying or sitting to a standing position

(4) Assess for symptoms of right- and left-sided heart failure

3. Calcium channel blocking agents—block influx of calcium into cells by way of the slow channels

  a. Expected effects

    (1) Decreased HR; slows tachycardic dysrhythmias

    (2) Decreased myocardial contractility; prevents angina pectoris

    (3) Decreased BP owing to arteriolar vasodilation

    (4) Prevention of coronary artery spasm

  b. Commonly given drugs

    (1) Nifedipine (Procardia)

    (2) Verapamil hydrochloride (Calan, Isoptin)

    (3) Diltiazem hydrochloride (Cardizem)

  c. Nursing considerations

    (1) Hold drug for HR less than 50 beats per minute; notify physician within 2 to 3 hours

    (2) Assess for orthostatic hypotension

    (3) Assess for symptoms of right- and left-sided heart failure

    (4) Note that the action of these drugs is potentiated when used with beta-blockers

4. Nitrates—dilate vascular smooth muscle

  a. Expected effects

    (1) Peripheral vasodilation, especially venous capacitance and arterial resistance vessels, leads to pooling of blood in the peripheral circulation. Pooling of blood decreases the amount of blood returned to the right side of the heart, and thus decreasing heart preload and workload.

    (2) Collateral circulation of the heart is dilated with higher doses of IV NTG; increased oxygen is delivered to the myocardium

  b. Commonly given drugs

    (1) Nitroglycerin (Tridil)—IV drip preparation given for acute anginal attacks; clients cardiac status must be to be monitored

    (2) Nitroglycerin (Nitrostat)—sublingual preparation given for acute anginal attacks

    (3) Nitroglycerin (Nitro-Bid)—oral preparation given to prevent anginal attacks

    (4) Nitroglycerin (Transderm-Nitro)—transdermal preparation given to prevent anginal attacks

  c. Nursing considerations

    (1) BP of less than 90/60 mm Hg, hold medication and contact physician

    (2) Assess for orthostatic hypotension

(3) Remove old patches, wash site to remove all medication

(4) Rotate sites of transdermal preparations

(5) IV preparation must be mixed in a glass IV bottle; use only polyethylene tubing to prevent absorption of drug into tubing

5. Antidysrhythmic drugs—suppress or obliterate impulses originating in the **conduction** pathway and competing with the SA node; in the subclassifications of these drugs, different mechanisms occur to suppress or obliterate dysrythmias

a. Expected effects—decreased HR, regulated regular heart rhythm

b. Commonly given drugs

(1) Lidocaine (Xylocaine)—IV only; first sign of toxicity is confusion; severe toxicity causes seizures

(2) Quinidine polygalacturonate—major side effect is diarrhea

(3) Procainamide hydrochloride (Pronestyl)—major concern with IV administration is hypotension; major concerns with oral administration are rash and arthralgia

(4) Bretylium tosylate (Bretylol)—major concerns are hypotension, nausea, and vomiting after rapid IV infusion

c. Nursing considerations

(1) Monitor for bradycardia and heart block

(2) Assess for central nervous system abnormalities

6. Antihyperlipidemics (lipoprotein lowering drugs) lower serum lipoprotein levels by a decrease in their production or by a removal of lipoproteins from the body

a. Expected effect—decreased risk of developing atherosclerosis

b. Commonly given drugs

(1) Gemfibrozil (Lopid) inhibits synthesis of lipoproteins

(2) Lovastatin (Mevacor) inhibits synthesis of lipoproteins

c. Nursing considerations

(1) May elevate creatine phosphokinase (CPK) levels

(2) Administer with food to decrease gastric irritation

(3) Monitor liver function periodically for increases in alanine aminotransferase (ALT) and aspartate aminotransferase (AST)

(4) Teach client that excess cholesterol will be eliminated by way of the bowel and may cause increased flatus or change in stool consistency

B. Procedures

1. Electrocardiogram (EKG, ECG)—a record of the electrical activity of the heart. Six limb leads and six precordial leads depict the transmission of impulses down through the conduction system. Abnormal electrical activity may indicate impaired impulse transmission through the heart, which could be caused by ischemic, injured, or infarcted cardiac tissue.

2. Stress test—an ECG tracing, done while the client exercises on either a stationary bike or treadmill, to evaluate the myocardial response to an increased oxygen demand. This tests helps diagnose

preinfarction angina. For clients unable to exercise, a dipyridamole (Persantine) thallium stress test can be performed. The injected (IV) dipyridamole dilates the coronary arteries and increases oxygen demand; the thallium shows the well-perfused areas of the heart.

3. Echocardiography—ultrasound technique used to evaluate the internal structure and function of the heart muscle and valves. This technique evaluates cardiac chamber size, wall action, ejection fraction, and presence of cardiac effusions.

4. Cardiac catheterization and coronary angiography—invasive procedures used to evaluate ejection fraction and filling pressures of the heart ventricles, that usually are performed by way of the femoral or anticubital artery (left heart cath) or vein (right heart cath). Patency of the coronary arteries is also evaluated through the use of fluoroscopy during dye injection. Dye injection results in diuresis, therefore, monitor and replace fluids after the procedure.

5. Serum cardiac markers—proteins released into the blood after heart muscle damage
   a. Cardiac enzymes: cellular enzymes released into blood when cardiac cells die
      (1) CPK
      (2) Lactate dehydrogenase (LDH)
      (3) Isoenzymes—are more specific to cardiac cell injury; fractionation of CPK and LDH
         (a) CK-MB (creatine kinase isoenzyme containing M and B subunits) elevates to peak within 24 to 48 hours of the myocardial infarction (MI)
         (b) Level of LDH_1 greater than that of LDH_2, increases in 24 to 48 hours after an MI and peaks in 2 to 3 days to return to normal in approximately 5 to 10 days
         (c) Elevation of enzyme levels indicates MI
         (d) Note: alphabetically C comes before L, thus it is easy to remember that CK-MB peaks first—within 24 hours—before LDH changes
   b. Troponin level—myocardial muscle protein is elevated in the face of myocardial injury—highly specific for myocardial damage from 24 hours up to 1 week; Troponin I and T
   c. Myoglobin level—increases within 3 hours of an MI. A history of trauma, inflammation, and ischemic changes to the noncardiac skeletal muscles needs to be ruled out because these also can cause elevated levels of myoglobin.

C. **Psychosocial concerns**
   1. Denial—the most common and earliest response to chest pain. Clients frequently attribute chest pain to indigestion or stress and thus may delay treatment
   2. Anxiety—an uncomfortable feeling associated with an unknown direct cause. Many clients are unable to discuss their feelings of anxiety; however, they do feel uneasy about what may happen

3. Fear—an uncomfortable feeling associated with real danger
4. Anger—normal sequence of feelings in the cardiac client when lifestyle changes occur. The anger, sometimes aimed at caregivers, usually is a reaction to required lifestyle changes as a result of the client's illness
5. Lifestyle changes—directly related to the degree of incapacitation and mainly revolve around diet, activity, type of work, personal habits, and environment

  D. **Health history—question sequence**
1. What symptoms are you having that have made it necessary for you to seek assistance?
2. Are you currently being treated by a physician for any other problems?
3. Have you ever been treated for any injuries or illnesses in the past?
4. Is there a family history of cardiac disease?
5. Are you presently taking any prescription or over-the-counter drugs? If so, what are they?
6. Are you following a diet prescribed by a physician?
7. Do you follow a specific diet?
8. Do you smoke or have you ever smoked? If yes, how much?
9. Do you drink alcohol, coffee, soft drinks, or tea? If yes, how much?
10. What is your usual activity level? Do you exercise and how much?
11. Do you live a stressful lifestyle, either in the home or at work?

  E. **Physical examination—appropriate sequence**
1. Vital signs—ABCs
2. Chest pain evaluation—scale of 0 to 10
3. Skin color, temperature, moisture, turgor—compare central versus peripheral
4. Arterial pulses
5. Jugular vein distention—evaluate with the client positioned with the head of the bed elevated to at least a 35-degree angle
6. Inspection of the chest for chest wall movement and pulsations
7. Palpation of the chest for point of maximal impulse (PMI) and chest wall pain (Figure 2-1). Use the mitral valve area to palpate the PMI.
8. Auscultation of heart sounds (Figure 2-1)
   a. Diaphragm of stethoscope for S_1 and S_2, high-pitched murmurs
   b. Bell of stethoscope for S_3 and S_4, low-pitched murmurs
9. Auscultation of lung sounds—use stethoscope diaphragm

IV. Pathophysiologic disorders
  A. **Coronary artery disease**
1. Definition—a disorder of diminished blood flow to the coronary arteries. The heart is starved of blood flow, and thus of oxygen and nutrients
2. Pathophysiology—atherosclerotic plaque lines the walls of the coronary arteries. Plaque continues to grow over the years, resulting

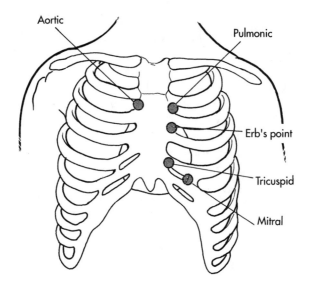

Figure 2-1 Cardiac auscultatory areas. (From Price SA, Wilson LM: *Pathophysiology: clinical concepts of disease processes,* ed 5, St. Louis, 1997, Mosby.)

in decreased lumen size. The overall effect is an imbalance between the amount of oxygen supplied to and required by the myocardium.

3. Etiology—contributing factors
   a. Heredity
   b. Age
   c. Gender
   d. Hypertension
   e. Hyperlipidemia
   f. Obesity
   g. Diabetes
   h. Smoking
   i. Sedentary lifestyle
   j. Coronary artery spasm—coronary artery spasm is one of the etiologies of CAD—unknown why it occurs—causes severe decreased blood flow to the heart due to spasm
4. Incidence—leading cause of death in the United States. Approximately 500,000 deaths a year occur from coronary artery disease. It is estimated that close to 5 million people have coronary artery disease.
5. Assessment
   a. Questions to ask
      (1) Where is the pain? Can you point to the pain with one finger?
      (2) How long have you had the pain?
      (3) On a scale of 0 to 10, which number would you assign to your pain? (1 is mild pain; 10 is the most severe)

      (4) Does the pain radiate? If so, where?

      (5) How would you describe your pain?

      (6) What were you doing just before the pain started?

      (7) Did you do anything that made the pain better or worse?

b. Clinical manifestations

  (1) Angina pectoris—myocardial ischemia

     (a) Chest pain, tightness, or heaviness

     (b) Relieved quickly: 3 minutes to a maximum of 15 minutes by rest or by sublingual nitroglycerin (NTG)

     (c) Physical exertion or stress initiates symptoms

     (d) Radiation of pain may or may not be present

  (2) *Prinzmetal's angina* is chest pain that occurs during rest or sleep caused by coronary artery spasm

  (3) Myocardial infarction (MI)—myocardial necrosis

     (a) Severe crushing, stabbing chest pain—more severe than angina

     (b) Not relieved by rest or NTG

     (c) Pain lasts much longer than angina: longer than 20 minutes

     (d) Frequently associated with shortness of breath (SOB), nausea, and diaphoresis

     (e) May or may not have radiation of pain

c. Abnormal laboratory findings

  (1) Angina pectoris

     (a) Lipid levels—may be elevated, indicating atherosclerotic involvement

  (2) Prinzmetal's angina

     (a) Lipid levels—may be elevated, indicating some associated atherosclerosis

  (3) MI

     (a) Enzymes—elevated levels of troponins, myoglobin and CK-MB, $LDH_2 > LDH_1$ indicate myocardial necrosis

     (b) CBC—elevated leukocyte count (WBC)

d. Abnormal diagnostic tests

  (1) Angina pectoris

     (a) ECG—ST-segment elevation and T-wave inversion are more common in unstable angina. During pain-free periods, ST segment and T waves most often are normal

     (b) Exercise stress test—during test: chest pain, ST-segment elevation, bradycardia, or exaggerated tachycardia are exhibited

     (c) Echocardiography—may show abnormal wall motion and decreased ejection fraction, less than 50%

     (d) Cardiac catheterization—shows impaired blood flow, partial obstruction or narrowing of coronary arteries

(2) Prinzmetal's angina
  (a) ECG—ST-segment elevation occurs before or during pain then returns to normal when pain is relieved. Dysrhythmias are not uncommon during pain.
  (b) Exercise stress test—helps distinguish between Prinzmetal's angina and angina pectoris. In Prinzmetal's angina, the results would be normal.
  (c) Cardiac catheterization—coronary artery spasm can be induced during test to differentiate between types of angina

(3) MI
  (a) ECG, specific leads
    (i) ST-segment elevation—injured cardiac tissue
    (ii) T-wave inversion—ischemia, seen in the acute stages
    (iii) Q waves larger or wider than normal in specific leads—indicative of myocardial necrosis
  (b) Chest x-ray (CXR)—may show various degrees of left ventricular failure or pulmonary congestion
  (c) Echocardiography—identifies abnormal wall motion of ventricles, abnormal chamber size, septal abnormalities, valvular dysfunction, and reduced ejection fraction of less than 50%
  (d) Radionuclide blood pool imaging with radioactive technetium (^{99m}TC)—pinpoints infarcted tissue, size of infarct, and degree of ventricular dysfunction. Thallium-201 myocardial perfusion scintigraphy can detect ischemic tissue.

6. Expected medical interventions
  a. Angina pectoris
    (1) Nitrate therapy
    (2) Beta-blocker and calcium-channel blocker therapy to decrease oxygen consumption by the heart
    (3) Low-fat, low-cholesterol, calorie-controlled diet
    (4) Diagnostic studies to determine the extent of coronary artery impairment
    (5) Percutaneous transluminal coronary angioplasty (PTCA) to dilate coronary arteries if indicated
    (6) Intra-coronary artery stents—used to prevent closure of a coronary artery dilated by PTCA and to prevent restenosis of the artery
    (7) Coronary artery bypass graft (CABG) to occluded or partially occluded coronary arteries
  b. Prinzmetal's angina
    (1) Nifedipine (Procardia) to prevent coronary artery spasm
    (2) Change in lifestyle as deemed necessary

   c. MI

     (1) Admission to the hospital in a monitored unit, either telemetry or coronary care unit

     (2) Pain medication for chest pain relief

     (3) Maintenance of BP as needed

     (4) Thrombolytic therapy if chest pain lasts less than 6 hours, and the client has not had recent surgery, trauma, pregnancy, or a bleeding disorder or has not recently taken anticoagulants

     (5) Emergency heart catheterization followed by PTCA and stent placement or CABG surgery if indicated

     (6) Infusion of Abciximab (ReoPro), a platelet aggregate inhibitor—to prevent abrupt closure of a treated coronary artery by a fresh clot—use after PTCA

     (7) Antidysrhythmic therapy as needed

     (8) Bed rest, sedatives if necessary

7. Nursing diagnoses

   a. Chest pain related to imbalance between oxygen supply and demand of myocardium

   b. Anxiety related to threat of physical well-being

   c. Decreased CO related to cardiac rhythm disturbances

   d. Decreased CO related to decreased ventricular contractility

   e. Activity intolerance related to decreased cardiac contractility

8. Client goals

   a. Client will state chest pain is relieved

   b. Client will state feeling more relaxed and calm

   c. Client will exhibit vital signs that are within 10% of baseline

   d. Client will increase activity without associated symptoms by 5% each day (e.g., each day, 10 more feet walked, 5 more steps climbed, and so on)

9. Nursing interventions

   a. Acute care

     (1) Top priority—once ABCs have been stabilized, the priority is pain relief

     (2) Administer oxygen and other medications as directed

     (3) Monitor at least every hour for indications of decreased CO—sustained HR greater than 20 beats per minute over baseline, lowered BP, and decreased urine output

     (4) Monitor cardiac rhythm for premature ventricular contractions (PVCs), the most common dysrhythmia, and treat with Lidocaine

     (5) Monitor lung sounds for crackles, wheezes, and consolidation

     (6) Maintain a patent IV line

     (7) Maintain a restful environment

     (8) Give brief explanations for all procedures, tests, and equipment

     (9) Encourage verbalization of feelings

b. Home care regarding client education
   (1) How to administer and store short- and long-acting nitrates
      (a) Sublingual nitrates
         (i) Take sublingual nitroglycerin at pain onset, then two at 5-minute intervals. If the pain persists, call for assistance and transport to a hospital emergency room
         (ii) Store in dry, dark bottle
         (iii) Obtain a new bottle every 6 months because once opened, the shelf life is 3 to 6 months. A tingling under the tongue indicates potency of medication.
      (b) Transdermal nitrates
         (i) Rotate sites in less hairy areas above the knees or elbows
         (ii) Wash site after removal of patch
   (2) How to perform interventions for evaluation of medication effectiveness
      (a) How to take radial pulse daily; best before getting out of bed
      (b) Which adverse reactions require medical assistance, such as persistent anorexia, nausea, vomiting, or change in vision
   (3) How to increase activity level slowly
   (4) How to take weight daily: before breakfast, at the same time each day, using the same scale, and wearing the same amount of clothing; report losses or gains of over 2 lb/wk to physician
   (5) How to change diet to a low-fat, low-cholesterol, moderate-to-low salt diet
   (6) When sexual activity can resume; usually when client can climb a flight of stairs without SOB or chest pain
c. Home environment evaluation
   (1) Location of bedrooms, bathrooms, and kitchen
   (2) Need to walk steps
   (3) Roles of family members
   (4) Need for job counseling
10. Evaluation protocol
   a. How do I know that my interventions were effective?
      (1) Has the client's chest pain decreased?
      (2) Does the client feel any SOB or dizziness?
      (3) Does the client feel anxious right now?
   b. What criteria will I use to change my interventions?
      (1) Chest pain is not relieved or is not reduced to a comfortable level for the client
      (2) SOB is not relieved or is exacerbated
      (3) Client is unable to tolerate even simple activities, such as turning in bed or ambulating in a room, without SOB or diaphoresis

    c. How will I know that my client teaching has been effective?
      (1) Client will demonstrate correct technique for evaluating own pulse
      (2) Client will walk 10 feet further each day without chest pain or SOB
      (3) Client will take nitroglycerin when in pain, up to three tablets at 5-minute intervals

11. Older adult alert—as a normal course of aging, some similar characteristics are:
    a. Decreased renal excretion with an increased risk for digitalis toxicity
    b. Decreased skin turgor and dry mucous membranes; inspection of the tongue best indicates dehydration or decreased fluid volume
    c. Decreased CO

B. Cardiac dysrhythmias

1. Definition—a disorder of the electrical system of the heart, causing abnormal HR, rhythm, or both
    a. Most common effect—decreased CO
    b. Most severe effect—sudden cardiac death
    c. Most dangerous effect—ventricular dysrhythmia
    d. Least dangerous effect—atrial dysrhythmia
    e. Tachycardia is more dangerous than bradycardia because of the decreased coronary artery filling time associated with tachycardia. Clients are more likely to experience chest pain and SOB with tachycardia.

2. Pathophysiology—three mechanisms may trigger cardiac dysrhythmia
    a. Reentry mechanism—the conducted impulse is permitted to enter into a rapid circular motion through conduction pathways that result in tachycardia
    b. Increased automaticity—the electricity required to stimulate a cell to depolarize is reduced. The cell is easily stimulated, allowing for abnormal impulse formation that results in premature beats.
    c. Impaired conduction—the impulse is either slowed or blocked in conduction pathways, usually resulting in bradycardia or atrioventricular (AV) heart block—first, second, or third degree. The most common site for impaired conduction is the AV node.

3. Etiology—most commonly arise from the following
    a. Myocardial cellular hypoxia, from a cardiac, hematologic (anemia), or respiratory disorder
    b. Electrolyte imbalance
    c. Drug toxicity

4. Incidence—major cause of death in the client with an acute MI

5. Assessment
    a. Questions to ask
        (1) Have you felt any palpitations or a feeling as if your heart is flipping over in your chest?
        (2) Have you felt dizzy or light-headed?
        (3) Have you had blurred vision?
        (4) Have you had any chest pain or SOB?
    b. Clinical manifestations
        (1) Irregular heart rhythm with a rate over 100 or under 60 beats per minute
        (2) Pale skin color, diaphoresis
        (3) Feeling of increased anxiety, nervousness leading to confusion, lethargy, and comatose state
        (4) Hypotension, BP less than 90/60 mm Hg
    c. Abnormal laboratory findings
        (1) Arterial blood gases (ABG)—hypoxemia: partial pressure of oxygen in arterial blood (PaO_2) of less than 80 mm Hg; acidosis with a pH of less than 7.35
        (2) Electrolytes—severe high or low levels, especially potassium, magnesium, or calcium
        (3) Toxicology studies—elevated levels
    d. Abnormal diagnostic tests
        (1) ECG—conclusive evidence of the type of dysrhythmia; should be obtained when client is symptomatic
        (2) Holter monitor, 24-hour ambulatory ECG—gives information regarding dysrhythmia, in relation to client activity, especially if dysrhythmia is intermittent. It is very important for client to maintain an activity log during monitoring
        (3) Electophysiologic studies (EPS)—in the hospital, dysrhythmia is medically induced for an accurate diagnosis of the site of origin and effectiveness of selected drugs
6. Expected medical interventions
    a. Cardioversion or defibrillation for life-threatening dysrhythmia as indicated
    b. Antidysrhythmic drugs
    c. Pacemaker insertion, temporary and/or permanent as indicated
7. Nursing diagnoses
    a. Decreased CO related to ineffective cardiac rhythm
    b. Activity intolerance related to ineffective CO
    c. Anxiety related to change in health status
8. Client goals
    a. Client will have appropriate CO as evidenced by HR within 10 to 20 beats per minute of baseline and rhythm without ectopy; BP systolic within 20 mm Hg of baseline

   b. Client will increase activity without associated symptoms by 5% each day (e.g., each day, 10 more feet walked, 5 more steps climbed, and so on)
   c. Client will state feeling more relaxed and calm
9. Nursing interventions
   a. Acute care
      (1) Monitor cardiac client in a critical care or telemetry unit
      (2) Initiate prompt treatment for life-threatening dysrhythmias—lidocaine for PVCs and ventricular tachycardia; pacemaker for third-degree heart block
      (3) Monitor lung sounds, evaluate for left ventricular failure
      (4) Administer antidysrhythmic drug therapy and evaluate for adverse reactions
   b. Home care regarding client education
      (1) Explain the adverse reactions, desired effects, and symptoms to report from medication therapy
      (2) Encourage the client to cease any activity if dysrhythmic symptoms occur and take peripheral pulse for 1 minute at that time—note the rate and regularity
      (3) Explain dietary restrictions because of the stimulant effect of, for example, coffee, tea, and chocolate products
      (4) Discourage smoking
10. Evaluation protocol
   a. How do I know that my interventions were effective?
      (1) Client will not have symptoms of heart rhythm problem
      (2) Client will not feel SOB
   b. What criteria will I use to change my interventions?
      (1) Increased or sustained symptoms associated with dysrhythmia
      (2) Decreased BP with a change in level of consciousness (LOC)
      (3) Evidence of SOB at rest
   c. How will I know that my client teaching has been effective?
      (1) Client uses decaffeinated coffee and tea, and is not eating chocolate
      (2) Client reports no difficulties taking scheduled medication and has noted no side effects
      (3) Client states that if palpitations or dizziness occur a rest period of at least 15 to 30 minutes is required, with the radial pulse taken at the beginning and end of the rest period
11. Older adult alert
   a. Older adult clients have a decreased CO as a normal course of aging. Thus it is imperative to have baseline vital signs to determine changes after medication is begun
   b. Because renal excretion in older adult clients is decreased, they are more vulnerable to drug toxicity from the antidysrhythmic drugs

    c. Quinidine, a common antidysrhythmic drug, is known to cause severe watery diarrhea. In older adult clients this could quickly lead to metabolic acidosis, electrolyte imbalance, and water dehydration from the loss of potassium and buffers.

C. **Congestive heart failure (CHF)**
  1. Definition—heart is unable to produce sufficient CO to meet the metabolic demands of the body
  2. Pathophysiology—there are many causes of CHF, most of which fit into two categories
    a. The etiologies that cause a decrease in contractility of the myocardium
    b. The etiologies that cause the myocardium to work harder
    c. Cardiac compensatory mechanisms—to improve CO
      (1) Tachycardia
      (2) Ventricular dilation
      (3) Ventricular hypertrophy
    d. Left ventricular failure is manifested first in most clients
      (1) Left ventricle is unable to propel blood in a forward motion into the arterial circulation
      (2) Blood that cannot be propelled forward will back up into the left atrium and then into the pulmonary vessels and lung fields
      (3) Pulmonary vessels become engorged with blood, and plasma begins to leak out of the vessels into the interstitial and alveolar spaces
      (4) The life-threatening form is referred to as acute pulmonary edema and exhibits frothy pink sputum and severe gas exchange abnormalities
    e. Right ventricular failure is commonly caused by overwork of the right ventricle attempting to pump blood into greatly engorged pulmonary vessels. Because blood cannot be propelled forward, it backs up into the systemic circulation (not considered a life-threatening situation).
  3. Etiology—many conditions can cause CHF, including MI, systemic and pulmonary hypertension (increased afterload), valvular abnormalities, and myocarditis
  4. Assessment
    a. Questions to ask
      (1) Are you having difficulty breathing?
      (2) Does minimal activity make it even more difficult to breathe?
      (3) When you sleep, how many pillows do you place under your head?
      (4) Do you ever wake up feeling as if you are smothering?
      (5) Do your ankles or feet swell? At what time of day does this occur?
      (6) Do you feel fatigued or tired on a daily basis?

b. Clinical manifestations
   (1) Left-sided failure—think left, lung
       (a) Dry cough, eventually productive
       (b) Fatigue
       (c) Dyspnea on exertion, then at rest
       (d) Crackles or rales in lung fields, usually bilaterally at the bases
       (e) Orthopnea—unable to sleep flat
       (f) Paroxysmal nocturnal dyspnea (PND): awakens from sleep with a smothering feeling
       (g) S_3 heard over left ventricle
   (2) Acute pulmonary edema
       (a) Profound dyspnea, progressing to respiratory failure and arrest
       (b) Pink, frothy sputum production
       (c) Crackles in all the lung fields
       (d) Respiratory acidosis, hypoxemia
       (e) Metabolic acidosis
   (3) Right-sided failure
       (a) Jugular venous distention
       (b) Easily fatigued
       (c) Hepatomegaly—enlarged liver
       (d) Dependant, pitting edema—if on bed rest, sacral edema; if ambulatory, ankles and feet edematous
       (e) S_3 heard over right ventricle
c. Abnormal laboratory findings
   (1) ABG—hypoxemia equals a PaO_2 of less than 80; hypercapnia equals a partial pressure of carbon dioxide in arterial blood ($PaCO_2$) of greater than 45
   (2) Electrolytes—low sodium from vascular fluid overload; low potassium and magnesium from diuretic therapy
   (3) Liver function studies—slight elevation in levels of AST, bilirubin, and alkaline phosphatase from hepatomegaly
d. Abnormal diagnostic tests
   (1) CXR—left-sided failure only: pulmonary congestion and interstitial edema
   (2) ECG—changes indicative of hypertrophy of the left or right ventricle; would also be diagnostic for dysrhythmias
   (3) Echocardiogram—left-sided failure: abnormal wall movement, may be hypokinetic; diminished ejection fraction of less than 50%

5. Expected medical interventions
   a. Digitalis preparations to increase pumping capability of the myocardium
   b. Diuretics to decrease fluid load in the interstitial spaces
   c. Oxygen as SOB and fatigue become more of a problem

6. Nursing diagnoses
   a. Decreased CO related to poor left or right ventricular pumping capability
   b. Fluid volume excess in interstitial spaces related to increased vascular pressure and shifting of fluid into interstitial spaces
   c. Impaired gas exchange related to fluid layer in the alveoli and small airways
   d. Activity intolerance related to decreased oxygenation of body tissues from decreased CO
   e. Anxiety related to SOB and fatigue, secondary to decreased oxygenation of the body tissues
7. Client goals
   a. Client will exhibit vital signs that are within 10% of baseline
   b. Client will exhibit decreased crackles in the lung field by 10% within 2 hours
   c. Client will exhibit a decrease in the circumference of edematous extremities by 1 inch within 2 days of the initial therapy
   d. Client will maintain a PO_2 of 80 to 100 mm Hg and a partial pressure of carbon dioxide (PCO_2) of 35 to 45 mm Hg; in chronic obstructive pulmonary disease (COPD), both PO_2 and PCO_2 are maintained at 60 mm Hg, plus or minus 5 mm Hg
   e. Client will increase activity without associated symptoms by 5% each day (e.g., each day—10 more feet walked, 5 more steps climbed, and so on)
   f. Client will state feeling less anxious; facial features will exhibit a relaxed look
8. Nursing interventions
   a. Acute care
      (1) Left-sided failure
          (a) Give medications by IV route
          (b) Evaluate heart and lung sounds initially and then every 30 minutes after initial therapy. When sounds are clear, evaluate at least every 2 to 4 hours
          (c) Administer oxygen as ordered or during periods of SOB or during activity
          (d) Maintain head of bed with an elevation of at least 40 to 60 degrees, mid-to-high Fowler's position
          (e) Balance rest and activity to meet client needs
      (2) Right-sided failure
          (a) Weigh client daily before breakfast—same time, same scale, same amount of clothing; expect a loss initially; report any daily weight changes when client is on diuretic therapy
          (b) Elevate edematous extremities above the level of the heart when in bed; in chair, elevate to prevent dependency of lower legs below knee level; monitor edema for a decrease

        (c) Turn and reposition at least every 2 hours; use skin protective devices (heel protectors); consider use of air pressure beds or mattresses

        (d) Ambulate client or move from bed to chair at least three times a day to promote circulation and prevent venous stasis

    b. Home care regarding client education

        (1) Proper weight monitoring—client should take weight daily, write weight on calendar, and report any weight gain or loss of 2 lb/wk or more to physician

        (2) Limit salt in diet by cooking without salt, and add salt at table only to maintain a sodium restricted diet. Caution client about the use of salt substitutes because some contain high levels of potassium.

        (3) Pulse monitoring done daily either before getting out of bed or at rest if taking digitalis preparations. If experiencing extreme dyspnea or frothy sputum, take pulse and notify physician.

        (4) Potassium replacement in diet required if taking nonpotassium-sparing diuretics such as furosemide (Lasix) and bumetanide (Bumex). Increase intake of foods such as oranges, prunes, bananas, watermelon, potatoes, and beans

9. Evaluation protocol

    a. How do I know that my interventions were effective?

        (1) Is the client's fatigue less?

        (2) Does the client feel any dizziness?

        (3) Has the client's SOB lessened?

        (4) Has the swelling in the client's ankles and feet decreased?

    b. What criteria will I use to change my interventions?

        (1) Sustained or increased fatigue and intolerance to activity with therapy

        (2) Visible SOB; a client who reports increased SOB, especially at rest

        (3) Client reports dizziness, and a systolic BP having dropped more than 10% of baseline

        (4) Client reports that swelling in ankles and feet has increased with or without weight gain

    c. How will I know that my client teaching has been effective?

        (1) Client will take a 20-minute rest after any activity that increases the RR or effort in breathing

        (2) Client will maintain daily weight at plus or minus one pound, with an average weekly gain or loss of no more than 2 pounds

        (3) Client will sustain daily HR between 60 to 100 beats per minute, either before getting out of bed or at rest

        (4) Client will not add salt to food, except at the table

10. Older adult alert
    a. Older adult clients with a susceptibility to orthostatic hypotension have increased risk for falls when taking diuretics or anti-dysrhythmic drugs
    b. Hypotension may be a dysfunction even more profound in older adult clients. Normal expectation in the aging process is an increased BP.
    c. Older adult clients are at even greater risk for skin breakdown because their skin tends to be thin and fragile. This risk is greatly increased in clients with peripheral edema, poor circulation, and poor nutritional status.

D. **Valvular heart disease**
   1. Definition—a dysfunction of one or more of the cardiac valves
      a. Stenosis—restriction of blood flow in a forward motion through the heart
      b. Regurgitation—unpredictable blood flow through the heart. Some blood moves forward, and some blood regurgitates back into the previous chamber.
   2. Pathophysiology—two fundamental irregularities
      a. Stenosis
         (1) Significantly decreased valve lumen from thickened or calcified leaflets
         (2) Restricted blood flow through the lumen
         (3) Reduced blood output from the chamber attempting to push blood through the stenotic lumen
         (4) Hypertrophy, which eventually occurs from an increase in chamber pressure
         (5) Right- or left-sided heart failure, depending on the valves affected, is the end result
      b. Regurgitation or insufficiency
         (1) Leaflets of valve unable to close completely from scarring, calcium deposits, or papillary muscle dysfunction
         (2) Reduced blood output from the chamber attempting to empty blood is the result. Some blood is ejected forward, and some blood is ejected backward.
         (3) Regurgitated blood eventually is added to blood already present in the chamber, which then increases the pressure and workload
         (4) Hypertrophy of the walls of the affected chambers
         (5) Symptoms of right- or left-sided failure eventually occur, depending on the valve affected
   3. Etiology—valvular heart disease is most commonly acquired from rheumatic fever, bacterial endocarditis, MI, and congenital disorders

4. Incidence—the incidence of the illnesses is different for each valvular condition
   a. Mitral abnormalities
      (1) Stenosis is more common in females
      (2) More common in the population younger than 45 years
   b. Aortic abnormalities
      (1) More common in males
      (2) Aortic stenosis is the most common valvular abnormality in the older adult population
5. Assessment
   a. Questions to ask
      (1) Are you having any chest pain? If yes, where?
      (2) Do you have any SOB?
      (3) Do you have SOB only with exercise or all the time?
      (4) Do you feel very tired? If yes, describe pattern.
   b. General clinical manifestations with any valve dysfunction
      (1) Fatigue
      (2) Dyspnea on exertion
      (3) Chest pain on exertion
      (4) Orthopnea
      (5) Palpitations
      (6) Heart murmur (different with each valve abnormality)
   c. Abnormal laboratory findings—there are no specific laboratory studies used to diagnose valvular heart disease
   d. Abnormal diagnostic test results
      (1) Echocardiogram—allows most accurate diagnosis because it allows visualization of valve movement and impairment, such as poor ejection fraction
      (2) ECG—most changes are associated with chamber enlargement. Atrial dysrhythmias are common as are AV blocks.
      (3) CXR—chamber enlargement and pulmonary congestion
      (4) Cardiac catheterization
         (a) Pressure increased in the affected chambers—pressure in chambers affected by valve dysfunction is higher than normal
         (b) Less than 50% *ejection fraction,* which is the percentage of blood ejected from the chambers; 60-75% ejection fraction is the normal range for healthy individuals
         (c) Dye injected into an affected chamber is regurgitated backward into the associated heart structure (chamber or vessel)
6. Expected medical interventions
   a. Treat findings as they occur
      (1) Digitalis preparations, diuretics for findings associated with CHF
      (2) Antidysrhythmic drugs for atrial dysrhythmias

b. Valvuloplasty to repair leaflets
c. Valvular commissurotomy to free fused leaflets
d. Valvular replacement
e. Oral anticoagulants for life after mechanical valvular replacement surgery

7. Nursing diagnoses
   a. Fatigue related to poor tissue perfusion
   b. Ineffective breathing pattern related to fluid in airways
   c. Activity intolerance related to poor tissue perfusion and oxygenation

8. Client goals
   a. Client will state fatigue has decreased
   b. Client will demonstrate a RR of 18 to 22 breaths per minute and of normal depth at rest
   c. Client will increase daily activity without associated symptoms by 5% each day (10 more feet walked, five more steps climbed)

9. Nursing interventions
   a. Acute care
      (1) Assess lung sounds for crackles and heart sounds for murmurs or increased intensity of murmur at least every 2 hours
      (2) Administer oxygen during acute episode of SOB or cardiac dysrhythmias
      (3) Balance rest and activity—45- to 60-minute rest period after meals or a bath; no activity longer than 15 to 20 minutes
   b. Home care: regarding client education
      (1) Antibiotic prophylaxis required before any invasive procedure or dental work to prevent bacterial endocarditis
      (2) Daily weight taken in the morning on rising to evaluate fluid status: before breakfast, at the same time each day, using the same scale, and wearing the same amount of clothing; report losses or gains of over 2 lb/wk to physician
      (3) Expected effects and side effects of medication therapy
      (4) Low-salt diet; minimal caffeine

10. Evaluation protocol
    a. How do I know that my interventions were effective?
       (1) Does the client feel more energetic?
       (2) How many pillows is the client sleeping on?
       (3) Does the client report that breathing is comfortable?
       (4) Was the client able to ambulate further today before becoming short of breath?
    b. Which criteria will I use to change my interventions?
       (1) Client indicates that fatigue is no better or worse
       (2) Client's RR is rapid and labored at rest or with minimal activity

        (3) Client is unable to increase activity level by any amount before becoming short of breath

        (4) Client sleeps on three or more pillows or with head of bed above 60 degrees

    c. How will I know that my client teaching has been effective?

        (1) Client will obtain a prescription for antibiotics before dental work, and so on

        (2) Client takes daily weight in the morning before breakfast, at the same time, with the same scale, and with the same amount of clothing

        (3) Client is not putting salt on food until after it is prepared

        (4) Client takes diuretics in the morning or afternoon rather than at night

11. Older adult alert

    a. Many of the drug therapies for older adults may cause orthostatic hypotension. As a result of the aging process, these clients are more prone to orthostatic hypotension.

    b. Older adult clients sent home on anticoagulants must be reminded to have prothrombin times done periodically through the physician's office, initially weekly, then monthly as values stabilize.

    c. The vascular tone in older adult clients is not as responsive to cardiovascular stress. Thus clients may not respond appropriately to fluids or medications in the face of hypotension.

E. Inflammatory heart disorders

1. Definition—a group of cardiac disorders involving an inflammatory process of the layers of the heart

    a. Endocarditis—an inflammation of the endocardium, the innermost layer of the heart that may include the cardiac valves and papillary muscles

    b. Myocarditis—an inflammation of the myocardium, the actual heart muscle

    c. Pericarditis—an inflammation of the visceral and parietal pericardium, the outermost layer of the heart

2. Pathophysiology

    a. Endocarditis

        (1) Acute—develops on normal valves, progresses rapidly, causes severe destruction, and may be fatal without treatment

        (2) Subacute—occurs on damaged heart valves, progresses slowly, and survival is possible without treatment

        (3) In both the acute and subacute forms, bacteria in the circulation are attracted to the sluggish blood in the atrial floor or to the damaged areas of the heart, most frequently on the valves

        (4) Vegetations result from clumped bacteria

        (5) Vegetations erode and destroy cardiac and valvular tissue, leading to impaired pumping efficiency and eventually to intractable heart failure

        (6) Vegetation growth produces fragile cardiac lesions that can break off, embolize, cause ischemia, and infarct organs; most common is in the brain

  b. Myocarditis

        (1) Insidious process that does not resemble an MI; either diffuse or local damage to the myocardium may occur from a pathogen or toxin

        (2) May take one of three paths

           (a) No signs of heart failure

           (b) Latent period of approximately 1 year, then findings of heart failure

           (c) Rapid onset of heart failure

  c. Pericarditis

        (1) Acute—the two layers of the pericardium are inflamed and roughened. Friction between the layers may result in increased fluid production in the space between the two layers. A dry form, fibrinous pericarditis, lasts less than 6 weeks. Adhesions form between the sac layers, restricting heart filling and pumping.

           (a) Cardiac tamponade—complication with fluid buildup. Serous purulent, or hemorrhagic pericardial effusion will occur. A point of increased pressure on the heart results in ineffective pumping.

              (i) Treatment immediately required because pericardiocentesis leads to the withdrawal of the fluid from the pericardial sac

              (ii) Pericardiotomy—incision or window in the pericardium will prevent further occurrences of cardiac tamponade

        (2) Chronic—constrictive pericarditis. From the recurrence of a preexisting condition the two layers of pericardium eventually become thickened, fused, and scarred together. The pericardium then will act as a large band surrounding the heart, constricting the pumping action of the heart and leading to minimal cardiac filling and output. Treatment involves imperative removal of the pericardium to restore appropriate cardiac pumping.

 3. Etiology

  a. Endocarditis—entry of pathogens during dental work, IV drug use, or any invasive procedure; bacteria is the most common pathogen

  b. Myocarditis—most common infecting agent is a virus; bacteria, protozoal, and rickettsial diseases are less common

    c. Pericarditis—causes
       (1) Infectious—most common source is viral or idiopathic (unknown)
       (2) Noninfectious—after an acute MI, trauma, and uremia: Dressler's syndrome: 1 to 4 weeks after MI
       (3) Autoimmune—rheumatic disease and systemic lupus erythematosus

4. Incidence
    a. Endocarditis—5 of every 1000 clients admitted to hospitals have infective endocarditis. The mean age is 50 years, and the ratio of men to women is 2 to 1. A decrease in the number of cases caused by streptococcal infections has occurred; however, there has been an increase in the number caused by atypical organisms such as yeasts and fungi.
    b. Myocarditis—impossible to evaluate because the incidence changes within age groups and within groups affected by different etiologies
    c. Pericarditis—far more common in the male population

5. Assessment
    a. Questions to ask
       (1) Do you have chest pain? Where is it?
       (2) Have you been running a fever? What is the highest temperature you have had?
       (3) Have you been experiencing flu-like symptoms?
       (4) Do you have a prosthetic valve?
       (5) Have you had any infections or have you had any dental work or invasive procedures performed?
    b. Clinical manifestations (Table 2-1, p. 70)
    c. Abnormal laboratory findings (Table 2-2, p. 71)
    d. Abnormal diagnostic tests (Table 2-3, p. 71)

6. Expected medical interventions
    a. Endocarditis
       (1) Parenteral antibiotic therapy for 4 to 6 weeks
       (2) Antipyretics and analgesics
       (3) Valvular surgery if needed, usually at a later date
    b. Myocarditis
       (1) Supportive treatment
       (2) Dysrhythmias are as they occur
       (3) Antibiotics: organism can be identified
    c. Pericarditis
       (1) Anti-inflammatory agents; nonsteroidal anti-inflammatory agents are the drugs of choice
       (2) Analgesics and antipyretics—aspirin is the drug of choice
       (3) Pericardiocentesis for cardiac tamponade—removal of pericardial fluid by needle insertion into the epigastric area

TABLE 2-1	Clinical Manifestations of Inflammatory Heart Disorders		
Assessments	**Endocarditis**	**Myocarditis**	**Pericarditis**
Unique findings	Splinter hemorrhages of nail beds Petechiae—common around conjunctiva, mucous membranes	History of a viral syndrome within weeks, common in spring and fall Sudden unexplained heart failure	Pericardial friction rub
Pain	Not common	Chest pain: pericardial	Chest pain: pleuritic, increased when lying flat or with deep breaths, decreased when upright and leaning forward; may radiate to neck, shoulder, back, and arms— common between shoulder and base of neck; exaggerated with inspiration and body movements
Heart sounds	Heart murmur— present or intensified	None specific	Distant muffled heart sounds
Pertinent findings	Fever acute; high, over 101° F. Subacute: low grade of 99 to 100° F Fatigue, malaise	Malaise, easily fatigued Exertional dyspnea	Fever Malaise, fatigue Anxiety Nonproductive cough, orthopnea

    (4) Pericardial window—open chest drainage of pericardial fluid; pericardium left open to prevent future episodes of cardiac tamponade

    (5) Pericardiectomy—removal of both layers of pericardium for fibrous pericarditis or constrictive pericarditis

  7. Nursing diagnoses

    a. Chest pain related to cardiac inflammatory process

    b. Decreased CO related to poor contractile state of the myocardium

    c. Altered body temperature related to cardiac inflammatory process

TABLE 2-2 Abnormal Laboratory Findings of Inflammatory Heart Disorders

Laboratory Effects	Endocarditis	Myocarditis	Pericarditis
CBC—WBCs	↑	↑	↑
ESR	↑	↑	↑
Blood culture	Positive for infecting organism	Not done	Not done
Rheumatoid factor	Present in 50% of clients	Negative	Negative
Cardiac enzymes	May be ↑	↑	May be ↑

↑ = increased

TABLE 2-3 Abnormal Diagnostic Tests of Inflammatory Heart Disorders

Diagnostic Tests	Endocarditis	Myocarditis	Pericarditis
ECG	Normal initially, later conduction abnormalities, cardiac dysrhythmias	ST-segment and T-wave abnormalities, Q-wave appearance	Elevated ST segment in all leads
Echocardiogram	Identify vegetation on cardiac structures and valvular abnormalities	Dilated ventricles, poor wall contraction	Pericardial fluid present, decreased wall motion during systole, abnormal septal movement
Other Tests	CXR—cardiomegaly	Endomyocardial biopsy—inflammatory process in myocardial cells, myocardial necrosis CXR—cardiomegaly	CXR—enlarged cardiac silhouette

8. Client goals
   a. Client will state that chest pain is decreased or relieved
   b. Client will exhibit BP and HR within 20% of baseline
   c. Client will exhibit body temperature of 37° C, or 98.6° F, or baseline for the client
9. Nursing interventions
   a. Acute care
      (1) Endocarditis
         (a) Evaluate for CHF changes and evidence of embolization

        (b) Administer antipyretics as needed for temperature elevation; administer antibiotics as ordered

        (c) Evaluate for improvement of murmurs and activity intolerance

    (2) Myocarditis

        (a) Monitor for changes indicating CHF

        (b) Offer pain relief for chest discomfort

        (c) Evaluate for less fatigue and exertional dyspnea

    (3) Pericarditis

        (a) Offer pain relief for chest pain

        (b) Administer fever-reducing agents for temperature elevation

        (c) Evaluate frequently for complications

            (i) Cardiac tamponade—distended neck veins that remain distended during inspiration, which is *Kussmaul sign,* and SOB

            (ii) Pericardial effusion—increased anxiety and restlessness, dyspnea, hypotension, and muffled heart sounds

  b. Home care regarding client education

    (1) Endocarditis

        (a) Home administration of IV antibiotics

            (i) Importance of evaluating IV access before each administration

            (ii) Findings associated with infection in IV access

            (iii) Importance of giving medications on time and not missing a dose

        (b) Gradual increase of activity

            (i) Balance rest and activity

            (ii) Frequent rest periods

            (iii) No activity lasting longer than 15 to 20 minutes

            (iv) Increase activity by 5 minutes per day

            (v) Stop activity when fatigued or experiencing SOB

        (c) Avoidance of persons with upper respiratory infections

        (d) Careful adherence to antibiotic prophylaxis for dental and invasive procedures

    (2) Myocarditis

        (a) Monitoring techniques for any changes, especially in HR or rhythm, and flu-like symptoms. Immediately report any of these changes to physician.

        (b) How to monitor for findings associated with heart failure

        (c) Need for family members to learn cardiopulmonary resuscitation techniques in cases of life-threatening dysrhythmia

(3) Pericarditis
   (a) Seek help immediately
      (i) Chest pain, eased by an upright, leaning forward position
      (ii) Sudden SOB
   (b) Wear a medical alert bracelet or necklace with indicated condition
   (c) Avoid fatigue
10. Evaluation protocol
   a. How do I know that my interventions were effective?
      (1) Has client's chest pain gone away or improved?
      (2) Does client feel warm? If yes, check temperature.
      (3) Does client feel less short of breath or have less or no swelling in ankles or feet?
   b. Which criteria will I use to change my interventions?
      (1) Client indicates chest pain has become worse or has not decreased in intensity
      (2) Client states a feeling of being warm with a temperature elevation
      (3) Client exhibits sudden sustained SOB, audible crackles in the lungs, increased anxiety and restlessness, jugular venous distension at a 35-degree angle or higher, or has developed edema of the ankles or feet
   c. How will I know that my client teaching has been effective?
      (1) Client and family are able to demonstrate the correct technique for taking a pulse and identify correct criteria for calling physician
      (2) Client and family are able to demonstrate the correct technique for home IV antibiotic administration
      (3) Client and family are able to correctly identify circumstances that require prophylactic antibiotic administration
11. Older adult alert
   a. The inelastic vascular systems of older adult clients will not respond as quickly or as effectively to the situations of inflammatory heart disorders. Little compensation will occur for a sudden decrease in CO. Thus clinical findings may be more acute.
   b. Older adult clients with prior angina may attempt to treat pain associated with inflammatory heart disorders as if it were angina pectoris

WEB Resources

http://www.americanheart.org/
   American Heart Association National Center
http://www.nhlbi.nih.gov/
   National Heart, Lung, and Blood Institute (NHLBI)

REVIEW QUESTIONS

1. During client assessment the nurse identifies jugular venous distention at a bed elevation of 35 degrees. The evaluation of this finding is that the client may be manifesting
   1. Left-sided heart failure
   2. Right-sided heart failure
   3. Pulmonary hypertension
   4. Pulmonary congestion

2. When assessing a female client's chest pain, she indicates that it has a sharp character. She points to her sternum when asked where her pain is located and indicates that it radiates up into her neck. What other information is needed to distinguish this pain from a possible MI? The client
   1. Took two nitroglycerin tablets at home without relief of pain
   2. States the pain is accompanied by nausea
   3. Has a family history of coronary artery disease in women
   4. Took a third nitroglycerin in the car at the hospital parking lot, which relieved her pain

3. The priority assessment in the client experiencing an acute MI would be
   1. Peripheral pulses
   2. Heart rate
   3. Respiratory effort
   4. Chest pain

4. Which ordered intervention for a client hospitalized for cardiac dysrhythmias of premature ventricular beats and for complaints of difficulty breathing would be done first?
   1. Give the ordered morphine
   2. Place oxygen on the client
   3. Start an IV
   4. Call the physician for premature ventricular contractions greater than 6 per minute

5. The client describes a nightly ritual of going to bed, lying flat in bed, and waking up around 2 o'clock in the morning feeling as if he is smothering. The home care nurse would document this as
   1. Orthopnea
   2. Dyspnea
   3. Paroxysmal nocturnal dyspnea
   4. Nocturnal dyspnea

6. The most appropriate nursing intervention for the client being treated with chemotherapy agents and with complaints of intermittent exertional dyspnea would include
   1. Instruct the client to take frequent rest periods
   2. Ask the client to describe the activities during the periods of dyspnea
   3. Instruct the client in the use of inhalers as needed (prn) with spacers
   4. Instruct the client not to walk more than 20 steps then to rest for a few minutes

7. A client is in pulmonary edema. Which one of the following STAT physician orders is most appropriate to do last?
   1. ABG evaluation
   2. IV digoxin, 0.25 mg
   3. IV Lasix, 40 mg
   4. Oxygen at 4 L/min by way of nasal cannula

8. A client with mitral valve disease requires more teaching when the client tells you
   1. "I take my penicillin only when the dentist has to drill a tooth."
   2. "I take my penicillin before each dentist visit."
   3. "I weigh myself at 7 o'clock every morning with my pajamas on, before I eat breakfast."
   4. "I have removed the salt shaker from the stove so I can't add salt as I cook."

9. A teaching priority for clients returning home after a brief hospitalization for bacterial endocarditis is
   1. Monitor daily weight because weight fluctuations are important
   2. Balance rest and activity with expected changes in both areas
   3. Avoid persons with upper respiratory infections when not on an antibiotic regimen
   4. Learn IV antibiotic administration technique for home administration

10. A client with a history of pericarditis should be alerted to which assessment finding?
    1. Sudden palpitations
    2. Sudden sustained SOB
    3. Progressive lethargy
    4. Subtle sleeplessness

ANSWERS, RATIONALES, AND TEST-TAKING TIPS

Rationales	Test-Taking Tips

1. Correct answer: 2

Jugular venous distention is a result of the backflow of blood from a failing right ventricle. For option 1, left-sided heart failure, to be correct the given assessment findings would have to be associated with abnormal lung findings—rales, rhonchi, wheezing, and crackles. Pulmonary hypertension and pulmonary congestion, options 3 and 4, may eventually result in a situation of right-sided heart failure. However, the question asks for the primary cause, not a secondary cause of neck vein distention.

Cluster and eliminate options 1, 3, and 4 because they deal with the lung. If you had difficulty with this question, it indicates that you need to review the anatomy and physiology of the heart. Practice drawing the chambers, and on each side write what happens when they fail. Then, on any similar test question, always draw your heart picture before you make a choice of the best answer.

2. Correct answer: 4

The fact that the third nitroglycerin tablet relieved the client's pain is important because she is within the criterion of three nitroglycerin tablets allowed for angina before further intervention. The key term in the question is "distinguish the pain." The only way to differentiate angina from MI pain is to evaluate the effects of sublingual nitroglycerine tablets, that is, one tablet taken 5 minutes apart for a total of three tablets. If the pain is not relieved after three tablets, an MI is suspected; however, if the pain is relieved after one, two, or three tablets the conclusion is the pain was an angina attack. Option 1 is a

A word of caution to those of you who selected option 1 and did not read the remaining options. To prevent your knee-jerk reaction in the future, use the process of reading all the options when you "think that you know" option 1 is the correct answer. After you have read option 1, go ahead and select it. Then skip down to option 4 and read it, then read option 3; then read option 2; and last, reread option 1. See if you still agree with your first choice, option 1. Select it, and go on to the next question. Only then will you have given yourself every opportunity to choose the correct answer. Remember that when you do not read all of the options you are limiting your ability to pass a test.

correct answer but not the best answer of the four options. If option 4 were not listed, then option 1 would be the best answer. In option 2, nausea is not exclusively associated with an acute MI. Nausea accompanies many pathologic conditions. In option 3, a family history of coronary artery disease in a man or woman contributes only to *a high-risk category* and not to a differentiation between angina and an MI.

3. Correct answer: 3

Content associated with the airway is a priority of assessment in any client. Note that the option is not "respiratory rate" but rather, "respiratory effort." *Respiratory effort* is the amount of energy used to breathe and the degree of difficulty in breathing. If the respiratory effort is great, the client most likely is having a complication, such as left-sided heart failure, from the MI in progress. Option 1 would be done last. Peripheral pulse strength may act as an indirect indicator of effective or ineffective CO. Options 2 and 4 are appropriate but not the priority. They would be done after evaluation of the respiratory effort, with the HR checked first and then the chest pain. In the same sense, if the HR is abnormally high or low, this finding may indicate a complication. Note that in this situation, the MI is in progress.

The ABCs guide the priority assessments in most situations. Remember to select the answer that supports what you know—not what you do not know. If you have no idea of the correct answer, cluster options 1, 2, and 4 with the theme "cardiac." The clue is that the client is "experiencing an acute MI." Select option 3, which is the odd man out because it is associated with "pulmonary." This is an action to evaluate for complications of the MI, left-sided heart failure.

Rationales	Test-Taking Tips

As with any other acute condition, respiratory status takes precedent. Also, option 4—chest pain—is a global answer without parameters such as the intensity, location, initiation, or relief.

4. Correct answer: 2

Placing oxygen on a client who is short of breath is the first action to do of the ordered interventions. With the given information this takes priority over starting an IV, giving morphine, or calling the physician. Option 1, to give morphine, would be a first action if the information included that the client had chest pain or other suspected cardiac pain such as pain in the left arm, or pain radiating up into the neck or down into the abdomen. Morphine might also be given first if the client has acute pulmonary edema. Morphine would have overall effectiveness as compared with oxygen. Morphine has a greater and quicker effect to pool the blood, dilate the bronchioles, and calm the client than does the administration of oxygen, which usually takes a minimum of 30 minutes to effect a change in the levels of blood gases. Option 3, to start an IV sounds like a good answer. However, it is not the first action to take in this situation because the vital signs and other assessment data are unknown, with no indication of

The most common error on this question is to "read" into the situation more information than is given in the stem. Most test-takers read into the question and give the client pain, frequent PVCs, acute CHF, or an acute MI. Be aware that as you read the options there is a tendency to add more information than given in the question. To prevent this error, simply make a few notes on scrap paper next to your test of what information is given—PVCs and difficulty breathing. Yes, that is it. Using this approach allows the question to fall into the easier category of selecting option 2, which is directed at treating the breathing problem.

a need for immediate IV medications or fluids. Option 4 is a third action after oxygen and an IV is started and only if the client has no pain. If the information in the stem stated the number of PVCs were more than 6 per minute *and* the client had pain, then this option would be the last action to complete of the 4 options.

5. Correct answer: 3

Going to bed in a flat position but waking up in the middle of the night feeling as if you are smothering is referred to as paroxysmal nocturnal dyspnea (PND). Orthopnea, option 1, is difficulty breathing when lying down. Dyspnea, option 2, is difficulty breathing. Nocturnal dyspnea is difficulty breathing at night without a determination of how the difficult breathing happens. Options 1, 2, and 4 describe the situation but are too general for this particular question.

If you have no idea of a correct answer or you think that all of the options are correct, use common sense. Narrow the selections to 3 or 4 because the event happens at night. Then, narrow them down further with the use of common sense. The situation happens suddenly. The word, *paroxysmal* means a sudden event or outburst. Another common use of paroxysmal is paroxysmal atrial tachycardia (PAT) in clients diagnosed with prolapsed mitral valve.

6. Correct answer: 2

The best response here is to use the nursing process with the need for further assessment before giving interventions to the client. Option 1 is too general of a selection. Ask yourself "when" regarding "frequent rest periods" because insufficient information is given. In option 3, the use of an inhaler may be appropriate for intermittent exertional dyspnea. However, more information is needed in the stem for this option to be the best answer. Does the client

Avoid reading into the given situation, especially after reading the options that might introduce new, logical, and familiar information. To prevent this, simply read the question at least two more times after the initial read. Read the question a second time as you narrow the options to two. And then reread the question followed by your selected option. If they do not fit, you will know. The more times you read the question the greater chance you will have to pass. Remember the question has the clues that lead you to the correct answer.

Rationales	Test-Taking Tips

have a history of asthma? Option 4 sounds good for a general guideline of dyspnea with walking but it introduces new information into the situation—the dyspnea is from walking. That is an incorrect conclusion from the data in the stem. No description of the "exertional activity " is stated.

7. Correct answer: 1

A client in pulmonary edema must have IV Lasix to bring about quick diuresis and IV digoxin to increase contractility of the heart. Both have the expected result of decreased fluid in the lungs. The result of option 4 would be to increase the oxygen delivery from about 21% to 25%. The blood gas evaluation, ABGs, would be done last because the diagnosis is known. Pulmonary edema is a medical emergency that requires immediate treatment before performing any type of evaluation. It is inappropriate in the given situation to withhold therapy until baseline ABG results are obtained.

The key term "pulmonary edema" guides you to determine that the left heart has acutely failed and cannot get blood into the systemic circulation. Note that options 2, 3, and 4 are actions to treat the acute pathologic condition. Option 1, the ABGs, is an action for the evaluation of therapy or for getting a baseline assessment. In this situation, a baseline assessment becomes secondary to treatment of the acute clinical condition that is an emergency.

8. Correct answer: 1

The client must be taught to take prophylactic antibiotics before any dental work or invasive procedure or therapy. Prophylactic antibiotics prevent bacterial endocarditis after such invasive actions. All other statements are correct actions for clients with mitral valve problems.

The word "only" in option 1 makes the client response too narrow. This word alerts you to use common sense. You should suspect that there are other precautions that clients with mitral valve disease would need to follow such as restricting caffeine ingestion, maintaining regular dental hygiene, and knowing the expected effects and side effects of prescribed medications.

9. Correct answer: 4

The priority teaching need for a client going home after hospitalization for bacterial endocarditis is how to administer the IV antibiotics at home. They will be required for 4 to 6 weeks. Options 1, 2, and 3 are appropriate to include in the discharge teaching but are not the priority.

The key word "brief" alerts the reader that longer treatment for an infection, endocarditis, at home would be needed. Recall that most infections require a 10- to 14-day regimen of therapy. Note the question is asking about a "priority." This should tell you that all the options are correct. You have to determine which one is to be taught first or is most important to include. If you read the options and looked for one correct answer, you most likely made a wrong choice. Remember that the question holds the clue to the correct option.

10. Correct answer: 2

Sudden sustained SOB is the best option, given that the client has a history of pericarditis. The finding in option 2 is indicative of cardiac tamponade, a life-threatening complication of pericarditis. These clients should be taught that this finding requires immediate attention at the nearest hospital emergency room. Option 1 is a classic finding in mitral valve dysfunction. Options 3 and 4 with the focus, a decreased LOC, are indicative of an increased $PaCO_2$ (over 45) or increasing intracranial pressure from infection or a history of head trauma.

Of the given options, the ABCs—airway, breathing, and circulation—take priority and guide nursing assessments and interventions. Thus, option 2, associated with respiration, is the correct answer over option 1, which relates to circulation factors. If you have no idea of the correct answer, use actions to figure it out. Note that options 1 and 2 are sudden. Options 3 and 4 indicate a longer time for the findings to occur. Therefore, decide between options 1 and 2. Progressive means ongoing or worsening over a period of time. Subtle means insidious, indirect, sneaky, or roundabout. It is likely that both of the findings in options 3 and 4 would not be noticed quickly by the client.

3

The Vascular System

FAST FACTS

1. Any agent that causes vasodilation of the blood vessels causes a subsequent initial slight increase in HR and a decrease in BP.
2. Any agent that causes vasoconstriction of the blood vessels causes a subsequent increase in BP and cool extremities.
3. Pain and anxiety can cause a sympathetic response.
4. A sympathetic response causes the following: (1) release of two catecholamines, epinephrine and norepinephrine, which are potent vasoconstrictors; (2) subsequent increase in BP; and (3) an increase in the serum glucose for energy.
5. Venous congestion results in ankle edema, brownish discoloration, and venous ankle ulcers that are very difficult to heal.
6. Arterial insufficiency results in gangrene, which starts at the tips of the toes or fingers as a bluish-black discoloration, then causes a shriveling effect on the digits.
7. **Afterload** of the left ventricle is the systemic vascular resistance (SVR), or the impedance to blood flow out of the left ventricle.
8. Afterload involves three factors: aortic pressure, vessel size, and blood viscosity.
9. Most clinical situations require that the afterload be decreased to facilitate left ventricular emptying.
10. The lymphatic system is part of the vascular system with these three functions: (1) removing fluid and protein from the interstitial space, (2) returning this fluid into the vascular space by way of the thoracic ducts to the subclavian veins, and (3) transporting immune components back into the circulatory system.

CONTENT REVIEW

I. The vascular system—has many functions

A. **System responsibilities**
1. Carries oxygenated blood and nutrients to tissues and cells
2. Carries deoxygenated blood back to lungs for reoxygenation
3. Carries waste materials away from tissues and cells, back to organs of excretion

B. **The lymph system—part of the vascular system**
1. System responsibilities
   a. Removes fluid and proteins from interstitial space
   b. Returns fluid and proteins to the circulating fluid volume
   c. Similarly, transports immune components back into the circulatory system by way of the lymph system

II. Structure and function

A. **Arteries**
1. Carry oxygen and nutrient rich blood away from the heart to tissues and cells by way of the aorta
2. Arteries have a very muscular, thick wall structure composed of three layers
   a. Outer layer—tunica adventitia
   b. Middle layer—tunica media
   c. Inner layer (in contact with blood flow)—tunica intima
3. The smallest branches of arteries, connecting to capillaries, are called *arterioles*
4. The pulmonary artery is the exception because it carries unoxygenated blood away from right side of heart to lungs

B. **Veins**
1. Carry unoxygenated blood back to right side of the heart for reoxygenation and waste removal
2. Veins have thinner walls than arteries, allowing for easier contraction and expansion
3. Vein walls contain the same three layers as arteries
4. They are unique because veins contain valves at various intervals to ensure blood flow will continue in a forward motion toward the heart. This flow is driven by the pumping of skeletal muscle and suction generated by respiratory movements, especially inspiration.
5. The smallest branches of veins, connected from capillaries, are called *venules*
6. The pulmonary vein is the exception because it carries oxygenated blood back to left side of the heart away from the lungs

C. **Capillaries or capillary bed**
1. Definition—Microscopically small vessels connecting arterioles and venules

    2. Sites of transfer of nutrients, fluids, and gases into the tissues

    3. Collect waste from excretory organs

D. Lymph vessels

    1. Components of the capillary bed

    2. Are similar to veins in structure and flow, with the same three layers and intermittent valves to propel lymph fluid forward

    3. Collect fluid and proteins from the interstitial space and return them to the circulating blood volume by way of the thoracic ducts to the subclavian veins

    4. Introduce important elements of the immune system such as antibodies and lymphocytes into the circulating blood volume

    5. The lymphatic structures are comprised of the tonsils, spleen, and thymus

E. Sequence of flow—blood and lymph

Outlet of the left ventricle

Aorta, 100 mm Hg
Highest pressure in the vascular system

Arteries

Arterioles

Capillaries ➤ Small lymphatics

Venules   Larger lymphatics

Veins   Thoracic ducts

Inferior vena cava   Subclavian veins at the junction of the subclavian and internal jugular veins

Superior vena cava ◄ ◄

Right atria 0 to 5 mm Hg
Lowest pressure in vascular system

Right ventricle

Pulmonary artery

Lungs

◄ ◄ ◄ Left atria

III. Targeted concerns

A. **Pharmacology—priority drug classifications**

1. Antihypertensive drugs
   a. Beta-adrenergic blockers (Chapter 2, p. 47)
   b. Calcium-channel blockers (Chapter 2, p. 48)
   c. Angiotensin-converting enzyme (ACE) inhibitors—interrupt the renin–angiotensin-aldosterone system; prevent formation of angiotensin II, a potent vasoconstrictor from angiotensin I; and inhibit aldosterone release
      (1) Expected effects—a decrease in the release of aldosterone with subsequent decrease in sodium and water retention because of decreased circulating blood volume. A decrease in vascular tone results in vasodilation.
      (2) Commonly given drugs
         (a) Captopril* (Capoten)
         (b) Enalapril maleate* (Vasotec)
      (3) Nursing considerations
         (a) Administration should occur at the same time each day, 1 hour before meals
         (b) Rebound hypertension occurs if the drug is abruptly stopped
         (c) Monitor the following
            (i) Laboratory results for electrolytes; for elevated levels of creatinine, AST, and ALT; for slight elevation of potassium; and for diminished WBC counts
            (ii) BP—monitor carefully with initiation or change of therapy
            (iii) For volume-depletion because it may cause a profound decrease in BP or sustained orthostatic hypotension
            (iv) For orthostatic hypotension, which is common with the first dose
            (v) For the major side effects: proteinuria, renal failure, agranulocytosis, and neutropenia
   d. Alpha–adrenergic receptor blockers inhibit the action of the sympathetic nervous system at some point along the system
      (1) Expected effects—venous and arteriolar vasodilation, lowered BP or sustained orthostatic hypotension
      (2) Commonly given drugs
         (a) Clonidine hydrochloride (Catapres)
         (b) Methyldopa (Aldomet)
         (c) Prazosin hydrochloride (Minipress)

---

*The generic names of ACE inhibitors end in "pril."

(3) Nursing considerations

    (a) Because any sympathetic inhibitor can cause orthostatic hypotension, taking lying and standing BPs is imperative. Check these at least daily. If dosage is changed, check these before administration.

    (b) Renal monitoring is imperative, such as levels of creatinine and blood urea nitrogen (BUN), as is strict input and output monitoring. All of these drugs may cause decreased renal blood flow.

    (c) BP should be monitored carefully and frequently if there are findings associated with dehydration

    (d) Monitor for the more common side effects

        (i) CNS depression

        (ii) Impotence

        (iii) Psychotic disturbances such as nightmares, depression, and delirium

    (e) Monitor for the major side effects

        (i) Aldomet: thrombocytopenia and leukopenia

        (ii) Catapres: CHF

e. Direct smooth muscle relaxants—directly dilate the arterioles

  (1) Expected effects—decreased peripheral resistance, afterload, and decreased BP

  (2) Commonly given drugs

    (a) Hydralazine hydrochloride (Apresoline)

    (b) Minoxidil (Loniten)

  (3) Nursing considerations

    (a) Laboratory tests must be performed before starting drug therapy: CBC, creatinine, LE prep (Anti-nuclear Antibody Screen, serum), ANA (Anti-nuclear Antibody) titer, and electrolytes

    (b) Because severe rebound hypertension can occur if the drug therapy is discontinued without weaning, warn the client not to do so without physician's orders

    (c) Teach client to rise slowly from chairs or the bed because of the risk of orthostatic hypotension

    (d) Monitor the BP carefully, especially after the first dose and with any changes in dosage; for Minoxidil, check HR before dose for reflex tachycardia

    (e) Note that Minoxidil can be used topically for alopecia

f. Diuretic agents—induce excretion of water, sodium, or potassium from the body

  (1) Expected effects—reduction in circulating blood volume, preload, and decreased BP

  (2) Commonly given drugs

    (a) Hydrochlorothiazide (Hydrodiuril)—potassium lost, thiazide diuretic

        (b) Furosemide (Lasix)—potassium lost, loop diuretic

        (c) Bumetanide (Bumex)—potassium lost, loop diuretic

        (d) Spironolactone (Aldactone)—potassium saved

     (3) Nursing considerations

        (a) Monitor sodium, potassium, magnesium, and chloride levels; check baseline levels before initial dose is given

        (b) Teach client to evaluate his or herself for the following

           (i) Daily weight: client should report a sharp loss or gain of more than 2 lb/day to physician

           (ii) Postural hypotension from loss of fluid

           (iii) Symptoms of electrolyte imbalance

        (c) Monitor for metabolic alkalosis from loss of chloride—circumoral and extremity numbness and tingling, feeling of lightheadedness, apprehension, irritability, disorientation, confusion, or more severe findings of hypocalcemia such as seizures or tetany

  g. Drugs used for hypertensive crisis—given only by IV; cause potent, rapid vasodilation of arteriolar bed

     (1) Expected effect—rapid decrease of BP, within minutes

     (2) Commonly given drugs

        (a) Nitroprusside (Nipride)—IV drip only

        (b) Diazoxide (Hyperstat)—IV bolus only

     (3) Nursing considerations

        (a) Monitor BP continuously, every 1 to 10 minutes if using a noninvasive BP monitoring system

        (b) Use arterial pressure line—best evaluation for continuous monitoring

2. Anticoagulant agents—interfere with coagulation pathway at some point

  a. Expected effect—prevent the blood from clotting

  b. Commonly given drugs

     (1) Oral anticoagulant—most common

        (a) Warfarin sodium (Coumadin)—fully therapeutic in 2 to 3 days; lasts about 7 to 10 days after final dose

        (b) Antidote—vitamin K (phytonadione; Aquamephyton), given IM, and by IV slowly

     (2) Parenteral anticoagulant—most common

        (a) Heparin sodium—immediate effect; lasts about 4 hours after final dose

        (b) Antidote—protamine sulfate, given IV slowly

  c. Nursing considerations

     (1) Monitor activated partial thromboplastin time (aPTT) for heparin administration; on the average, normal level is 30 seconds for aPTT; on heparin therapeutic goal is 1½ to 2 times normal

      (2) Monitor prothrombin time (PT) for warfarin administration; on the average, normal level is 15 seconds. For international accuracy, PT's are now reported as International Normalized Rates (INR)—normal should be 1-2; on oral anticoagulants therapeutic goal is an INR of 2-3.

      (3) Do not administer aspirin to patients taking oral anticoagulants

      (4) Evaluate all urine, stool, and vomitus for blood

      (5) Institute bleeding precautions—soft toothbrush, avoid IM injections, and evaluate venipunctures for bleeding

      (6) Note that the therapeutic level for both oral and parenteral drugs is 1.5 to 2 times the normal control levels

      (7) Monitor side effects

         (a) Coumadin—nausea, vomiting, and anorexia

         (b) Heparin—alopecia with long-term use

      (8) Note that the major toxic effect of both preparations is bleeding

3. Antiplatelet agents—prevent aggregation of platelets

  a. Expected effect—decrease thrombus formation

  b. Commonly given drugs

    (1) Aspirin

    (2) Dipyridamole (Persantine)

    (3) Ticlopidine (Ticlid)

    (4) Clopidogrel (Plavix)

    (5) Abciximab (ReoPro)—IV preparation used after angioplasty to prevent reocclusion of the artery

  c. Nursing considerations

    (1) Caution clients against the use of aspirin for more than 24 hours to treat fever and chills; the effects of aspirin may mask a serious infection or blood dyscrasia

    (2) Instruct client not to take aspirin with coumadin; results would enhance the effect of coumadin, with increased bleeding risk. Coumadin may be given with dipyridamole (Persantine) after valve replacement.

4. Thrombolytic agents—dissolve a thrombus or embolus

  a. Expected effects—return of blood flow to vessel obstructed by a thrombus; stop the showering of emboli

  b. Commonly given drugs

    (1) Streptokinase (Streptase)

    (2) Alteplase (Activase, t-PA, tissue plasmin activator)

  c. Nursing considerations

    (1) Clients must be started on heparin drip concurrently with thrombolytic agent to prevent more thrombus formation

    (2) Monitor client for excessive bleeding, and all body excrement for blood

    (3) Institute bleeding precautions—soft toothbrush, no IM injections, and evaluate all venipunctures for bleeding

(4) Assess client carefully for severe allergic reaction and anaphylaxis, which are most commonly seen with streptokinase

5. Sympathomimetic agents—these vasopressors mimic the effects of stimulation of organs and blood vessels by the sympathetic nervous system
   a. Expected effect—elevated BP
   b. Commonly given drugs
      (1) Dopamine hydrochloride (Intropin)
      (2) Dobutamine (Dobutrex Solution)
      (3) Ephedrine
   c. Nursing considerations
      (1) For best results, blood volume must be adequate before starting IV drip; there is minimal or no effective response in clients who are dehydrated
      (2) It is imperative to continuously monitor BP—every 2 to 5 minutes
      (3) An arterial line is the best way to evaluate BP
      (4) Drug must be titrated carefully to prevent hypertension
      (5) IV sites must be monitored carefully for infiltration; drug may cause sloughing of tissue
      (6) A central line is the best administration method

B. Procedures
1. Doppler ultrasonography—noninvasive test that identifies the presence of a decrease in arterial blood flow by evaluating audible arterial signals: arterial flow, intermittent solid sounds; venous flow, and more continuous swish sound
2. CT scan—permits visualization of arterial walls and adjacent structures, and thus is helpful in the diagnosis of aortic aneurysms
3. Angiography (arteries) and venography (veins)—invasive tests in which contrast medium is injected into the artery or vein. X-ray studies of the area injected are done. The actual obstruction can be visualized.

C. Psychosocial concerns
1. Noncompliance—a major concern in clients with hypertension because of the lack of symptoms associated with hypertension. Symptoms tend to remind clients to take their medication.
2. Fear—a major concern in many clients with vascular disease that is directly related to danger of death or loss of limb
3. Lifestyle changes—a major issue in patients with arterial occlusive disease, which may eventually end in limb amputation. Other issues considered are the need for dietary changes and exercise, along with cessation of smoking and caffeine use.

D. Health history—questions and sequence
1. What symptoms are you having that have made it necessary for you to seek assistance?

2. Are you being treated for other disorders?
3. Is there a family history of vascular disease?
4. Are you presently taking any prescription or over-the-counter medications?
5. Have you noticed a change in your weight? Either a loss or gain? How much and over what period of time?
6. Do you smoke? How much and for how long?
7. Do you use alcohol? How much and for how long?
8. Are you presently following a special diet? What kind?
9. Do you have a history of high cholesterol or triglycerides?
10. Do you exercise? How much and how often?
11. Do you have pain in your legs when walking? How far are you able to walk before the pain begins?
12. Do you live or work in a stressful environment? How do you cope with this stress?
13. Do you have headaches? How often? How do you relieve them?

E. **Physical examination—questions and sequence**
   1. ABCs—vital signs
   2. Examination for LOC—awake, alert, and oriented; pupillary response
   3. Examination of skin color, temperature, moisture, and turgor; mucous membranes
   4. Examination of neck for distended veins
   5. Inspection of the chest—bilateral chest movements and abnormal chest movements
   6. Palpation of the chest for tenderness and growths
   7. Auscultation of heart sounds
   8. Inspection of the abdomen for pulsations and asymmetry
   9. Auscultation of the abdomen for abnormal sounds and bruit
   10. Palpation of the abdomen
   11. Examination of the peripheral pulses, especially the feet

IV. Pathophysiologic disorders
A. **Shock**
   1. Definition—insufficient tissue perfusion. If left untreated or if treatment is resisted the result will be inadequate tissue oxygenation and cellular death
   2. Pathophysiology—shock is the state in which one of the three important functions of the circulatory system have been lost: circulating blood volume, a balance between **vasoconstriction** and **vasodilation,** or a competent pumping action of the heart. Clients pass through several stages of shock regardless of the cause of the syndrome
      a. Stage I, compensated shock—body uses compensatory mechanisms: increased HR, vasoconstriction of peripheral and GI vessels to maintain near normal CO and BP

   b. Stage II, decompensated shock—beginning of decrease in CO and BP
      (1) Massive vasoconstriction, which causes vasodilation of the microcirculatory system (capillary circulation)
      (2) Extensive pooling of blood in capillaries of the microcirculatory system
      (3) Transfer of fluid from blood into the interstitial space and edema
      (4) Drastic reduction in venous return with a significant decrease in BP
      (5) Lack of cellular oxygenation because of the decrease in capillary blood flow
      (6) Lactic acidosis production because cells are functioning in anaerobic metabolism
   c. Stage III, progressive shock
      (1) Occurs if tissue perfusion is not improved
      (2) Becomes more profound with cell necrosis
      (3) Causes eventual organ death and client demise
3. Etiology
   a. Hypovolemic shock—lack of adequate circulating blood volume frequently from blood loss with trauma, plasma loss as in burns, and dehydration syndrome with fluid loss such as with GI losses
   b. Cardiogenic shock—severely decreased CO from poor pumping capability of the heart; more common after an extensive myocardial infarction (MI) or with chronic cardiomyopathy
   c. Distributive shock—blood vessels dilate throughout the vascular bed causing a redistribution and pooling of blood; also termed *vasogenic shock*
      (1) Three types
         (a) Anaphylactic shock—allergic or hypersensitive reaction to an allergen; clients also manifest bronchial constriction with acute respiratory distress or arrest
         (b) Neurogenic shock—inability of the nervous system to control dilation of the blood vessels. This type of shock is most common after spinal cord injury, spinal anesthesia, and severe vagal stimulation induced by pain, trauma, or stress.
         (c) Septic shock—pathogenic organisms present in the blood lead to a release of vasoactive materials, such as histamine, prostaglandins, bradykinins, and leukotrienes, causing massive vasodilation
4. Assessment
   a. Questions to ask
      (1) What is your name? Where are you? Do you know the day and year?
      (2) Do you feel weak or nauseated?

(3) Do you feel short of breath?

(4) Clinical manifestations (Table 3-1)

   b. Abnormal laboratory findings (Table 3-2)

   c. Abnormal diagnostic study results

     (1) ECG—tachycardia, also may show ischemia and dysrhythmias

     (2) CXR—pulmonary congestion in later stages, especially in cardiogenic shock

5. Expected medical interventions

   a. Fluid replacement as necessary with crystalloids (normal saline or lactated Ringer's solution); colloids (hetastarch or human albumins) or other plasma expanders; and blood (packed cells may be given more than whole blood)

   b. Fluid volume monitoring with central venous pressure (CVP) line, or pulmonary artery line; keep CVP above 8 cm H_2O, systolic pressure above 90 mm Hg, and mean arterial pressure (MAP) between 70 and 90 mm Hg

   c. Oxygen to improve tissue oxygenation

   d. Mechanical ventilation as necessary to maintain respiratory status

   e. Vasopressors to maintain BP

TABLE 3-1   Clinical Manifestations of Shock

Assessment Findings	Hypovolemic	Cardiogenic	Distributive
Respiratory	Rapid, shallow	Same	Same
Cardiovascular	Rapid, weak, thready pulse, hypotension	Same	*Anaphylactic*—same *Neurogenic*—bradycardia, hypotension *Septic*—same
Integumentary	Cool, clammy, pale skin	Cool, clammy, pale skin	*Anaphylactic and neurogenic*—dry, cool, pale skin *Septic*—early: warm, dry, flushed skin; late: same as hypovolemic
Neurologic	Anxiety, irritability, nervousness, restlessness, leading to confusion and LOC	Same	*Anphylactic*—same *Neurogenic*—same *Septic*—drowsiness leading to stupor then coma
GI and genitourinary	Decreased bowel sounds, oliguria	Same	Same

TABLE 3-2	Abnormal Laboratory Findings in Shock

Laboratory Findings	Hypovolemic	Cardiogenic	Distribution
Hemoglobin and hematocrit	Decreased	Within normal range	Within normal range
WBC	Increased	Increased	Increased
ESR	Increased	Increased	Increased
Blood cultures	Negative	Negative	Positive for growth of causative agent, most common gram negative and gram positive; only about 50% of clients who are septic have positive blood cultures
Electrolytes	Potassium increased from cellular death	Same	Same
BUN	Increased from dehydration, blood loss, breakdown of old blood in gut, decreased renal perfusion	Increased from decreased renal perfusion	Increased from decreased renal perfusion
Creatinine	Increased related to decreased renal perfusion	Same	Same
Blood glucose	Increased in response to stress	Same	Same
Prothrombin time, partial thromboplastin time	Increased	Increased	Increased
Platelets	Decreased	Decreased	Decreased
AGBs	Hypoxemia, metabolic acidosis, respiratory alkalosis	Same	Same

    f. Laboratory test results monitoring for evaluation of the treatment of abnormalities

    g. Nutritional support by enteral or parenteral routes

6. Nursing diagnoses

    a. Impaired gas exchange related to diminished circulation

    b. Altered tissue perfusion (GI, cerebral, cardiac, pulmonary, renal) related to impaired circulation

    c. Decreased CO related to poor cardiac pumping capability, inadequate blood volume, and vascular pooling

    d. Fluid volume deficit related to blood loss and fluid shift into the interstitial spaces and tissues

7. Client goals

    a. Client will maintain PaO_2 of over 80 mm Hg, pH between 7.35 and 7.45, and $PaCO_2$ between 35 and 45 mm Hg

    b. Client will maintain adequate tissue perfusion of all organs as evidenced by minimal adequate functioning of those organs. That is, clients can state their own name, location, and correct date or year. Bowel sounds present which is indicative of mesenteric perfusion. Diarrhea may indicate hypoxic mesentery.

    c. Client will keep BP and HR within 20% of baseline

    d. Client will maintain adequate fluid volume as evidenced by urine output of at least 30 ml/hr

8. Nursing interventions

    a. Acute care

        (1) Maintain patent airway while monitoring breathing patterns for tiring and increased respiratory effort

        (2) Monitor circulatory parameters every 10 to 15 minutes until stable

        (3) Maintain at least one large-bore IV—16- or 18-gauge—for fluid and blood product administration

        (4) Be prepared to utilize a modified Trendelenburg (body flat, legs elevated) position to maintain organ perfusion when therapy is begun or when therapy is ineffective

        (5) Give all medications by IV route

    b. Home care regarding client education

        (1) If shock has been induced by an allergen, the client must be instructed to wear a medical-alert bracelet to alert health care personnel to allergy. Facilitate the client obtaining and learning how to use an epinephrine kit, which must be carried with the client at all times.

        (2) A client who has experienced a critically ill situation such as shock may leave the hospital confused and somewhat disoriented or forgetful. The client will need help at home to reorganize thinking processes and bring this aspect of the illness to completion.

9. Evaluation protocol
   a. How do I know that my interventions were effective?
      (1) Does the client know his or her own name? Where he or she is? The date or year?
      (2) Does the client feel dizzy or weak?
      (3) Is the client experiencing SOB?
   b. Which criteria will I use to change my interventions?
      (1) Client is confused as to person, place, and time
      (2) Client indicates being dizzy and feeling weak even in a flat or modified Trendelenburg position; assessment findings indicate vital signs are not stabilizing
      (3) Client indicates having SOB with assessment findings that indicate increased respiratory effort, shallow respirations, and no energy to breathe deeply
   c. How will I know that my client teaching has been effective?
      (1) Client describes the situation that would require use of an epinephrine kit and demonstrates use of the kit
      (2) Client orders a medical-alert bracelet
      (3) Client states feeling less anxious, with fewer periods of confusion or forgetfulness at home, and is progressing to a state of normalcy experienced before the illness
10. Older adult alert
    a. Older adult clients have increased **peripheral vascular resistance** as a normal change of aging. Thus, little compensation is available for those in shock. Vital signs will change more rapidly than in younger adults.
    b. Older adults have decreased elasticity of blood vessels, resulting in a decrease in the normal compensatory mechanism for vasoconstriction as seen in younger adults
    c. Older adult clients may have a higher BP than younger clients as a result of increased vascular resistance. Therefore, when evaluating vital signs, keep in mind the client's baseline. Older adults may tend to have a higher baseline BP than younger clients. Be aware that a decrease in BP of more than 20 mm Hg may have significant effects, especially on the renal glomerular filtration rate; do not wait for a decrease to 100/60 mm Hg systolic to seek intervention.
    d. If on cardiac medication, older adult clients will have inhibition of the normal compensatory action, that is, increased HR of over 100 beats per minute. Look for a sustained increase in HR of over 20 beats per minute above baseline. Consider this increase to be a possible sign of shock.

B. **Atherosclerosis**
   1. Definition—one type of arteriosclerosis that represents a broad class of arterial wall changes associated with decreased elasticity.

Atherosclerosis is an occlusive arterial disease that mainly affects the coronary, cerebral, and femoral arteries as well as the aorta

2. Pathophysiology—involves the accumulation of cholesterol and lipids, called *lesions,* in the walls of affected arteries
   a. Layer of the wall most commonly affected is the intima rather than the medis or adventia
   b. Progression of lesions
      (1) Start with a fatty streak
      (2) Progress to a fibrous plaque
      (3) Proceed to a lesion made up of the fibrous plaque, calcium, and a thrombus
      (4) Progress over many years, eventually occluding the affected artery to as much as 100% of the lumen
3. Etiology—many factors characterized as nonmodifiable and modifiable are believed to precipitate the onset of atherosclerosis
   a. Nonmodifiable factors
      (1) Heredity
      (2) Age
      (3) Gender
      (4) Race
   b. Modifiable factors
      (1) Environment, including dietary factors
      (2) Smoking
      (3) Hypercholesteremia
      (4) Hypertension
      (5) Diabetes
      (6) Obesity
      (7) Stress
      (8) Sedentary lifestyle
4. Incidence—underlying cause of most cardiac and vascular diseases
5. Assessment—widely variable depending on the vessels affected. The various disorders that can occur will be discussed in detail within the chapter in which the disorder belongs, for example, coronary artery disease is discussed in Chapter 2, The Cardiac System.

C. Hypertension
1. Definition
   a. A consistent elevation of BP on three or more checks
   b. Systolic greater than 140 mm Hg, diastolic greater than 90 mm Hg, or both
   c. Hypertensive crisis is an acute increase in BP to a life-threatening level, greater than 200 mm Hg systolic and greater than 110 mm Hg diastolic
2. Pathophysiology—changes and circumstances increase BP
      (a) Changes
            (i) Change in hormones that regulate BP, such as aldosterone, renin, and antidiuretic hormone

(ii) Increase in circulating blood volume

(iii) Increase in HR

(b) Circumstances

(i) Those that cause vasoconstriction

(ii) Those that stimulate the sympathetic nervous system

3. Etiology

a. Most clients (90%) are classified as having primary or essential hypertension, meaning the cause is unknown

b. The remaining (10%) have secondary hypertension, meaning hypertension is from a known cause, for example, renal disease and pregnancy

4. Incidence—over 85 million Americans have hypertension, and nearly half are unaware

5. Assessment

a. Questions to ask: Remember—hypertension is asymptomatic in most clients. These questions are meant for clients who are beginning to have symptoms.

(1) Do you have trouble remembering?

(2) Do you ever have dizzy spells or a feeling of light-headedness?

(3) Do you feel tired quite often?

(4) Do you suffer from headaches? If yes, when do they occur most often? Is there a pattern to the headaches?

(5) Do you ever have nosebleeds?

(6) Do you feel as if you have a lot of stress in your life, and if so how do you handle it?

b. Clinical manifestations

(1) Usually none in clients with mild to moderate hypertension

(2) Moderate to severe

(a) Difficulty remembering

(b) Headaches, common on waking

(c) Palpitations

(d) Epistaxis—very common in hypertensive crisis or very high, undiagnosed hypertension

(3) BP greater than 140/90 mm Hg on three separate occasions

c. Abnormal laboratory findings—with renal involvement

(1) Urinalysis—proteinuria and hematuria

(2) Elevated creatinine

(3) Elevated BUN

(4) Elevated cholesterol and lipid levels

d. Abnormal diagnostic test results

(1) ECG—left ventricular hypertrophy

(2) CXR—left ventricular enlargement

6. Expected medical interventions
   a. Weight reduction as necessary
   b. Encouragement for cessation of smoking
   c. Implementation of a low-salt diet
   d. Restriction of caffeine and alcohol in diet
   e. Encouragement for increased exercise
   f. Administration of antihypertensive medication if lifestyle alterations are ineffective at least 6 months after implementation
7. Nursing diagnoses
   a. Knowledge deficit regarding medical regimen related to incomplete client teaching
   b. Risk for noncompliance to medical regimen related to asymptomatic illness and side effects from medication regimen
8. Client goals
   a. Client will explain individualized medical regimen
   b. Client will follow medical regimen as evidenced by controlled BP and loss of weight
9. Nursing interventions
   a. Acute care—hypertensive crisis
      (1) Monitor BP every 5 to 15 minutes until stable and controlled
      (2) Maintain cardiac monitoring for dysrhythmias
      (3) Evaluate neurologic status every 30 to 60 minutes for changes
      (4) Maintain IV access for antihypertensive drug therapy
      (5) Monitor laboratory values—creatinine, electrolyte, and hematocrit and hemoglobin (H&H) levels for hydration status and renal function
   b. Home care regarding client education
      (1) Instruct client on low-sodium, low-fat, limited-caffeine, and possibly reduced-calorie diet
      (2) Instruct client on expected effectiveness of medications ordered, possible side effects, and to report side effects to physician
      (3) Instruct client to monitor BP frequently and to schedule follow-up examinations with physician
      (4) Discuss with client the relationship between exercise, diet, medications, weight loss, and BP control
      (5) Caution client on use of over-the-counter substances such as cold medications and their ability to increase BP
10. Evaluation protocol
    a. How do I know my interventions were effective? Note: Acute care interventions are best evaluated by objective data
       (1) BP is maintained at a level compatible with organs not being compromised
       (2) Neurologic status is stable and minimal or no deficit is noted
       (3) Cardiac dysrhythmias are not apparent

    b. What criteria will I use to change my interventions?

      (1) Unstable BP

      (2) Neurologic deficit or deterioration noted in assessment

      (3) Significant cardiac dysrhythmias present

    c. How will I know that my client teaching has been effective?

      (1) Client uses small amounts of salt at the table only

      (2) Client reads labels before buying groceries and prepares low-fat foods

      (3) Client maintains appropriate weight as directed by physician

      (4) Client can describe method of taking medication, pattern of BP, and side effects necessary to alert physician

      (5) Client knows the frequency of physician visits and the time of the next appointment

  11. Older adult alert

    a. Owing to decreased vascular elasticity seen normally in older adult clients, it is likely that BP readings will be labile

    b. It would not be uncommon for these clients to suffer adverse hypotension from antihypertensive medications, especially if they have volume depletion

D. Peripheral arterial occlusive disorders

  1. Definition—a group of disorders that causes a decrease in lumen diameter, damage to the wall of the lumen, or both; three of the more common disorders

    a. Arteriosclerosis obliterans

    b. Raynaud's disease

    c. Thromboangiitis obliterans (Buerger's disease)

  2. Pathophysiology

    a. Arteriosclerosis obliterans (partial obstruction) caused by atherosclerotic plaque—vessel diameter becomes progressively smaller; skin color of extremity is usually pale

      (1) Collateral circulation increases blood flow to the area that may be affected

      (2) In time, collateral vessels will not be sufficient to feed affected area with oxygen and nutrients

      (3) Ischemic tissue will eventually turn into necrotic tissue without medical intervention

      (4) Process can take many years before the client begins to have symptoms

      (5) Formation of a fresh thrombus in an affected vessel may lead to acute necrosis of the affected area

      (6) Arteries most commonly affected—carotid, iliac, and femoral

    b. Raynaud's disease—vasospasm of the small arteries or arterioles in the hands and fingers. Skin color of digits— whiteness to cyanosis. With spasm as artery relaxes, color

changes to rubor, or redness, with throbbing or burning pain from reactive hyperemia, which indicate greater artery relaxation
(1) Often aggravated from a response to cold, stress, or use of vibrating tools
(2) Tobacco is thought to be a major precipitating factor
c. Buerger's disease—thromboangiitis obliterans, significant inflammatory occlusive changes in the peripheral arteries and veins of hands and feet. Skin color of extremity is usually reddened—rubor.
(1) Possibly related to an autoimmune response
(2) Untreated can lead to necrosis and loss of extremities
(3) Tobacco is thought to be a major contributing factor
3. Etiology
a. Atherosclerosis
b. Autoimmunity
c. Inflammation
d. Thrombus
e. Trauma
f. Vasospasm
4. Assessment
a. Questions to ask
(1) Do you have pain in your calf when you walk? This is called intermittent claudication.
(2) Does your leg pain stop when you stop walking?
(3) Do you have pain in your legs or hands when you are resting?
(4) Do your feet or hands feel cold to you?
(5) Do you ever have changes in your eyesight or hearing for a brief period of time?
(6) Do you ever have a time when you feel like you cannot think clearly? Does this occur when you are stressed?
b. Clinical manifestations (Figure 3-1, Table 3-3)

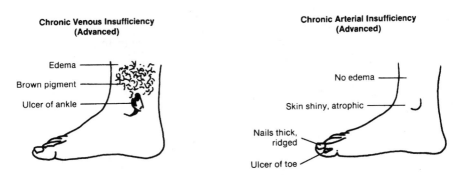

Figure 3-1 Common manifestations of chronic arterial and venous peripheral vascular problems. (From *AJN/Mosby Nursing board review,* ed 9, St. Louis, 1994, Mosby.)

TABLE 3-3	Clinical Manifestations of Peripheral Arterial Occlusive Disorders	
Disorders	**Primary Manifestations**	**Secondary Manifestations**
Carotid occlusion	Visual or auditory disturbances, headache	Slowed mental processes, seizures
Femoral—iliac occlusion	Intermittent claudication—pain in calf of legs on walking, pain in extremity at rest	Cool extremities, poor peripheral pulses, hypertrophied toenails, capillary refill takes greater than 3 sec
Raynaud's disease	Paleness of the digits, then cyanosis, cold, numbness (which is the vasospastic period)	Previous symptoms are followed by an extreme rubor in the extremity with throbbing or burning pain (blood reenters the extremity)
Buerger's disease	Intermittent claudication first felt in arch of foot then calf, pain in the extremity at rest, sparse hair distribution	Ischemic digits, parathesias, dependant rubor in the extremity, capillary refill takes greater than 3 sec

  c. Abnormal laboratory findings—none specific
  d. Abnormal diagnostic test results
   (1) Noninvasive
    (a) Doppler ultrasonography—demonstrates degree of ischemia experienced by patient
    (b) Plethysmography—indicates decline in peripheral circulation
   (2) Invasive—angiography—circulation with occlusions are visualized with a contrast dye
 5. Expected medical interventions
  a. Nitrates or calcium-channel blockers to dilate collateral circulation
  b. Weight reduction
  c. Smoking cessation—"cutting down" is ineffective
  d. Anticoagulant and antiplatelet drugs
  e. Peripheral angioplasty
  f. Thrombolytic therapy
  g. Bypass grafting
  h. Endarterectomy, surgical or laser
  i. Extra-anatomic bypass grafting
  j. Amputation as necessary
 6. Nursing diagnoses
  a. Altered peripheral tissue perfusion related to impedance of flow in the vessels

    b. Pain related to decline in oxygenation secondary to decreased blood flow to the affected area

    c. Risk for impaired skin integrity related to poor tissue oxygenation, secondary to a decline in peripheral circulation

7. Client goals

    a. Client will exhibit an increase in peripheral tissue perfusion as evidenced by warmth in the affected area

    b. Client will state pain is minimal or relieved in affected area

    c. Client will not lose skin integrity to the affected area

8. Nursing interventions

    a. Acute care—may be a postsurgical period

        (1) Follow guidelines for care of the client after surgery

        (2) Avoid strain over the incision to prevent graft dislodgement or incisional disruption

        (3) Monitor for hemorrhage—arterial bleeding; check underneath the client's extremity

        (4) Administer ordered anticoagulants

        (5) Place client in reverse Trendelenburg if ordered by the physician to increase blood flow to lower extremities; avoid extremity elevation

        (6) Evaluate neurovascular status of affected extremity with each check of vital signs

            (a) Pulses distal to site

            (b) Skin temperature and color as compared with unaffected extremity

            (c) Sensation

            (d) Movement

    b. Home care regarding client education

        (1) Emphasize need to eliminate nicotine and caffeine

        (2) Discourage use of any heat products to area; encourage a warm living environment

        (3) Instruct the client to seek physician's advice for any skin breakdown of the lower extremities

        (4) Encourage a mild exercise program—walking, interspersed with adequate rest and relaxation exercises

            (a) Lying flat in bed with legs elevated above heart for 2 to 3 minutes

            (b) Dangling on side of bed with legs relaxed for 2 to 3 minutes

            (c) Exercising feet—flex, extend, invert, and evert; hold each position for 30 seconds

            (d) After exercise, lying flat in bed with legs at heart level and covered with blanket for 5 minutes

        (5) Instruct client to wear warm socks and gloves when entering a cold weather environment

        (6) Instruct client on technique for capillary refill checks and for skin and foot care

9. Evaluation protocol
   a. How will I know that my interventions were effective? The acute care interventions are best evaluated by objective data.
      (1) Vital signs are stable
      (2) No bleeding noted from incision
      (3) Neurovascular status is intact and unchanged from baseline after surgery
      (4) Pain is controlled
   b. What criteria will I use to change my interventions?
      (1) Bleeding noted at the dressing site, sustained elevated HR of greater than 20 beats per minute over baseline, decrease in systolic BP of greater than 20 mm Hg from baseline
      (2) Loss of peripheral pulses distal to the surgical site
      (3) Loss of sensation, warmth, movement, or change in color of extremity distal to the surgical site
      (4) Change in neurologic status
   c. How will I know that my client teaching has been effective?
      (1) Clients will state they have stopped smoking cigarettes and drinking caffeinated beverages
      (2) Clients will state homes are heated at 72 degrees in winter and that they always wear warm clothing on hands and feet when outside
      (3) Clients indicate they have been walking a half a block more each day without pain, followed by 30 minutes of rest and a relaxation exercise
      (4) Clients will have minimal or no break in skin integrity on lower extremities
10. Older adult alert
    a. Realize that tissue perfusion in older adult clients may be even more compromised from poor vascular elasticity
    b. A positive note: Because older adult clients have had many years to develop their obstructive disorder, reliable collateral circulation may be present
    c. The perceptions of pain by an older adult client may be altered by decreased nerve ending functioning and by concurrent disorders such as arthritis; therefore, pain assessment may be more difficult

E. Peripheral venous disorders
   1. Definition—disorders that decrease normal venous return from the peripheral circulation to the heart
      a. Chronic venous insufficiency—poor venous return, with venous stasis and eventual venous status ulcer
      b. Deep vein thrombosis—inflamed deep vein of leg or pelvis with a thrombus in the area of inflammation

2. Pathophysiology
   a. Chronic venous insufficiency
      (1) Valves in the veins have become incompetent
      (2) Blood pools in the vessels of the lower extremities
      (3) Venous pressure in these areas increases
      (4) Blood pooling hinders efficient oxygen and nutrient exchange in the capillary area
      (5) Area becomes edematous, brown in pigmentation, and stasis ulceration is inevitable
      (6) Stasis ulcers are difficult to heal as a result of poor oxygenation and nutrition to the tissue areas involved
   b. Deep vein thrombosis
      (1) Common in clients likely to have venous stasis, such as those on strict bed rest or with sedentary jobs
      (2) Stasis of blood facilitates thrombus formation
      (3) States of hypercoagulability—either increased clotting factors or increased viscosity of the blood, that is, increased H&H levels or severe dehydration—allow for clumping of erythrocytes and platelets, with thrombus formation beginning
      (4) Any injury to a vessel wall causes platelets and blood debris to be attracted to the area and clots to form easily
3. Etiology
   a. Chronic venous insufficiency—caused by nonfunctioning valves in the veins of the lower extremities; gravity allows blood to pool in lower vasculature
   b. Deep vein thrombosis—occurs in response to hypercoagulability, venous stasis, or actual injury to a vessel wall
4. Incidence
   a. Chronic venous insufficiency
      (1) Follows an episode of deep vein thrombosis
      (2) May take many years to manifest
   b. Deep vein thrombosis
      (1) More common in the female population
      (2) Found in one third of all patients who have had major surgery or a major illness
5. Assessment
   a. Questions to ask
      (1) Do you have any pain in either of your legs? Do you have pain when in a relaxed position? Do you have pain when you point your toes toward your head?
      (2) Is there any swelling in either of your legs?
      (3) Do you feel any warm areas in your legs?
   b. Clinical manifestations
      (1) Chronic venous insufficiency (see Figure 3-1, p. 101)
         (a) Chronically edematous limbs—usually around the ankles; commonly bilateral

       (b) Thick, rough, brownish-colored skin around the ankles
       (c) Venous stasis ulcers—more common by the ankles
     (2) Deep vein thrombosis
       (a) Pain at the site of thrombus
       (b) Swelling at the site of thrombus, usually in one
          leg only
       (c) Redness and warmth at the site of thrombus

> ⚠ **Warning!**
>
> Clients must be monitored very carefully for the onset
> of **sudden respiratory distress.** This change in status
> can be indicative of an acute pulmonary embolism
> caused by the clot in the leg breaking away and
> traveling to the lungs.

  c. Abnormal laboratory findings—none that are specific
  d. Abnormal diagnostic test results
     (1) Doppler ultrasonography—documents diminished
       circulation to an area and impedance to venous blood flow
     (2) Plethysmography—documents diminished circulation to
       the area
  6. Expected medical interventions
    a. Chronic venous insufficiency
     (1) Elevate leg as much as possible
     (2) Wear knee length support hose
     (3) Use wet saline dressings for stasis ulcers
    b. Deep vein thrombosis
     (1) Bed rest and affected limb elevated at least 4 to 6 inches in
       the acute phase
     (2) Heparin drip for approximately 7 days
     (3) Coumadin for 3 to 6 months
     (4) Thrombolytic drug therapy
  7. Nursing diagnoses
    a. Impaired skin integrity related to poor venous return and
      venous pooling
    b. Impaired tissue integrity related to poor venous return and
      venous pooling
    c. Pain related to inflammation in the area of the thrombus or
      ulceration
  8. Client goals
    a. Client will exhibit that skin impairment will not increase in size
      and begin granulation healing
    b. Client will exhibit that tissue integrity improves as evidenced
      by decreased ankle edema by ¼-in/wk
    c. Client will state that the pain has been relieved by measures
      instituted

9. Nursing interventions
   a. Acute care—deep vein thrombosis
      (1) Monitor vital signs at least every 2 to 4 hours until stable
      (2) Monitor for sudden changes in respiratory effort or lung sounds, which may be indicative of pulmonary embolism
      (3) Maintain patent IV for heparin drip
      (4) Monitor for therapeutic aPTT, which may be 1.5 to 2 times normal
      (5) Maintain bed rest for 5 to 7 days
      (6) Elevate legs above the level of the heart to enhance venous return while on bed rest
      (7) Maintain warm, moist compresses to affected legs
   b. Home care regarding client education
      (1) Instruct client on how to take oral anticoagulant drugs, how often to have APTT studies drawn, and how to institute bleeding precautions
      (2) Emphasize need to eliminate tobacco and substances with caffeine
      (3) Instruct client not to wear restrictive clothing around lower extremities and not to cross legs at the knee
      (4) Instruct client to consult with gynecologist about using birth control medications if relevant because they often are associated with venous thrombosis
      (5) Avoid standing or sitting for periods longer than 1 hour
      (6) Need to elevate legs above the level of the heart for at least 8 hours each day in the acute stage
10. Evaluation protocol
    a. How do I know that my interventions were effective?
       (1) Has the client's leg pain improved?
       (2) Has swelling in the client's leg decreased?
       (3) Is the client having any SOB?
    b. What criteria will I use to change my interventions?
       (1) Changes in client's vital signs of more than 20% from baseline
       (2) Findings associated with pulmonary embolism
       (3) Pain in client's extremity
       (4) Minimal or no decrease in the size of extremity swelling
    c. How will I know that my client teaching has been effective?
       (1) Client has an aPTT drawn every week in physician's office
       (2) Client raised foot of bed 6 inches for sleeping with legs elevated
       (3) Client, if female, no longer wears tight undergarments such as garters
11. Older adult alert
    a. As a normal course of aging the venous valves in the blood vessels become inefficient; older adult clients are at great risk for venous insufficiency

b. Older adults are at greater risk for venous occlusion from decreased CO and changes in vein wall integrity, decreased mobility, and a tendency to dehydrate from lack of sufficient fluid intake

F. Aortic aneurysm
1. Definition—a dilation of the aorta
2. Etiology—most common pathology
   a. Atherosclerosis
   b. Hypertension—plays a key role in the development
3. Incidence—more common in the male population, usually those over 50 years of age
4. Pathophysiology
   a. Abdominal aortic aneurysms
      (1) More common than thoracic aortic aneurysms
      (2) Walls of aorta are under high pressure owing to pressure directly exerted on them with each ventricular ejection
      (3) For this reason, and as a result of changes associated with atherosclerosis, the media of the aorta wall begin to weaken and bulge outward
      (4) Pressure continues on the walls, and eventually the intima tears
      (5) The tear allows blood to be diverted into the wall of the aorta—this is referred to as a *false aneurysm*
      (6) The wall fills with blood, which then clots
      (7) The wall now bulges outward and into the lumen; this increases both BP and **peripheral vascular resistance**
      (8) Over a period of time the outer wall may tear, allowing for rupture of the aneurysm. This is a medical emergency and requires immediate surgery.
5. Assessment
   a. Questions to ask
      (1) Have you experienced any pain in your groin or along your sides?
      (2) Have you been experiencing lightheadedness?
   b. Clinical manifestations
      (1) Most are asymptomatic until they dissect or rupture in which case the pain is severe
      (2) Thoracic aneurysms—pain between the shoulder blades
      (3) Abdominal aneurysms—flank or groin pain
         (a) Pulsatile mass in midabdominal area
         (b) Decreased peripheral pulses—unilaterally or bilaterally
         (c) Bilateral pale, lower extremities
   c. Abnormal laboratory findings: CBC—in an acute rupture may indicate decreased H&H, several hours after incident
   d. Abnormal diagnostic test results
      (1) CXR and abdominal X-ray—may show calcification of the aneurysm and highlight its outline

(2) CT scan—documents the size of the aneurysm

(3) Aortography—with contrast medium can delineate aneurysm and determine if there are other compromised arteries

6. Expected medical interventions

    a. Medications to decrease BP to lowest point tolerable for client

    b. Surgical repair with graft if aneurysm is larger than 6 cm

7. Nursing diagnoses

    a. Decreased CO related to alternate flow of blood into the wall of the aorta

    b. Alteration in peripheral tissue perfusion related to blood pooling in the arterial wall

    c. Severe anxiety related to fear of death

    d. Pain related to the effects of aortic changes

8. Client goals

    a. Client will maintain BP and HR within 20% of baseline

    b. Client will exhibit palpable peripheral pulses and warm extremities

    c. Client will show decrease in anxiety as evidenced by relaxed facial features

    d. Client will state that measures used to relieve pain have done so

9. Nursing interventions

    a. Acute care

        (1) Take vital signs every 5 to 15 minutes

        (2) Monitor neurologic signs at least every 30 minutes

        (3) Monitor lung and heart sounds at least every hour

        (4) Prepare the client physically and mentally for surgery

        (5) Medicate for pain as vital signs permit

        (6) Monitor lower extremities for changes in neurovascular status

        (7) Measure abdominal girth every hour, before and after surgery; do not palpate site of aneurysm

    b. Home care regarding client education

        (1) If the client has an aneurysm that must be evaluated every 6 months by ultrasonography, he or she must be taught the importance of those follow-up visits

        (2) Instruct client on postoperative home care

            (a) On a return visit, have the client demonstrate incision care

            (b) Inform the client about activity restrictions

                (i) Teach the client that lifting usually is not permitted for at least 6 weeks; afterward only 2 lb can be lifted, with a gradual increase

                (ii) Teach the client how to avoid a pulling or straining situation

(iii) Inform the client that driving usually is restricted until at least the first postoperative visit with the physician

10. Evaluation protocol
    a. How do I know that my interventions were effective?
       (1) Has the client's pain improved with pain medication? Rate on a scale of 0 to 10.
       (2) Does the client know his or her own name? Where he or she is? The date and year?
       (3) Are the client's vital signs within 20% of baseline?
       (4) Are the peripheral pulses present? Are the extremities warm and of normal color for the client?
    b. What criteria will I use to change my interventions?
       (1) Unstable vital signs
       (2) Rapidly changing neurologic signs
       (3) Change in neurovascular status in lower extremities indicating impairment
       (4) Abdominal girth is increasing
       (5) Pain is unrelieved or becoming more severe
    c. How will I know that my client teaching has been effective?
       (1) Client demonstrates the correct technique for incisional care
       (2) Client plans for a friend to drive to physician's office for follow-up visit
       (3) Client identifies how to avoid exertion while at home and how to rest at least 3 times a day

11. Older adult alert
    a. Owing to the decreased cardiovascular status of older adult clients, decreased CO and decreased vascular elasticity, these clients usually are unable to withstand the trauma of aortic rupture. Periodic checkups should be encouraged to identify aortic aneurysms in their intact state so that surgical repair can be offered.
    b. The suddenness and life-threatening nature of the illness make it imperative that clients and significant others have time together before surgery and as much time as possible after surgery. Many times they have been together for over 30 years and need that time to adjust and support one another.

WEB Resources

http://www.proed.net/ecc/ECC_home.htm
   ECC Home (Emergency Cardiac Care)

http://pharminfo.com/disease/cardio/HT_info.html
   Hypertension Information Center

REVIEW QUESTIONS

1. The most effective method of monitoring fluid volume in the client with refractory hypovolemic shock is
    1. BP trends
    2. HR comparisons
    3. CVP trends
    4. Arterial line comparisons

2. The client with cardiogenic shock will show evidence of improved tissue perfusion by a
    1. Change in LOC
    2. Increased urine output
    3. Decreased $PaCO_2$
    4. Change in the oxygen saturation in arterial blood (SaO_2) from 84% to 88%

3. The appropriate body position for a client in hypovolemic shock with compromised vital signs is
    1. Positive tilt
    2. Reverse Trendelenburg
    3. Modified Trendelenburg
    4. Trendelenburg

4. At a health screening fair a nurse has identified a client with a BP of 200/100 mm Hg. The intervention at this point would be to
    1. Retake the BP immediately to verify the reading
    2. Refer the client to their physician for further evaluation within the next 24 hours
    3. Refer the client to their physician for further evaluation within 1 week
    4. Ask the client to have a family member take the client to the nearest hospital emergency room within the next hour

5. The client is told that he or she has a 100% occlusion of the left femoral artery. The assessment of the left lower extremity reveals a warm, pink foot, with appropriate blanching, sensation, and movement. The nurse is aware that the reason for appropriate neurovascular status is
    1. The client's daily walking periods of 30 minutes
    2. The use of special high cotton socks at all times
    3. The venous circulation that has assumed the roles of the arteries
    4. The presence of effective collateral circulation

6. During an initial assessment, a client indicates the inability to walk as far as he used to owing to pain in the right calf. Which of these questions would the nurse want to ask the client initially to confirm a suspicion and establish the direction of the remaining questions?

1. How often do you have your discomfort?
2. How far can you walk before you have pain?
3. Does your pain stop when you stop walking?
4. When does your pain start?

7. The purpose of a heparin drip in a client with deep vein thrombosis is to
   1. Prevent further clot formation in the leg
   2. Dissolve the clots in all affected veins
   3. Minimize general clot formation
   4. Decrease the risk of pulmonary embolism

8. A client is started on coumadin after being on a heparin for 3 days. What injectable agent should be available in case of a bleeding emergency the next day?
   1. Vitamin C
   2. Protamine sulfate
   3. Aquamephyton
   4. Vitamin B_{12}

9. An imperative assessment factor of highest priority in the postoperative client for thoracic aortic aneurysm repair is
   1. Urine output
   2. Bowel sounds
   3. Neurologic status
   4. Lower extremity pulses

10. When assessing a client with an intact abdominal aortic aneurysm, the nurse identifies that the lower extremities are cool to the touch but the pulses are palpable. This is a result of
   1. Poor venous return from the lower extremities
   2. Peripheral edema from the increased interstitial pressure
   3. Poor cardiac output in the lower extremities
   4. Loss of cardiac output in false channels of the aorta

ANSWERS, RATIONALES, AND TEST-TAKING TIPS

Rationale	Test-Taking Tips

1. Correct answer: 3

Central venous pressure monitoring tends give the best information about fluid volume changes in clients. If the CVP is low, less than 5 cm H_2O, the client has hypovolemia; if the CVP is over 12 cm H_2O, the client has hypervolemia. The initial CVP reading provides the baseline from which fluid therapy is initiated and changed as a specific condition changes. Option 1, BP trends, is not a *direct* indicator of volume changes in clients and, therefore, option 1 is not the best answer.

In option 2, HR comparisons are most important when clients are in the *initial* stage of shock or situations of volume changes. Arterial line comparisons, option 4, indicate changes in afterload or the resistance to function. Cluster these two and eliminate them as possible choices. Heart rate can be dependent on fluid balance—the HR increases with over- or underhydration. However, this is not the most effective method for fluid volume evaluation. A clue in the stem is "refractory hypovolemic" shock. This provides the focus of volume changes.

2. Correct answer: 2

The only criterion listed that shows improvement in tissue perfusion is increased urine output. This indicates an increase in renal function, which indirectly reflects more fluid and oxygen to the kidney. Option 1 is a correct answer but is not the best answer because it contains the word "change" without a given direction of the change in the LOC. Has it increased or decreased? If the question had stated an increased LOC, this would have been the best answer rather than urine output increased. Findings from changes in tissue oxygenation are manifested more quickly in the brain than in the kidney.

Think about it. For a determination in changes of urine output, it typically takes an hour. Changes in mental status occur over a time period of minutes rather than hours. Option 3 and option 4 have no direct relationship to tissue perfusion changes.

Rationale	Test-Taking Tips

3. Correct answer: 3

A modified Trendelenburg position is the upper body in a supine type position and the legs elevated above the level of the heart. This position increases blood flow to vital organs but does not induce cerebral congestion and edema. Use common sense. In shock, the brain needs arterial circulation and venous drainage, not arterial and venous congestion. A positive tilt is associated with a reverse Trendelenburg position (the opposite of Trendelenburg), which has the client with the head of the bed elevated and the legs in a downward position. In this position the brain has minimal blood flow and the legs get good arterial blood flow, with the risk of pooled blood in the veins. A Trendelenburg position, the head down and the legs elevated, results in the congestion of blood in the brain because the cerebral veins cannot drain. A Trendelenburg position is preferred with pregnant women in the event of a prolapsed cord and for clients before and during central venous catheter insertion into the subclavian or jugular vein.

The basic body position of Trendelenburg is supine. An easy way to remember modified Trendelenburg is to associate the "T" in Trendelenburg with the "T" in the tail of the body, or the legs. This position is used when clients are pale—raise their tail first—elevate the legs and do not lower the head. Common sense helps you to figure out that a modified Trendelenburg is different.

4. Correct answer: 2

The best response is to have the client contact the physician within the next day. The physician then decides when a

This question falls into the harder question category because each of the options could be the correct answer. A clue in each option is the

further workup is required. The BP is high enough to be considered a higher risk for the complications of stroke or heart attack. Recall that hypertensive crisis is a systolic over 200 mm Hg and a diastolic of over 110 mm Hg. Option 1, an immediate repeat BP is not the best action. The BP may be elevated from the anxiety of being informed of the first reading. So a recheck may not be therapeutic or accurate. Option 3 is a correct answer but not the best of the given options. Within 1 week's time this client may have further pathologic deterioration. Option 4 is not indicated because no other findings are given in the stem. If findings of dizziness, headache, or visual problems were given, then option 4 would be the best answer.

time. In option 1, an immediate recheck is inappropriate. Rechecks of BP are more accurate if done 5 to 10 minutes after the client sits quietly. Given the data of only a BP reading, the time in option 3 is too long and the time in option 4 too short. Option 1 is most appropriate in the given situation.

5. Correct answer: 4

Collateral circulation is feeding the lower extremities to a point of maintaining an adequate neurovascular status at this point. Collateral circulation is the development of a blood pathway through enlargement of secondary vessels after the obstruction of a main vessel. The client's walking, in option 1, may help support the physiologic changes in the circulation of the leg. However, it could be a secondary and not the primary reason for the findings. Even though option 2 sounds good, it is unreasonable for the client to wear special socks "all" the time. Option 3

The use of common sense will guide the correct selection. Daily walks improve all circulation, not just to the left leg. To have "warm" socks on "all" the time would be impossible. Note that when absolute words such as "all" are included in an option, it is usually not the correct answer.

is a false statement. Venous circulation will not assume the role of arterial circulation.

6. Correct answer: 4

Asking when the pain occurs opens up the conversation to discuss the pain and does not lead the client to answer questions in any certain direction. The questions in options 1, about the frequency, and option 2, about normal walking, could be subsumed under the question in option 4 of when the pain starts. To ask about when the pain stops, option 3, logically follows the question about when the pain starts.

This question falls into the harder question category because all of the options are correct answers. The clue of time in the question, "ask . . . initially," guides you to think logically. After you have read all of the options, put them into a sequence from a start to finish. Remember that this questioning sequence can be used for other conditions with pain.

7. Correct answer: 1

Heparin therapy is used in clients to prevent further clot formation. Anticoagulants do not dissolve clots. Thrombolytics, such a streptokinase, dissolve clots. Option 3, to minimize general clot formation, could be a correct answer for a different question such as the purpose of low-dose heparin therapy. However, this question is specific for deep vein thrombosis, that is, clot formation in the legs. Option 4 is a secondary benefit from heparin therapy in deep vein thrombosis. It is not the primary reason for the heparin drip. Other actions can decrease the risk of pulmonary embolism such as adequate fluid intake and the

Cluster options 2, 3 and 4 because of the words "decrease," "dissolve," "minimize," and eliminate these as possible answers. Recall that to dissolve clots the therapy is given in several doses of a medication rather than a drip in the acute phase within 24 hours.

minimization of movement of the affected extremity in the acute stage.

8. Correct answer: 2

Protamine sulfate is the antidote for heparin. Vitamin C helps in the healing process. Aquamephyton or Vitamin K is the antidote for increased levels of coumadin. Vitamin B$_{12}$ is required for many neurologic and hematologic functions.

This type of question with two different medications and a timeframe is a more difficult type of question. First you have to establish which drug the question is about—heparin. Because coumadin was just initiated, its effect is minimal at the timeframe that is in the question. Coumadin has a peak or therapeutic action within 48 to 72 hours after the daily doses are given. Thus, it is unlikely to be the cause of a bleeding emergency within 24 hours of the initial dose.

9. Correct answer: 3

Neurologic status is imperative after thoracic aortic aneurysm repair because cerebral arteries that feed the brain flow off of the thoracic aorta. After abdominal aneurysm repair the priority is urine output because the renal arteries flow from this part of the aorta. Assessing bowel sounds is a secondary factor after abdominal aneurysm repair. Monitoring heart sounds has no direct value after aneurysm repair.

If you have no clue as to the correct response, try a cluster approach. Cluster options 1, 2, and 4 under the category of specific assessments as compared with option 3, which is a more general or global response. Select the one that is different.

10. Correct answer: 4

Some of the blood flow is trapped in the false channels of the aortic aneurysm, causing a decrease in peripheral vascular pressures and status. More information would need to be given in the stem to support the selection of the other options.

Beware of question hangover. This situation is before surgery. The important term in the stem is "intact abdominal aneurysm." Recall that the aneurysm pathology may result in false channels that defer some of the blood. You may want to look at a picture in your Med-Surg Text to help you remember and differentiate between the types of aneurysms.

4

The Hematologic System

FAST FACTS

1. Sluggish blood flow accelerates clot formation by allowing clotting factors to reach levels high enough for the initiation of a clotting reaction.
2. Higher H&H levels and severe dehydration result in thicker blood and a sluggish flow, for example, in clients with chronic lung diseases.
3. Rough surfaces found in the lumen of blood vessels or in wounds activate platelet aggregation, with the result of clotting.
4. Blood proteins such as albumin, which are responsible for the colloid osmotic pressure, help hold plasma in the vascular space.
5. A decreased amount of serum albumin allows plasma to leak out of the vascular space into the interstitial spaces, with the result of generalized massive edema called *anasarca*.
6. Plasma protein levels effect some drug actions and levels of toxicity, such as digoxin.

CONTENT REVIEW

I. **The hematologic system is responsible for the following**
   A. Transporting oxygen
   B. Transporting nutrients to the cells of the body
   C. Transporting waste to the kidneys, skin, and lungs
   D. Transporting hormones to the tissues of the body
   E. Protecting the body from life-threatening microorganisms
   F. Facilitating heat transfer from the body

II. **Structure and function**
A. Blood volume is 55% plasma and 45% cells
B. Blood is composed of three types of cells—erythrocytes (RBCs), platelets, and WBCs
C. Plasma is a pale-yellow liquid composed of water, blood proteins, and other dissolved solutes
D. The part of the blood volume that is made up of cells is called the *hematocrit* and is largely composed of RBCs. The hematocrit is expressed as a percentage.
E. RBCs house hemoglobin, necessary for carrying oxygen
F. Platelets become sticky when they come into contact with a foreign substance or a damaged blood vessel
G. WBCs are responsible for fighting disease in the body; there are several divisions of WBCs
   1. Granulocytes—granules in cytoplasm
     a. Neutrophils
     b. Basophils
     c. Eosinophils
   2. Agranulocytes—no granules in cytoplasm
     a. Lymphocytes
     b. Monocytes

III. **Targeted concerns**
A. Pharmacology—priority drug classifications
   1. Hemostatic agents—inhibit plasminogen activator and have antifibrinolytic action
     a. Expected effect—control excessive bleeding
     b. Commonly given drugs
       (1) Aminocaproic acid (Amicar)
       (2) Thrombin (Thrombinar)
     c. Nursing considerations
       (1) Urine will turn reddish brown
       (2) Postural hypotension may occur
   2. Antihemophilic agents—synthetic factor VIII
     a. Expected effect—treatment of hemophilia A to enhance the clotting process
     b. Commonly given drugs
       (1) Human antihemophilic factor (synthetic factor VIII)
       (2) Factor IX complex (Konyne 80)—increases blood levels of clotting factors II, VII, IX, and X
     c. Nursing considerations
       (1) Infuse at manufacturer's prescribed rate
       (2) Monitor for decreased HR, increased BP, and RR, which may indicate an allergic reaction
   3. Vitamins—essential for normal cell reproduction
     a. Expected effect—maturation of RBCs

   b. Commonly given drugs
      (1) Cyanocobalamin (vitamin B_{12})
      (2) Folic acid (vitamin B_9, folvite)
   c. Nursing considerations
      (1) Give with food
      (2) Educate client about the risks of vitamin overdose. A potential overdose is more of a problem with fat-soluble vitamins because they accumulate in the tissues; excess water-soluble vitamins are normally excreted through the kidney.
4. Plasma and volume expanders—increase the colloidal osmotic pressure
   a. Expected effect—expands volume to maintain **cardiac output**
   b. Commonly given drugs
      (1) Human albumin (salt poor albumin which is low in sodium content)
      (2) Dextran 40 (Rheomacrodex)
      (3) Hetastarch (Hespan)
      (4) Plasma protein factor (Plasmanate)
   c. Nursing considerations
      (1) Monitor for signs of hypervolemia
      (2) Monitor vital signs for increases during administration
5. Colony-stimulating factors (CSFs) and colony-stimulating modifiers—stimulate production of several types of hematopoietic precursor cells
   a. Expected effects—increase RBC production; stimulate neutrophil production
   b. Commonly given drugs
      (1) Epoetin alfa (Epogen)—for increase in RBCs
      (2) Recombinant human granulocyte colony-stimulating factor, filgrastim (Neupogen)—for increase in neutrophils
   c. Nursing considerations
      (1) Monitor BP every 2 to 4 hours, and monitor labs daily
      (2) Do not shake vial because doing so may cause deactivation of drug
B. Procedures
   1. CBC and differential—provide information about cells in the hematologic system
   2. Hemoglobin electrophoresis—identifies abnormal hemoglobin
   3. Erythrocyte sedimentation rate (ESR)—elevated level indicates inflammatory, neoplastic, or necrotic processes, or a combination of any of these
   4. Peripheral blood smear—all three types of blood cells can be identified
   5. Reticulocyte count—evaluates bone marrow function
   6. Iron level and total iron-binding capacity—detect abnormal level of iron and iron-binding capacity

7. **Serum** ferritin level—identifies iron-deficiency anemia
8. Platelet count—actual count of platelets
9. Bone marrow examination—evaluates hematopoiesis
10. Lymphangiography—x-ray examination of the lymph system using radioactive dye to determine that the lymphatic system is not obstructed
11. Lymph node biopsy—identifies metastatic involvement

C. **Psychosocial concerns**
1. Anxiety—an uncomfortable feeling associated with an unknown cause; common in clients treated for a malignancy
2. Fear—an uncomfortable feeling associated with a known cause; also common in clients diagnosed with a malignancy. The fear is most often the fear of death.
3. Denial—may be seen in clients with a malignancy as a stage of grieving
4. Lifestyle—baseline of activities to evaluate need for change
5. Activities of daily living (ADL)—ability to perform

D. **Health history—question sequence**
1. Which problems would you like to discuss with the physician?
2. Which symptoms have you been experiencing?
3. Are you presently being treated for any illnesses?
4. Have you been treated for other illnesses in the past?
5. Have you had any surgical procedures?
6. Have you ever received a blood transfusion? For what reason?
7. Did you have an adverse reaction to your blood transfusion? If so, what was the reaction?
8. Which prescription and over-the-counter medications are you currently taking?
9. Do you have any allergies?
10. Is there a family history of any blood disorders?
11. What is your occupation?
12. Are you following any special diet?
13. Do you use alcohol?
14. Have you lost any weight lately?

E. **Physical examination—appropriate sequence**
1. ABCs—vital signs
2. Inspect skin, hair, and nails
3. Inspect and palpate lymph nodes—head-to-toe approach (Figure 4-1)
4. Inspect, palpate, and auscultate the cardiovascular system
5. Inspect, palpate, percuss, and auscultate the respiratory system
6. Assess neuromuscular function
7. Assess sensory function
8. Evaluate pain history
9. Inspect, auscultate, percuss, and palpate the abdomen
10. Inspect and palpate the genital system

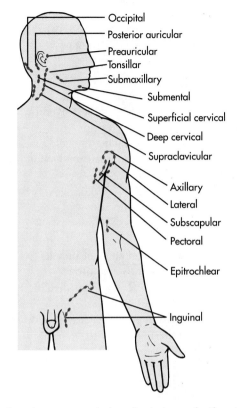

Figure 4-1 Lymph nodes to assess during physical examination. (From Lewis SM, Heitkemper MM, Dirksen SR: *Medical-surgical nursing: assessment and management of clinical problems,* ed 5, St. Louis, 2000, Mosby.)

IV. Pathophysiologic disorders
A. Anemia
1. Definition—decrease in RBC count, function or structure, with a subsequent decrease in oxygen-carrying capability of the blood
   a. Types
      (1) Pernicious anemia—vitamin B_{12} deficiency from a lack of intrinsic factor in the stomach
      (2) Folic acid deficiency anemia—a lack of folic acid intake or absorption
      (3) Aplastic anemia—low RBCs caused by bone marrow abnormality
      (4) Iron-deficiency anemia—low hemoglobin in RBCs
      (5) Hemolytic anemia—caused by breakup of RBCs
      (6) Blood loss anemia—loss of RBCs
      (7) Sickle-cell anemia—abnormal hemoglobin; causes RBC to assume a sickle shape

2. Pathophysiology
   a. Bone marrow is producing an insufficient number of RBCs
   b. RBCs are not synthesized effectively as a result of a lack of essential factor
   c. Folic acid is lacking in diet or absorption is blocked, such as in clients with alcoholism
   d. Too many RBCs are being destroyed owing to hereditary factors or to an acquired disorder
   e. RBCs are being lost owing to acute or chronic bleeding
3. Etiology—blood loss, abnormal production of RBCs, or increased destruction of RBCs
4. Incidence—more common in older adult clients; also common in clients with poor nutrition
5. Assessment
   a. Questions to ask
      (1) Do you ever feel short of breath?
      (2) Do you frequently feel tired?
      (3) Do you ever feel your heart beating too fast?
      (4) Does the cold bother you?
      (5) Do you suffer from headaches or dizziness?
   b. Clinical manifestations
      (1) Moderate anemia
         (a) SOB
         (b) Fatigue
         (c) Palpitations
      (2) Severe anemia
         (a) Paleness
         (b) Feeling of exhaustion
         (c) Sensitivity to cold
         (d) Dizziness, headaches
   c. Abnormal laboratory findings
      (1) RBC count decreased
      (2) Hemoglobin decreased
      (3) Hematocrit decreased
   d. Abnormal diagnostic test results—bone marrow aspirate; identifies specific type of anemia
6. Expected medical interventions
   a. Identify cause
   b. Treat cause, if possible
   c. Give iron preparations, and explain diet management
   d. Administer folic acid and B_{12}
   e. Administer blood transfusions or fluid resuscitation
   f. Give oxygen therapy for severe anemia
7. Nursing diagnoses
   a. Decreased CO related to a decrease in circulating blood volume

    b. Activity intolerance related to reduced oxygen-carrying capacity of the blood

    c. Self-care deficit: reduced ability for bathing and hygiene related to fatigue secondary to decreased oxygenation

8. Client goals

    a. CO will be appropriate as evidenced by BP within 10% of baseline

    b. Client will increase tolerance to activity as evidenced by ADL for 15 minutes without SOB

    c. Client will bathe upper body without SOB

9. Nursing interventions

    a. Acute care

        (1) Transfusion therapy

            (a) Proper identification of blood product and recipient must be completed by two licensed nurses. FIRST! Most states require that a registered nurse spike the blood bag and start the flow.

            (b) Vital signs must be taken before administration, paying special attention to the temperature; report any elevation to physician

            (c) Blood infusion must have its own IV site, with at least a 20-gauge needle

            (d) Client must be monitored carefully during administration for transfusion reactions; the first 15 minutes is the most critical, and the nurse must be present in the room

                (i) Anaphalytic reaction: wheezing, tachycardia, tachypnea, hypotension, and cardiorespiratory arrest

                (ii) Allergic reaction: hives, itching, chills, and fever (febrile reaction)

                (iii) Hemolytic reaction: low back pain, chills, and chest pain

            (e) Blood transfusion must be stopped immediately in the event of a reaction. Hang new tubing and fluid, usually normal saline; inform physician; return blood bag and tubing to blood bank; and obtain urine sample and send to laboratory. Note if only a febrile reaction, defined as an increase of 1 degree in temperature, physician may order an antipyretic and an antihistamine such as Benadryl and continue the transfusion.

    b. Home care regarding client education

        (1) How to balance rest and activity effectively—prioritize activities

        (2) What foods to eat to increase RBC production—foods high in iron, folic acid, and vitamin B_{12}

10. Evaluation protocol
    a. How do I know that my interventions were effective?
       (1) Transfusion therapy completed without reaction
       (2) Transfusion reaction managed quickly and effectively
    b. What criteria will I use to change my interventions?
       (1) Transfusion reaction noted
       (2) Transfusion reaction managed in a less than timely manner
    c. How will I know that my client teaching has been effective?
       (1) Client demonstrates methods to balance rest and activity
       (2) Client produces a food diary indicating food choices that are appropriate to increase RBC production
11. Older adult alert
    a. Older adult clients are very prone to vitamin B_{12} deficiency anemia from either a lack of vitamin B_{12} intake or an intrinsic factor. The nurse must assess clients for this anemia. It is best to be alert for clients with poor nutritional intake, a history of gastric ulcers, or gastric resection. Monitor the H&H of older adult clients.

B. Acute leukemia

1. Definition—an overgrowth of immature white blood cells of the bone marrow
   a. Acute myelogenous leukemia (AML)—overgrowth of the primitive cells from the myeloid stem cell line
   b. Acute lymphocytic leukemia (ALL)—proliferation of primitive lymphocytes
2. Pathophysiology
   a. AML—malignant cell is an immature myeloblast; the cell generates and infringes on other normal components of the bone marrow
   b. ALL—malignant cell is an immature lymphoblast; as in AML, the malignant cell infringes on the other normal components of the bone marrow
3. Etiology
   a. AML
      (1) Genetic abnormalities
      (2) Ionizing radiation
      (3) Viruses
      (4) Immunosuppressive agents
      (5) Chloramphenicol
      (6) Chemotherapeutic agents
   b. ALL
      (1) Radiation exposure
      (2) Genetic abnormalities
4. Incidence
   a. AML—adults over the age of 60; over 6000 new cases a year
   b. ALL—a childhood illness; approximately 20% of adult cases; over 5000 new cases a year

5. Assessment
    a. Questions to ask
        (1) Do you suffer from frequent infections?
        (2) Do you feel fatigued much of the time?
        (3) Do you bruise easily or bleed at unusual times?
        (4) Do you ever feel a deep pain in your bones?
    b. Clinical manifestations
        (1) Frequent or recurring infections
        (2) Fatigue and lassitude
        (3) Bruising and unusual bleeding (from low platelet counts)
        (4) Pale complexion
        (5) Enlarged lymph nodes
        (6) Enlarged spleen
        (7) Bone pain
        (8) AML may be preceded by an anemia
        (9) ALL has a rapid onset
    c. Abnormal laboratory findings
        (1) ALL—WBC over 10,000; increased lymphocytes
        (2) AML—WBC with myeloblasts present
    d. Abnormal diagnostic test results
        (1) Bone marrow aspiration
            (a) ALL— over 50% lymphoblasts
            (b) AML— over 50% myeloblasts
6. Expected medical interventions
    a. Chemotherapy to eliminate the malignant cell
    b. Bone marrow transplantation
7. Nursing diagnoses
    a. Pain related to increased production of leukemia cells in bone marrow
    b. Risk for infection related to ineffective, immature WBCs
8. Client goals
    a. Client will state that pain is decreased or relieved
    b. Client will be free of infective processes
9. Nursing interventions
    a. Acute care
        (1) Use of private room to prevent exposure to infection
        (2) Strict universal precautions; reverse isolation may be needed
        (3) Immediate evaluation of client for infection if a fever becomes apparent, a temperature over 99° F; blood cultures
    b. Home care regarding client education
        (1) Proper hand washing
        (2) Soft toothbrush with nonabrasive toothpaste
        (3) Use stool softeners for constipation and antidiarrheal agents for diarrhea to prevent skin breaks

(4) Maintenance of a minimal intake of 2000 to 3000 ml/day to prevent urinary stasis

10. Evaluation protocol
   a. How do I know that my interventions were effective?
      (1) Client does not have a fever
      (2) No other assessment findings are indicative of infection
   b. Which criteria will I use to change my interventions?
      (1) Elevated temperature
      (2) Positive cultures
   c. How will I know that my client teaching has been effective?
      (1) Client is using a soft toothbrush and has no bleeding from or infection in gums
      (2) Client states taking in more than 2000 ml/day in fluid with no findings of urinary infection

11. Older adult alert
   a. Bone pain may be confused with the pain of arthritis. A complete assessment of the pain reported by older persons needs to be performed.

C. Chronic leukemia

1. Definition—abnormal proliferation of *mature* WBCs
   a. Chronic myelogenous leukemia (CML)—increased production of the mature WBCs of the myeloid cell line
   b. Chronic lymphocytic leukemia (CLL)—increased production of poorly functioning mature lymphocytes

2. Pathophysiology
   a. CML—associated with a chromosome aberration, known as the Philadelphia chromosome; a translocation of the genetic material of chromosomes 9 and 22
   b. CLL—increased production of mature lymphocytes causing an impingement of other cells in the bone marrow

3. Etiology—most common is exposure to ionizing radiation and chemicals

4. Incidence—20% of all leukemias; more common in males over age 50

5. Assessment
   a. Questions to ask
      (1) Have you been losing weight?
      (2) Have you been feeling fatigued?
      (3) Do you have pain in your bones?
   b. Clinical manifestations
      (1) May be asymptomatic or symptoms may be vague
      (2) Fatigue
      (3) Weight loss
      (4) Bone pain
      (5) Splenomegaly
      (6) Lymphadenopathy

(7) Easy bruising

(8) Skin rashes or lesions

c. Abnormal laboratory findings

(1) CLL—in serum: increased mature WBCs, decreased platelets, and decreased RBCs

(2) CML—in serum: mature WBCs over 50,000

d. Abnormal diagnostic test results

(1) CLL—bone marrow in accelerated phase; large quantities of immature WBCs

(2) CML—bone marrow; large quantities of immature WBCs

6. Expected medical intervention

a. Chemotherapy—oral and IV

b. Bone marrow transplantation

7. Nursing diagnoses, client goals, nursing interventions, evaluations, and older adult alert—identical to the client with acute leukemia (p. 126)

D. Lymphoma

1. Definition—group of malignancies originating from the stem cell in the bone marrow; malignancy occurs in the lymphoreticular system

a. Two types

(1) Hodgkin's disease

(2) Non-Hodgkin's lymphoma

2. Pathophysiology

a. Hodgkin's disease—malignant cell origin has not been confirmed but theory suggests a B or T lymphocyte

b. Non-Hodgkin's lymphoma—the malignant cell is the lymphocyte at any stage of its development; this cell reproduces and then invades the bone marrow

3. Etiology

a. Hodgkin's disease—unknown; possible viral, genetic, or environmental factors have been investigated

b. Non-Hodgkin's lymphoma—high risk in clients with autoimmune illnesses and viruses such as Epstein-Barr

4. Incidence

a. Hodgkin's disease—over 7000 new cases a year. There is a greater incidence in the male population than in the female. The third and sixth decades are the two peak periods of incidence.

b. Non-Hodgkin's lymphoma—over 35,000 new cases per year. It is more common in males and after the age of 60

5. Assessment

a. Questions to ask

(1) Do you ever wake up at night soaked in sweat?

(2) Have you been losing weight?

(3) Have you noticed that you have been running fevers?

    b. Clinical manifestations—the two lymphomas are similar in manifestations
      (1) Night sweats
      (2) Fevers
      (3) Weight loss
      (4) Enlarged, painless lymph nodes
    c. Abnormal laboratory findings
      (1) CBC—mild anemia, increased WBC, decreased lymphocytes, increased ESR
      (2) Chemistries—increased alkaline phosphatase, increased gamma globulins
    d. Abnormal diagnostic test results
      (1) Lymph node biopsy—malignant
      (2) Lymphangiography—abnormal lymph nodes and possibly lymph vessel impairment
      (3) Bone marrow biopsy—abnormal cells
      (4) Staging laparotomy—lymph node site involvement
6. Expected medical interventions
    a. Staging laparotomy with splenectomy—splenectomy improves the effects of chemotherapy
    b. Chemotherapy
    c. External beam radiation therapy
7. Nursing diagnoses
    a. Pain related to the progression of the disorder to the bones
    b. Risk for infection related to an impaired immune system
    c. Altered nutrition—less than body requirements related to increased metabolic demands of the malignant disorder
8. Client goals
    a. Client will state that pain is improved or has been relieved
    b. Client will show no evidence of infection, that is, fever
    c. Client will lose no more weight but, rather, will increase weight by 0.5 kg per 2-week period
9. Nursing interventions
    a. Acute care
      (1) After the staging laparotomy clients must be cared for with all the routine nursing interventions discussed in Chapter 9, p. 311
      (2) After the staging laparotomy the client is at high risk for infection. Thus, nursing interventions must be aimed at rigorous prevention of postoperative infection.
    b. Home care regarding client education
      (1) Infection prevention actions
      (2) How to prepare medications if client is self-administering chemotherapy at home; techniques for preparation and administration must be discussed

(3) How to cope with the side effects of chemotherapy and radiation therapy
  (a) How to maintain hydration
  (b) How to administer antiemetics as needed
  (c) How to care for the skin during external radiation therapy
    (i) Not to wash area with soap
    (ii) Not to remove skin markings
    (iii) Not to apply creams or ointments to the skin unless specifically directed
  (d) How to recognize infection in the early stages
  (e) How to respond to hemorrhage if it occurs
10. Evaluation protocol
  a. How do I know that my interventions were effective?
    (1) Infection has been prevented
    (2) Infection has been identified early and treated effectively
  b. What criteria will I use to change my interventions?
    (1) Elevated temperature that is not responding to treatment; a temperature over 99° F is of concern in clients with immunosuppression
    (2) Overall status of client is deteriorating
  c. How will I know that my client teaching has been effective?
    (1) Client demonstrates ability to mix and administer chemotherapeutic drugs
    (2) Client can treat side effects of chemotherapy and external radiation therapy effectively
    (3) Client identifies appropriate skin care during radiation therapy
    (4) Client identifies assessment factors associated with infection to report to physician
    (5) Client identifies appropriate actions to treat hemorrhage occurring at home
11. Older adult alert
  a. Older adult clients have a greater risk for infection owing to the normal decrease in the immune response with age
  b. Evaluate older adult clients carefully for bone pain mistaken for arthritis

E. Multiple myeloma
  1. Definition—neoplasm of plasma cells
  2. Pathophysiology—plasma cells have transformed to a malignant form. An immunoglobulin M-protein is formed by the malignant plasma cells. M-protein is reproduced and prevents appropriate antibody production.
  3. Etiology—unknown; possibly viral or an inappropriate response to antigenic stimulation

4. Incidence—more than 10,000 new cases per year. This cancer is more common in the black population and is most common after the age of 60.
5. Assessment
   a. Questions to ask
      (1) Do you ever have pain deep in your bones?
      (2) Do you ever feel tired?
      (3) Do you have frequent infections?
   b. Clinical manifestations
      (1) Bone pain that increases with movement
      (2) Bone demineralization leading to hypercalcemia
      (3) Anemia
      (4) Renal insufficiency leading to renal failure
   c. Abnormal laboratory findings
      (1) Serum calcium elevated
      (2) Urinalysis—increased calcium
      (3) Serum electrophoresis—increased globulin
      (4) Serum creatinine elevated
   d. Abnormal diagnostic test results
      (1) Bone marrow aspiration—increased *immature* plasma cells
      (2) Skeletal x-ray films—demineralization of bone
6. Expected medical interventions
   a. Chemotherapy
   b. Radiation therapy—adjuvant therapy
   c. Bone marrow transplantation
7. Nursing diagnoses
   a. Pain related to bone demineralization and pathologic fractures
   b. Impaired physical mobility related to bone pain and pathologic fractures
   c. Altered nutrition—less than body requirements related to anorexia
8. Client goals
   a. Client will state that pain is relieved or decreased on a scale from 0 to 10
   b. Client will demonstrate ability to perform **range-of-motion** exercises at least twice a day to prevent muscle atrophy
   c. Client will maintain present weight, no further weight loss, or increase weight by 0.5 kg per 2-week period if indicated
9. Nursing interventions
   a. Position client for comfort—prevent pathologic fractures
   b. Encourage use of assistive devices
   c. Balance rest and activity
   d. Hydrate with over 3000 ml/day to treat hypercalcemia for the prevention of renal calculi

     e. Encourage high protein diet with appropriate vitamin intake, but not vitamins A and D—these facilitate absorption of calcium from the GI tract

     f. Utilize nursing measures outlined for clients with lymphoma

10. Evaluation protocol

     a. How will I know that my interventions were effective?

        (1) Client states comfort

        (2) Client exhibits no new pathologic fractures

        (3) Client has an appropriate diet—high protein and lacking in vitamins A and D

        (4) Client maintains urine output of at least 30 ml/hr

     b. What criteria will I use to change my interventions?

        (1) Client has unrelieved pain

        (2) Client has new pathologic fractures

        (3) Client cannot tolerate diet

        (4) Client's renal function is depressed; complaints of flank pain or other pain related to presence of kidney stones

     c. How will I know that my client teaching has been effective?

        (1) Client demonstrates appropriate fluid and food intake

        (2) Refer to evaluation protocol for lymphoma, p. 131

11. Older adult alert—same as for clients with lymphoma

WEB Resource

http://www.leukemia.org/index.html
Leukemia Society of America

REVIEW QUESTIONS

1. The client who is known to abuse alcohol will also suffer from a low folic acid level caused by
    1. Poor nutritional intake with minimal water intake
    2. Poor dentition with inadequate mastication of foods
    3. Absorption of folic acid being blocked by alcohol intake
    4. Increased motility in the bowel diminishing absorption time

2. Assessment findings commonly reported by the client with anemia are
    1. Fatigue, SOB with increased activity, and palpitations
    2. Tiredness, diarrhea, and muscle weakness
    3. Bone pain, SOB at rest, and early morning headaches
    4. Abdominal pain, SOB on exertion, and late evening headaches

3. Before initiating a blood transfusion the nurse must pay special attention to the baseline assessment of
    1. BP
    2. HR
    3. Temperature
    4. RR

4. A final nursing intervention in the face of a hemolytic blood transfusion reaction after the transfusion has been interrupted and replaced with an isotonic fluid must be
    1. Call the physician
    2. Administer IV antihistamine
    3. Increase IV normal saline fluid rate from a keep-the-vein-open (KVO) rate
    4. Obtain a urine sample

5. An initial manifestation of acute leukemia that would result in a client seeking health care is
    1. Fatigue
    2. Unusual bleeding
    3. Bruises from bumping into things
    4. Aching muscles and joints

6. A client with leukemia and a WBC count of over 30,000 mm^3 may be placed in a private room to
    1. Isolate other clients from this client's infection
    2. Prevent overfatigue from interaction with a roommate
    3. Facilitate the sleep of this client
    4. Minimize exposure of this client to common viruses and bacteria

7. The client receiving external radiation therapy must be taught how to care for the skin in the area of the therapy to prevent skin breakdown. Teaching must include
  1. The need to cleanse the skin thoroughly with non-antibacterial soap after treatments to prevent skin irritation and sloughing
  2. The application of baby oil to the area to prevent the drying effects of the therapy
  3. A caution for the client not to remove skin markings placed by the physician because they ensure consistent areas of therapy
  4. A suggestion that the client expose the radiated area to the air and the sun for at least two 10-minute periods per day

8. An assessment finding most often associated with Hodgkin's disease is
  1. Enlarged painful lymph nodes
  2. High fevers with severe dehydration
  3. Weight loss from frequent diarrhea
  4. Night sweats regardless of age

9. An important initial laboratory study in clients with multiple myeloma to support this diagnosis is
  1. Urinalysis with ESR
  2. CBC with differential
  3. Serum calcium level
  4. ABGs

10. A likely complication associated with multiple myeloma is
  1. Weight loss
  2. Urinary tract infection
  3. Pneumonia
  4. Pathologic fractures

ANSWERS, RATIONALES, AND TEST-TAKING TIPS

Rationales	Test-Taking Tips

1. Correct answer: 3

Alcohol prevents folic acid absorption. In option 1, the first part could be a correct answer. However, the second part of the option makes it incorrect. Option 2 may be a frequent finding in clients with alcohol abuse but is not directly associated with low folic acid levels. Option 4 is a true statement. Nevertheless, it has nothing to do with this situation in the question.

Because each of these options has two parts, avoid the tendency to carefully read the initial part of an option and then gloss over the second part. One technique is first to narrow the options to two. Then reread each option by reading the second part first and the first part second. Last, read the question one last time along with the option you have selected.

2. Correct answer: 1

A client who is anemic will typically have complaints of fatigue, SOB, and palpitations: "feeling that my heart is racing." In option 2, muscle weakness may be reported with low levels of potassium or phosphate, or high levels of calcium. In option 3, bone pain is typical in bone cancer. SOB at rest may occur in CHF or respiratory failure. The other findings listed have multiple causes.

Use a vertical technique to read and eliminate. Read down: Option 1, fatigue—yes; option 2, tiredness—yes; option 3 bone pain—no; and option 4, abdominal pain—no. Thus, with minimal reading time and effort, you can narrow the options to two, options 1 or 2. The next step is to compare the second item in each option: SOB with increased activity—yes, and option 2—diarrhea, usually is not found with anemia. The last step is to read the final item in the two options: palpitations are associated with anemia and muscle weakness—no. Select option 1.

3. Correct answer: 3

It is extremely important to obtain a baseline temperature before starting a blood transfusion because a fever is the more common initial finding of a reaction. The other assessments are important during blood

Note the key term in the stem, "special attention." A common sense approach is to identify that the HR, BP, and RR can vary to a greater degree and still be within normal range. However, temperature variation is more limited to minimal

administration in this order: RR, then the HR, and last the BP. In the event of an anaphylactic reaction to blood, clients will begin to wheeze with increased RR and respiratory effort. An increased HR during blood administration might indicate that the cardiac muscle is being stressed and the heart is in the initial stages of cardiac failure.

changes up or down and needs special attention.

4. Correct answer: 4

A final action is to have the urine checked for blood to see if the glomerular filtration system has been impacted by the reaction. Option 2, increasing the KVO rate, would be done after the blood was stopped and disconnected. Then the physician would be notified. An order for an antihistamine is most likely to be IV or PO, depending on the severity of the reaction. Epinephrine IV or Benadryl PO are commonly given for allergic reactions.

If you missed this question it was probably from a misreading of the question. Did you miss the key words: "final" and "intervention"? When a question provides a timeframe, it is essential to consider it as you read and select the best option.

5. Correct answer: 2

Bruising or unusual bleeding is the more common manifestation of acute leukemia and may be the finding that stimulates the client to seek a physician's evaluation. All of the other options may occur with acute leukemia. However, they are not commonly an initial problem that prompts the client to seek medical attention.

The key word "unusual" in option 2 hints that this is the correct option. The other options could be more common complaints of normal life or the results of sports activities or other physical exercises.

6. Correct answer: 4

Clients with leukemia are expected to have a high WBC

You may have narrowed the options to 1 and 4 based on the fact that an

Rationales	Test-Taking Tips

count. Yet, there is an inability to fight infection because the leukocytes are mainly immature forms. Thus, these clients must be protected from common infections and organisms. Clients with leukemia are not contagious to other persons. Option 2 introduces new information about interactions with an unknown type of roommate. Option 3 would be a good reason for a private room if the situation in the stem were about two clients, one of whom is hyperactive or manic.

increased WBC means infection. Yet you recall that the client with leukemia needs protection from others who may have an infection such as a cold. Go with what you know. That is, the safety of the client is a priority in this question because the question is about an individual and not about protection for a group or the general public. Select option 4 that has the focus on the individual client.

7. Correct answer: 3

The client should be warned not to remove skin markings so that therapy can be in a consistent area. They must not use any type of skin treatments unless instructed to do so by the physician. Soap will dry the skin. Baby oils may interfere with the actual radiation dose to increase or decrease the dosage. Exposure to the air is not harmful. However, exposure to the sun may cause detrimental effects on the skin in any area.

Because each of these options has two parts, avoid the tendency to carefully read the initial part of an option and then gloss over the second part. One technique is first to narrow the options to two. Then reread each option by reading the second part first and the first part second. Last, read the question one last time along with the option you have selected. If you have no idea of the correct answer, cluster options 1, 2, and 4 under the theme of "do something to the skin" and eliminate these. You could also eliminate option 4 because it is not a reasonable action. What would the client do if the sun were not out?

8. Correct answer: 4

Other pathologies that result in night sweats are acquired immune deficiency syndrome, or AIDS; tuberculosis; Non-Hodgkin's lymphoma;

Because each of these options has two parts, avoid the tendency to carefully read the initial part of an option and then gloss over the second part. One technique is first

menopause; and hypoglycemia. Read carefully. In Hodgkin's disease and Non-Hodgkin's lymphoma the lymph nodes are enlarged and painless. Option 1 states the nodes are painful. Other findings are a low-grade fever and weight loss. GI problems such as constipation and diarrhea are not common with this diagnosis.

to narrow the options to two. Then reread each option by reading the second part first and the first part second. Last, read the question one last time along with the option you have selected. Most test takers narrow these options to 1 and 4. Eliminate option 2 with the extremes of "high fever" and "severe dehydration." Recognize that option 3 is associated with the GI system, which is not a problem in immune system malfunctions such as Hodgkin's disease. If you read option 1 too quickly, you most likely missed the key word "painful." This option is like a two-part option, which you may want to read in reverse—painful and enlarged lymph nodes. Associate that acute infections result in painful lymph node enlargement. Remember the last time you had strep throat and your neck lymph nodes were enlarged and tender? Eliminate option 1, and select option 4.

9. Correct answer: 3

Clients with multiple myeloma, a neoplasm of the plasma cells, have hypercalcemia resulting from bone demineralization. Eliminate options 1 and 4 because the systems reflected are inappropriate to the given disease—the kidney and the lung. Option 2 is a more general laboratory test done to detect or confirm anemia, which is a lack of RBCs; polycythemia vera, which is an overabundance of RBCs; or viral and bacterial infections.

Because each of these options has two parts, avoid the tendency to carefully read the initial part of an option and then gloss over the second part. One technique is first to narrow the options to two. Then reread each option by reading the second part first and the first part second. Last, read the question one last time along with the option you have selected. Associate that potassium is imbalanced in most situations, except in multiple myeloma it is calcium. Recall tip—myeloma and calcium both have seven letters, so remember they have a relationship.

10. Correct answer: 4

It is common for clients with multiple myeloma to have pathologic fractures, which result from bone demineralization. Weight loss may occur but is not most likely to be considered a complication of the disease process. Options 2 and 3 are too narrow for a disease process that is extensive as is "multiple" myeloma.

Because each of these options has two parts, avoid the tendency to carefully read the initial part of an option and then gloss over the second part. One technique is first to narrow the options to two. Then reread each option by reading the second part first and the first part second. Last, read the question one last time along with the option you have selected. If you have no idea of the correct answer, use your common sense. This type of disease process is in multiple areas. Thus, eliminate options 2 and 3, which are in specific organ systems. Next, think about what you know of the two remaining options. Weight loss is commonly a diagnostic finding in a disease process. Pathologic fractures are more complex, spontaneous, and aligned to be considered a complication. Select option 4.

5

The Respiratory System

FAST FACTS

1. Dyspnea is the most common *subjective* assessment of patients who have a respiratory disorder.
2. Indication of whether dyspnea occurs at rest or with activity, which is called *exertional dyspnea,* is essential.
3. Accessory muscle use is the most common *objective* assessment in patients with dyspnea.
4. Respiratory arrest may be imminent when fatigue is evident and the abdominal, shoulder, and neck muscles are being used to breathe. Often patient goes into a tripod position, leans forward to rest on elbows.
5. Chest pain is not unusual in patients with respiratory difficulty and must be differentiated from cardiac chest pain. Identify whether the pain intensifies with the respiratory movement of inspiration or exhalation, or on external pressure exerted on the chest wall.
6. Cyanosis is very late evidence of hypoxemia.
7. Cyanosis rarely occurs in patients with anemia who turn dusky, grayish, or pallid rather than blue.
8. *Hypoxemia* is decreased oxygen driving pressure or tension in the *arterial blood.* Remember that "emia" means in the blood, for example, septicemia, anemia, and hyperkalemia.
9. *Hypoxia* is decreased oxygen driving pressure or tension at the *cellular level.* This leads to cellular deprivation of oxygen, resulting in a change to anaerobic metabolism with the production of lactic acid.
10. Hypoxemia leads to hypoxia if left untreated.
11. A respiratory rate over 24 breaths per minute results in severe fluid loss from the respiratory tract. For example, with a RR of 24 breaths per minute for a 24-hour period, 4 to 6 liters of fluid may be lost from the respiratory tract.

CONTENT REVIEW

I. **The respiratory system is responsible for the exchange of oxygen and carbon dioxide in the body, which takes place primarily in the alveoli of the lungs**

II. **Structure and function**
   A. Upper airways (nasal passages, pharynx, larynx)—warm, humidify, and filter inhaled air; also transport air to lower airways
   B. Lungs—two cone-shaped organs in the thoracic cavity on each side of the heart. The left lung has two lobes and 10 smaller partitions known as segments, and the right lung has three lobes and 10 segments.
   C. Lower airways (trachea, right and left mainstem bronchus, segmental bronchi, terminal bronchioles)—transport air to the alveoli
   D. Alveoli—found in the lung parenchyma. Gas exchange of oxygen and carbon dioxide occurs between the alveoli and pulmonary capillaries across the alveolar capillary membrane. Millions of alveoli exist in each lung.
   E. Alveoli walls contain type II pneumocytes that secrete surfactant which is responsible for decreasing surface tension of alveoli and maintaining alveolar patency

III. **Targeted concerns**
   A. Pharmacology—priority drug classifications
      1. Bronchodilators—relax bronchial tree and increase lumen size
         a. Expected effects—decrease RR and respiratory effort
         b. Commonly given drugs
            (1) Theophylline (Theo-Dur), oral (PO)
            (2) Albuterol (Ventolin), PO, inhalation
            (3) Aminophylline, IV
         c. Nursing considerations
            (1) Expected side effects—sinus tachycardia, palpitations, feelings of nervousness, and dizziness
            (2) Elevated HR—report and evaluate a HR of over 120 beats per minute
            (3) Toxic effects—nausea is the first sign of toxicity; also tremors and theophylline levels of over 20 μg/ml
            (4) Gastric distress—give with food or milk for prevention
      2. Mucolytic agents—cause a breakdown of secretions
         a. Expected effects—make expectoration of sputum easier for client; thin secretions
         b. Commonly given drugs
            (1) Acetylcysteine (Mucomyst)—given by aerosol
            (2) Water or appropriate hydration is best to thin secretions

c. Nursing considerations
   (1) Mucomyst is best administered as a nebulizer treatment for a respiratory effect. (Mucomyst also is given orally as an antidote for acetaminophen overdose. Multiple doses are given over a 3- to 4-day period.)
   (2) Client must be evaluated for bronchospasm during treatment, especially those with asthma
3. Expectorants—add bulk or fluid to sputum
   a. Expected effects—increased effectiveness of cough and soothing the mucosa of the bronchial tree
   b. Commonly given drugs
      (1) Guaifenesin (Robitussin)
      (2) Terpin hydrate (Terpinol)
      (3) Potassium iodide

> ⚠️ **Warning!**
>
> Clients must have adequate hydration for this drug classification to be effective.

   c. Nursing considerations
      (1) Client must have strong cough effort and energy to cough
      (2) There may be great controversy over clinical efficacy of this drug classification
4. Antitussive agents—narcotic and nonnarcotic cough suppressants
   a. Expected effect—relief of cough; used when coughing has become detrimental to a client's progress
   b. Commonly given drugs
      (1) Codeine (narcotic)
      (2) Dextromethorphan (Benylin DM Cough Syrup, a nonnarcotic)
   c. Nursing considerations
      (1) Evaluate lung sounds frequently to determine if secretions are being appropriately removed when cough is being suppressed
      (2) With narcotic preparations, monitor client for signs of respiratory depression and tolerance to drug
5. Corticosteroids—decrease the inflammatory response in the airway and decrease airway edema
   a. Expected effect—increased airway lumen size
   b. Commonly given drugs
      (1) Prednisone (Deltasone)
      (2) Methylprednisolone (Medrol)
      (3) Beclomethasone dipropionate (Vanceril)
   c. Nursing considerations
      (1) Doses must not be missed and must be tapered over a 4- to 5-day period. To prevent findings of adrenal insufficiency, do not stop drug therapy abruptly.

      (2) Drug must be given with food or milk to prevent gastric ulcers

      (3) Many preparations (such as intranasal) are prophylactic and not appropriate for acute attacks

6. Cromolyn sodium (Intal)—prevents release of histamine from the mast cells of the lungs

  a. Expected effect—prophylactically prevents bronchospasm caused by an allergen or exercise

  b. Nursing considerations

      (1) Administer by inhalation only

      (2) Caution client not to discontinue use without physician's order

      (3) Do not use for acute asthma episodes

7. Antimicrobial agents—used to treat respiratory infections. Specific agent is chosen based on the infecting pathogen.

  a. Expected effect—elimination of infection

  b. Commonly given drugs

      (1) Penicillins [penicillin G (Ledercillin), nafcillin (Nafcil), ampicillin (Omnipen), carbenicillin (Pyopen), ticarcillin (Ticar)]

      (2) Cephalosporins [cephalexin (Keflex), cefazolin (Kefzol), cefoxitin (Mefoxin)]

⚠ Warning!

Many clients who are allergic to penicillin also are allergic to the cephalosporins. The cephalosporin allergic reactions may not be as severe as those with penicillin.

      (3) Aminoglycosides [gentamicin (Tobramycin), streptomycin]

      (4) Tetracylines [doxycycline (Vibramycin)]

  c. Nursing considerations

      (1) Monitor for allergic reaction to antibiotic

      (2) Evaluate culture and sensitivity report to determine pathogen sensitivity to drug therapy

      (3) Ascertain specific nursing considerations for each antimicrobial group

8. Tuberculosis (TB) chemotherapy—bactericidal action against mycobacterium bacillus

  a. Expected effect—elimination of TB

  b. Commonly given drugs

      (1) First line drugs

         (a) Isoniazid

         (b) Ethambutol hydrochloride (Myambutol)

         (c) Rifampin (Rifadin)

         (d) Streptomycin

(2) Second line drugs
    (a) Capreomycin
    (b) Kanamycin sulfate (Kantrex)
    (c) Ethionamide
c. Nursing considerations
    (1) Pyridoxine (B_6) must be given with isoniazid to prevent neuritis
    (2) Rifampin may color urine and tears orange
    (3) Therapy may extend from 6 to 18 months. Liver function studies must be evaluated monthly for liver impairment.

B. Procedures
1. CXR—reveals abnormalities in lungs and thoracic cavity
2. CT scan—gives three-dimensional evaluation of thorax; abnormalities in lungs and thorax can be seen
3. Bronchoscopy—direct visualization of the inside of the bronchial tree using a flexible, lighted scope
4. Thorascopy—direct visualization of the pleura for disorders using a flexible, lighted scope. A chest tube is required after the procedure to reexpand the lung.
5. Pulmonary angiography—dye injected into the pulmonary vasculature to detect abnormalities such as clots in the vascular system of the lungs
6. MRI—use of magnetic fields to create an image of thoracic structures
7. Thoracentesis—drainage of fluid from the pleural space to decrease respiratory distress. Fluid is evaluated for abnormalities such as bacteria.
8. Sputum culture—provides evaluation of pathogens responsible for a respiratory illness
9. Pulmonary function testing—provides assessment of changes in lung volume and capacity to evaluate the presence and severity of lung disease
10. ABGs—sample of arterial blood evaluated for oxygen and carbon dioxide tensions, pH, bicarbonate level, and oxygen saturation; identify oxygen and carbon dioxide diffusion abnormalities and bicarbonate abnormalities (Table 5-1)
11. Ventilation-perfusion scan—imaging of the distribution of an inhaled radionuclide followed by imaging of lung perfusion by an injected radionuclide. This scintigraphic technique demonstrates perfusion defects in normally ventilated areas of the lung to diagnose pulmonary embolism.

C. Psychosocial concerns
1. Anxiety—a common finding in clients having difficulty breathing, which can exacerbate respiratory distress
2. Fear—respiratory distress produces great fear in clients. The fear of death is quite overwhelming in clients having difficulty breathing.

TABLE 5-1	Normal Arterial and Venous Blood Gas Values*

Arterial Blood Gases	Sea Level BP 760 mm Hg	1 Mile Above Sea Level (5280 ft) BP 629 mm Hg	Mixed Venous Blood Gases	Sea Level
Laboratory Value				
pH	7.35-7.45	7.35-7.45	pH	7.34-7.37
PaO_2	80-100 mm Hg	65-76 mm Hg	PvO_2	38-42 mm Hg
SaO_2	>95%†	>95%†	SvO_2	60%-80%†
$PaCO_2$	35-45 mm Hg	35-45 mm Hg	$PvCO_2$	44-46 mm Hg
HCO_3^-	22-26 mEq/L	22-26 mEq/L	$HCO3^-$	24-30 mEq/L

From Lewis SM, Heitkemper MM, Dirksen SR: *Medical-surgical nursing: assessment and management of clinical problems,* ed 5, St. Louis, 2000, Mosby.
*Assumes the patient is aged 60 years or younger and is breathing room air.
†The same normal values apply when SpO_2 (pulse oximetry) and SvO_2 are obtained by oximetry.
BP = barometric pressure
SaO_2 = arterial oxygen saturation
HCO_3^- = bicarbonate
PvO_2 = partial pressure of oxygen in venous blood
SvO_2 = venous oxygen saturation
$PvCO_2$ = partial pressure of carbon dioxide in venous blood

3. Depression—common in clients with long-term respiratory disease. The depression is related to decreased ability to care for themselves or to complete tasks as they had previously.
4. Denial—may be noted in respiratory clients up to the time when respiratory symptoms are severe and undeniable
5. Hopelessness—many clients experience this feeling due to the incurable nature of their illness
6. Social isolation—the physical incapacity of respiratory illnesses, as well as the frequent production of foul-tasting sputum, causes an isolation-type living situation for many clients

D. **Health history—question sequence**
   1. What symptoms are you experiencing?
   2. What causes your symptoms or makes them worse?
   3. What makes your symptoms better?
   4. When did you first notice these symptoms?
   5. Are you able to complete your own hygiene?
   6. Are you able to go to work or do work around the house?
   7. Do you find it necessary to stop and rest after activity? If so, how long must you rest before you can again become active? How long can you exert yourself before you must rest?

8. Is there a specific time of day when your symptoms are more noticeable?
9. Do you cough up a large amount of sputum? How often or how much? What does it look like?
10. Have you experienced fever, sweating during the night, or excessive fatigue?
11. Have you noticed a weight loss or gain recently?
12. Is there a family history of respiratory illness?

E. **Physical examination—appropriate sequence**
1. Patent airway
2. RR depth and effort
3. Inspection of client for the following:
   a. Accessory muscle use
   b. Cyanosis—circumoral, nail beds
   c. Jugular venous distension
   d. Chest size and configuration
4. Palpation
   a. Chest wall tenderness
   b. Subcutaneous emphysema
5. Percussion—at the lung bases bilaterally
6. Auscultation—the upper and lower lobes; especially the right middle lobe where aspiration is most common
   a. Normal lung sounds
   b. Adventitious lung sounds
      (1) Crackles
      (2) Rhonchi
      (3) Wheezes
      (4) Pleural friction rub

IV. Pathophysiologic disorders

A. **Laryngeal cancer**
1. Definition—cancer of the larynx or voice box
2. Pathophysiology—slow growing, starting as a squamous cell carcinoma; initially a small hard patch leading to ulceration and abscessing of the area
3. Etiology—most clients with laryngeal cancer have a history of smoking or of voice abuse
4. Incidence—men are more likely to develop than are women; over 10,000 cases per year
5. Assessment
   a. Questions to ask
      (1) Have you experienced any change in your voice?
      (2) Have you had a sore throat that would not go away? Any hoarseness?
      (3) Have you noticed any sores in your throat that would not heal?
      (4) Have you noticed any difficulty breathing or swallowing?

b. Clinical manifestations
(1) Hoarseness longer than 2 weeks
(2) Difficulty swallowing or breathing
(3) Persistent cough or sore throat
(4) Lump in throat or neck area
c. Abnormal laboratory findings—none specific
d. Abnormal diagnostic test results
(1) Laryngoscopy and biopsy—identifies tumor presence and vocal cord changes; biopsy specimen is positive for malignancy
(2) Laryngeal tomography—evaluates for extension of disease
(3) CXR—shows metastasis into lung
6. Expected medical interventions
a. Surgery—excision of small lesions; partial laryngectomy; total laryngectomy; radical neck dissection
b. Radiation therapy—may be primary intervention with small lesions or palliative with advanced lesions
7. Nursing diagnoses—postoperative
a. Ineffective airway clearance related to difficulty coughing effectively through artificial airway
b. Impaired verbal communication related to effects of recent surgery, presence of artificial airway
c. Anxiety related to altered communication and **ventilation**
8. Client goals
a. Client will maintain a patent airway at all times as evidenced by clear upper airway sounds
b. Client will make all needs known using alternative method of communication (writing notes)
c. Client will have relaxed facial features and indicate feeling less anxious
9. Nursing interventions
a. Acute care—postoperative
(1) Evaluate upper airway patency and suction tracheostomy as needed using strict sterile technique
(a) Hyperoxygenate by ambu bag with 100% oxygen with three to five breaths
(b) Instill catheter into tracheostomy (no suction) until client coughs or resistance is met
(c) Remove catheter and suction intermittently, rotating catheter; use continuous suction on removal if an inline suction catheter system is used
(d) Cleanse catheter with sterile saline
(e) Hyperoxygenate again, and repeat once if needed. Let the client rest for several minutes before suctioning again.
(f) Place client in high Fowler's position to decrease edema and facilitate breathing

(2) Administer humidified oxygen by tracheostomy collar or T-piece (a corrugated oxygen tubing attached to tracheostomy by a T connector)

(a) Monitor vital signs for shock

(b) Monitor neck dressings for bleeding and behind the neck for bloody drainage

(c) Monitor continuous portable suction devices, such as Jackson Pratt drains or hemovacs, for drainage. Empty when half full or every 8 hours, measure drainage, and record as output.

(d) Explore alternative means of communication (if not evaluated preoperatively), and implement those mutually agreed on

(e) Medicate for pain as needed

b. Home care regarding client education

(1) Discharge materials to include an extra tracheostomy tube and obturator that is used for insertion of the tracheostomy tube should it come out

(2) Teach client how to liquefy secretions with hydration and to use sterile saline if hydration is ineffective or a mucous plug is present

(3) Instruct client on the need for a bedside humidifier or vaporizer

(4) Teach client how to clean stoma; tracheostomy tube is not required after the stoma has healed

(5) Instruct client on how to use a stoma bib or a scarf to cover the stoma to protect from contaminants or to catch mucus

(6) Reinforce that speech therapy should continue, and advise client to join a support group

(7) Advise client on the need to wear a medical-alert bracelet

(8) Advise client on the need to continue with postoperative arm and shoulder exercises

10. Evaluation protocol

a. How do I know that my interventions were effective?

(1) Does client's breathing feel easy?

(2) Does client's tracheostomy tube need to be suctioned?

(3) Can client easily cough up secretions?

b. Which criteria will I use to change my interventions?

(1) Client reports feeling short of breath or increased SOB

(2) Client reports that secretions are too thick

(3) Client indicates a need for suctioning more often

c. How will I know that my client teaching has been effective?

(1) Client is wearing a medical-alert bracelet

(2) Client is following speech therapy interventions and attends support group meetings

(3) Client demonstrates appropriate stoma cleaning technique

11. Older adult alert
   a. Upper airway cilia are less efficient in older clients, making airways harder to clear
   b. Lungs are less elastic in older adult clients, and thus coughing may be more difficult. These clients may require a stimulus to cough.

B. Pneumonia

1. Definition—an acute inflammatory process of the parenchyma of the lung with a significant increase in interstitial and alveolar fluid
   a. Can involve one segment or several segments
   b. Can involve one lobe or several lobes
   c. Can involve one whole lung or both lungs
   d. Pneumonitis refers to the noninfectious inflammatory process of lung parenchyma
2. Pathophysiology—infecting organisms are typically inhaled. Organisms are transmitted to the lower airways and alveoli causing inflammation. Organisms can also be transmitted to the lungs by way of the circulatory system and then can become lodged in the lungs causing inflammation.
3. Etiology—may be caused by bacteria, virus, *Mycoplasma,* fungus, protozoa, or from aspiration or inhalation of chemicals or other toxic substances
4. Incidence—major cause of hospitalization and death in the United States; responsible for over 10% of hospital admissions
5. Assessment
   a. Questions to ask
      (1) Have you been experiencing difficulty breathing?
      (2) Are you having pain? Where?
      (3) Do you have a cough? If yes, are you coughing up anything from your lungs? What does it look like (consistency and color)?
      (4) Have you been running a fever? What is the highest your temperature has been?
      (5) Have you been feeling tired?
   b. Clinical manifestations
      (1) High fever—usually sudden increase to 102° F or higher, along with chills and diaphoresis
      (2) Sinus tachycardia
      (3) Dyspnea
      (4) Bronchial breath sounds over area of pneumonia
      (5) Cough and increased sputum production
      (6) Chest pain over area of pneumonia
      (7) Headache
      (8) Fatigue
   c. Abnormal laboratory findings
      (1) Sputum culture—positive for organism infecting the lungs
      (2) Blood cultures—may show organism in the blood if the client has progressed to a stage of bacteremia

(3) CBC—elevated WBC count, over 10,000

(4) ABGs—decreased PO_2

d. Abnormal diagnostic test results

(1) CXR—pneumonia appears as white opaque areas known as *areas of consolidation*

(2) Bronchoscopy—areas infected are directly visualized. Exudate can be cleared from area, and sputum cultures can be obtained.

6. Expected medical interventions

a. Antibiotic therapy based on sputum culture and sensitivity. Administer antibiotics known to be bactericidal to infecting bacteria.

b. Hospitalization only if client's health warrants in-hospital care

7. Nursing diagnoses

a. Ineffective airway clearance related to thick, tenacious sputum

b. Ineffective breathing pattern—tachypnea related to chest pain and airway inflammation

c. Impaired gas exchange related to exudate in alveoli

d. Activity intolerance related to **hypoxemia** and fatigue

8. Client goals

a. Client will maintain an open and clear airway as evidenced by clear upper airway sounds

b. Client will maintain RR between 14 and 20 breaths per minute

c. Client will maintain PO_2 above 80 mm Hg without supplemental oxygen

d. Client will complete physical care without frequent rest periods

9. Nursing interventions

a. Acute care

(1) Auscultate lungs every 2 hours for changes in lung sounds

(2) Assess any sputum expectorated for change in color, consistency, and odor

(3) Monitor ABGs or pulse oximetry for hypoxemia

(4) Elevate head of bed to improve respiratory excursion

(5) Ensure client turns, coughs, and takes deep breaths every 2 hours; ambulate as tolerated

(6) Position client on back and unaffected side to increase ventilation of affected lung

b. Home care regarding client education

(1) Continue coughing and deep breathing exercises every 2 hours

(2) Finish all antibiotics at prescribed intervals

(3) Call physician for new onset of fever, chest pain, or hemoptysis

10. Evaluation protocol

a. How do I know that my interventions were effective?

(1) Is client breathing easier?

(2) Has client's chest pain improved or been relieved?

(3) Is client coughing up thinner and less sputum, and has the color changed to be more clear?

(4) Other evaluations will be objective

(a) Lung sounds will improve, adventitious breath sounds will disappear, and lungs will be clear

(b) RR will decrease to 14 to 20 breaths per minute

(c) **Work of breathing** will decrease and accessory muscle use will disappear

(d) Temperature will return to normal

b. Which criteria will I use to change my interventions?

(1) Dyspnea has not improved or has increased

(2) Chest pain has not improved

(3) Sputum is increased in thickness or amounts, and color has not changed

(4) Tachycardia and febrile state continues

c. How will I know that my client teaching has been effective?

(1) Client is coughing and breathing deeply every 2 hours

(2) Client is taking antibiotics every 4 hours as ordered

(3) Client is able to state conditions that physician should be made aware of

11. Older adult alert

a. Older adults are at very high risk for pneumonia. Therefore, all concerns should be further evaluated.

b. Be concerned about any changes in orientation. This may be a first indication of pneumonia in older adults.

c. Be cautious in fluid administration. Hydrate older adults; however, do not overhydrate clients because doing so may initiate CHF.

C. **Tuberculosis**

1. Definition—a chronic, infectious, granulomatous pulmonary disease

a. Drug responsive strains

b. Drug resistant strains

2. Pathophysiology—the mycobacterium tubercle is transmitted in droplets expelled by an infected person during sneezing, coughing, or laughing. Client has inhaled the infected droplets, and the bacillus has invaded the lung tissue. Continued exposure usually is required for a client to become infected.

a. Primary infection—bronchopneumonia begins at area of bacillus invasion. Bacilli may spread by the lymphatic system. Necrotic degeneration, called *caseation,* occurs at the site of infection causing cavities filled with necrotic tissue to eventually liquefy. The liquefied material drains out of the cavity, leaving an air-filled cavity that calcifies and can be seen on CXR. The primary infection causes a sensitivity to the tuberculin bacillus that, in turn, causes an allergic reaction if the bacillus is reintroduced into the body.

b. Secondary infection—active TB. The primary infection sites may harbor latent bacilli for many years that become reactivated.

3. Etiology—inhalation of an acid-fast bacillus (AFB); *Mycobacterium tuberculosis*

4. Incidence—over 3 million new cases annually worldwide. A long decline occurred after the discovery of antitubercular drug therapy in the 1940s. A new resurgence has occurred with the immigration of people from Third World nations and with the outbreak of the human immunodeficiency virus (HIV).

5. Assessment
   a. Questions to ask
      (1) Are you suffering from night sweats?
      (2) Have you lost weight?
      (3) Have you been having low-grade fevers? (99° F to 100° F)
      (4) Have you been having increasing difficulty breathing?
      (5) Have you had chest pain? Where?
      (6) Have you been coughing? If yes, are you coughing up anything from your lungs? What does it look like?
   b. Clinical manifestations
      (1) Night sweats
      (2) Weight loss
      (3) Anorexia
      (4) Fatigue
      (5) Dyspnea
      (6) Productive cough
      (7) Pleuritic chest pain caused by inflammation of the pleura; felt in the outer aspects of the lungs
   c. Abnormal laboratory findings
      (1) Sputum culture—positive for acid-fast bacilli (AFB); takes about 2 to 3 weeks for results; the definitive diagnostic test
      (2) Skin testing—purified protein derivative (PPD) is the preferred method. Induration or wheal greater than 10 mm is a positive result. Checked 48 to 72 hours after placement of intradermal test on inner forearm. Indicates a person has been exposed to and ingested the bacilli without an active disease process.
      (3) CBC—WBC may be elevated
   d. Abnormal diagnostic test results
      (1) CXR—may see calcification of original site of infection; infiltrates in the parenchyma
      (2) Pleural needle biopsy—caseation necrosis; positive for granulomas

6. Expected medical interventions
   a. Preventative therapy: isoniazid therapy for 9 to 12 months in clients with positive PPD but no radiologic changes or symptoms
   b. Three or more TB chemotherapeutic drugs; combination of first and second line drugs; 9 to 12 months for responsive strains

  c. Five or more TB chemotherapeutic drugs for resistant strains; first and second line drugs for as long as 2 years

  d. Respiratory isolation until sputum cultures are clear of bacilli (approximately 2 weeks after medication is started). Note: Documentation of this diagnosis must be reported to the local public health department.

  e. Monitor monthly for an elevation in the liver enzymes which indicate a complication of the drug regimen

  f. Support the ingestion of foods high in B_6 to prevent peripheral neuropathies, which are side effects of the drugs

7. Nursing diagnoses

  a. Ineffective airway clearance related to thick, tenacious secretions

  b. Ineffective breathing pattern related to airway inflammation

  c. Altered nutrition—less than body requirements related to anorexia and fatigue

  d. Anxiety related to social isolation secondary to isolation protocols

8. Client goals

  a. Client will maintain clear airway as evidenced by clear upper airway sounds

  b. Client will maintain RR between 16 and 24

  c. Client will demonstrate weight gain of 0.5 lb/wk until ideal body weight is achieved

  d. Client will state that anxiety is decreased

9. Nursing interventions

  a. Acute care—infectious period

   (1) Maintain respiratory isolation

    (a) Private room with negative pressure ventilation—when door opens air rushes into the room instead of air rushing out of the room. This restricts bacilli to the room.

    (b) Increased air circulation in the room to dilute the number of airborne bacilli

    (c) Door to room must remain closed at all times

    (d) Personnel and visitors wear masks if client is coughing and does not cover mouth effectively

    (e) Gowns—only if anticipation for contamination of clothes with sputum

    (f) Articles in the room—rarely implicated in transmission but should be cleansed, disinfected, or discarded

    (g) Instructions for client to cover mouth and nose with a tissue when laughing, coughing, and sneezing. Discarded tissues should be burned.

    (h) Instructions for client to wear mask when removed from isolation and to change it frequently, usually every 2 hours

    (i) Sunlight should be allowed to enter the isolation room because it kills bacilli

   (j) Hands must be washed before and after entering room and certainly after direct client care

  (2) A chemotherapeutic drug regime should be instituted and the client educated about the medications

   (a) Instruct client to take all daily medication as ordered for the amount of time specified by physician in order to arrest the disease

   (b) Instruct client that medication must not be discontinued for any reason

   (c) Instruct client that all adverse reactions must be reported to physician

    (i) GI disturbances

    (ii) Stabbing pain or numbness in extremities

    (iii) Loss of vision

   (d) Instruct client not to allow themselves to run out of medication

  (3) Provide diversions while in respiratory isolation

 b. Home care regarding patient education

  (1) The importance of continuing medications that are ordered, exactly as they are ordered

  (2) Hands must be washed after handling anything in contact with sputum

  (3) Adequate nutrition must be maintained

  (4) Articles need not be discarded at home because although the disease is infectious, it is not transmitted by articles

> ### ⚠ Warning!
>
> **Clients must never have another PPD** because it could cause an anaphylactic reaction. Chest x-ray films should be used to evaluate the disease and usually are done every few years or when suspicious symptoms appear.

  (5) Medication can be obtained from the public heath department

10. Evaluation protocol

 a. How do I know that my interventions were effective?

  (1) Client stays in isolation room and wears mask when in contact with other people

  (2) Client covers mouth with tissue when coughing, laughing, or sneezing

  (3) Client indicates what medications should be taken and how often

 b. Which criteria will I use to change my interventions?

  (1) Client has visitors in the room and does not wear a mask, or does not wash hands after contact with sputum in the infectious stage

  (2) Client leaves room without wearing a mask

(3) Client states the medication needs to be taken for a few weeks

(4) Client asks to take all pills in the morning

  c. How will I know that my client teaching has been effective?

(1) Client demonstrates hand washing technique after handling anything coming into contact with sputum

(2) Client thoroughly cleans eating utensils; uses dishwasher if available owing to the need for long contact with very hot water to kill the bacilli

(3) Client describes adverse reactions that should be brought to the attention of physician or public health department

(4) Client shows nurse a chart with indicated times for medication administration

(5) Client indicates why it is important not to skip medication

(6) Client specifies where the medication can be obtained

11. Older adult alert

  a. Older clients may become confused with multiple drug therapies and may not follow the regimen correctly. These clients may need assistance to ensure proper administration.

  b. Nutrition and fluid intake should be assessed frequently to ensure anorexia has passed and client's nutrition is optimal

D. Acute respiratory distress syndrome (ARDS); noncardiogenic pulmonary edema

1. Definition—a disorder that follows direct insult to the body lungs

  a. Increased pulmonary capillary permeability, resulting in noncardiogenic pulmonary edema

  b. Massive interstitial fluid accumulation

  c. Atelectasis; decreased lung tissue compliance

2. Pathophysiology—lung injury leading to increased pulmonary capillary permeability. Fluid shifts from vascular space to alveoli, interstitial space, and pleural space (noncardiogenic pulmonary edema). Poor lung expansion, decreased lung compliance, and hypoxemia occur. Type II pneumocytes are damaged in the initial injury so that surfactant production is decreased (increased surface tension in alveoli) leading to atelectasis and subsequent hypoxemia

3. Etiology—two categories

  a. Pulmonary—aspiration; lung trauma; inhaled toxins; any type of pneumonia

  b. Nonpulmonary—multiple trauma, sepsis, any type of shock, fluid overload, eclampsia, head injury, pancreatitis, fat emboli, disseminated intravascular coagulation, transfusion reaction, high altitude, uremia

4. Incidence—over 100,000 cases each year, with most often a 40% to 50% mortality rate

5. Assessment
    a. Questions to ask
        (1) Are you having difficulty breathing?
        (2) What is your name?
        (3) Do you know where you are? Do you know today's date?
    b. Clinical manifestations
        (1) Changes in LOC or orientation; initially restlessness, anxiety, and irritability
        (2) Increased RR
        (3) Increased work of breathing; labored **respirations**
        (4) Use of accessory muscles, retractions
        (5) Crackles and rhonchi throughout lung fields (usually later in the process)
        (6) Cyanosis (late stage)
        (7) If on a ventilator, repeated high-pressure alarms without usual findings of increased resistance in airways from things such as increased secretions, fighting ventilator, or kinked tubes
    c. Abnormal laboratory findings—ABGs. Even with increased oxygen administration, PO_2 remains under 80 mm Hg. Respiratory alkalosis usually is indicated by a low PCO_2 (less than 35 mm Hg) owing to increased RR. Subsequently, as fatigue sets in, a high PCO_2 (over 45 mm Hg) will indicate respiratory acidosis. Metabolic acidosis will appear as hypoxemia progresses owing to anaerobic metabolism and lactic acid production.
    d. Abnormal diagnostic test results
        (1) CXR—may be normal initially, slowly changing to indicate progressive pulmonary infiltrates. Eventually CXR will show massive pulmonary infiltrates in the form of a "snowstorm" or "whiteout" effect, also called a "ground glass-like" appearance.
        (2) Pulmonary function studies—show decreased compliance or decreased elasticity of lungs
6. Expected medical interventions
    a. Mechanical ventilation with use of positive end expiratory pressure (PEEP) and positive pressure support (PPS) to increase oxygen exchange across alveolar membrane. PEEP may range from 5 to 20 cm; PPS usually is 5 cm.
    b. Medications—sedation and pharmacologic paralysis to maintain optimal mechanical ventilation
    c. Steroid use is controversial
    d. Nutritional support by enteral or parenteral routes
7. Nursing diagnoses
    a. Impaired gas exchange related to changes in alveolar capillary membrane and fluid in alveoli

    b. Ineffective breathing pattern related to decreased lung compliance

    c. Activity intolerance related to hypoxemia caused by changes in alveolar capillary membrane

    d. Fear related to unknown outcome, decreased ability to maintain adequate ventilation, and effects of therapy

8. Client goals

    a. Client will maintain PO_2 over 60 mm Hg and PCO_2 between 35 and 45 mm Hg

    b. Client will maintain RR between 18 to 22 with no accessory muscle use

    c. Client will tolerate moving in bed without causing a decrease in arterial oxygen saturation (SaO_2)

    d. Client will show relaxed facial expressions or indicate fear is decreased

9. Nursing interventions

    a. Acute care—clients are usually transferred to critical care and placed on mechanical ventilation to decrease the work of breathing and optimize oxygenation to tissues. Care of the client on mechanical ventilation includes the following:

        (1) Maintain the airway initially using an endotracheal tube, usually for 7 to 10 days, and then using a tracheostomy tube for long-term ventilator support

        (2) Maintain airway patency through suctioning as necessary. Use suction only when assessment indicates a need, for example, when client is unable to raise upper or lower airway secretions with coughing, or is having frequent nonproductive coughs.

        (3) Monitor lung sounds at least every 1 to 2 hours, especially at the posterior bases

        (4) Maintain ventilator settings as per physician's orders for tidal volume (V_T), RR, and fraction of inspired oxygen (FiO_2) also called oxygen percent, assist or controlled mode

        (5) Evaluate and support vital signs as necessary checking RR, HR, and BP hourly at a minimum. The client may require use of vasopressor therapy to maintain an optimal BP. The client must be turned every 2 to 4 hours.

        (6) Sedate and paralyze client as necessary—paralyzing agents such as vecuronium bromide (Norcuron) are used to decrease the amount of oxygen consumed by a client fighting to breathe

            (a) Note that paralysis is total—client will be unable to even open eyelids

            (b) Remember that when using any paralyzing agent, it is imperative to administer sedation at all times because these agents offer no sedation

        (7) Maintain nutritional status either through enteral feedings or total parenteral nutrition (TPN)

       (8) Provide and teach to family members alternate forms of communication while client is on ventilator, such as use of a writing board or alphabet board, for use after the paralyzing agent is removed

       (9) Communicate what is being done during paralytic therapy. Talk to these clients because they may be able to hear and must be informed of any actions, as well as events.

     (10) Restrain arms with wrist restraints to prevent dislodgment of the artificial airway. Obtain physician's order for renewal, and remove as per hospital policy to evaluate circulation and skin under the restraints.

     (11) Respond immediately to ventilator alarms to prevent injury to the client

     (12) Never turn off ventilator alarms

     (13) Monitor ventilator tubing for condensed water buildup, and remove as necessary by draining them as per hospital protocol

     (14) Undertake all nursing interventions necessary to prevent skin breakdown and the complications of immobility

  b. Home care—Clients' needs at home will be based on their specific condition. The major focuses will be education regarding the following.

      (1) Respiratory care

      (2) Medications

      (3) Nutritional support

10. Evaluation protocol

  a. How will I know that my interventions were effective?

      (1) Client will have improved ABG results

      (2) Client will exhibit a reduced work of breathing; decreased accessory muscle use

      (3) Client will exhibit stable vital signs with near normal baseline levels

  b. What criteria will I use to change my interventions?

      (1) ABG results are not within prescribed parameters

      (2) Work of breathing is increased or unchanged

      (3) Vital signs are below 20% of baseline

  c. How will I know that my client teaching has been effective?

      (1) Client effectively communicates needs

      (2) Client tries to work with the health care staff with things such as coughing

11. Older adult alert

  a. Older adults have decreased lung elasticity as a course of normal aging. ARDS will decrease elasticity even further and make the syndrome even more difficult to manage than in younger adults.

b. Many older adult clients have decreased auditory acuity. When intubated and on a ventilator, this decreased acuity will make communication even more difficult.

E. Chronic obstructive pulmonary disease (COPD)

1. Definition—a group of chronic, obstructive airflow diseases of the lungs. It involves four diseases; also called chronic airflow limitation (CAL)
   a. Chronic bronchitis
   b. Emphysema
   c. Asthma
   d. Bronchiectasis
2. Pathophysiology
   a. Chronic bronchitis
      (1) Hypertrophy and hypersecretion of mucous producing cells of the bronchi cause an increase in sputum production
      (2) Increased mucous causes a decrease in airway lumen size, and eventually this mucous becomes colonized with bacteria
      (3) Bronchial wall becomes scarred and fibrotic in response to chronic infection, leading to stenosis and airway obstruction
   b. Emphysema
      (1) Enlargement of air spaces distal to airways that conduct air to the alveoli
      (2) Enlarged spaces cause a breakdown in the alveoli walls, which causes an increase in airway size on **inspiration** but a decrease in alveolar membrane for gas exchange
      (3) Small airways collapse on **exhalation,** resulting in air being trapped in the alveolar spaces
      (4) These changes are products of the destruction of elastin in the distal airways and alveoli
   c. Asthma—two types, both resulting in bronchoconstriction
      (1) Intrinsic—no specific cause; usually adult onset
      (2) Extrinsic—response to specific allergen (Table 5-2)
   d. Bronchiectasis
      (1) Chronic dilation of the bronchi
      (2) Eventual breakdown of elastic and muscular layers of the bronchi
      (3) Seen as a result of chronic infection, inflammation, or both
3. Etiology
   a. Introduction of irritants (e.g., smoking or smoke from cigarettes), infections, and allergens into the respiratory system
   b. May be a genetic deficiency of alpha1-antitrypsin (responsible for preventing breakdown of lung elastin), which can lead to emphysema
4. Incidence—greater than 10% of the older adult population have some form of COPD

TABLE 5-2	Intrinsic versus Extrinsic Asthma		
Characteristic	**Extrinsic**	**Intrinsic**
Allergens as precipitants	Yes	No
Immediate skin test	Positive	Negative
Elevated immunoglobulin E	Common	Uncommon
Eosinophilia	Yes	Yes
Childhood onset	Common	Uncommon
Other allergies	Common	Uncommon
Family history of multiple allergies	Common	Uncommon
Hyposensitization therapy	Helpful	Equivocal
Typical attack	Acute and self-limiting	Often fulminant and severe
Relationship of attack to infection	May be present	Common

5. Assessment
   a. Questions to ask
      (1) Do you have difficulty breathing? Do you have difficulty all the time or is it caused by exertion?
      (2) Do you cough frequently? Do you bring up a large amount of sputum when you cough? How much? How thick is it? What does it look like?
      (3) Do you cough up more sputum when you are more active?
      (4) Have you noticed a weight loss over the past year?
      (5) Do you feel tired quite often?
      (6) Are your activities impaired by your SOB or fatigue?
      (7) Do you have many respiratory infections? Over what period of time?
   b. Clinical manifestations—all conditions are manifested by prolonged expiration; a change in the normal inspiratory-to-expiratory ratio from 1 to 2, to 1 to greater than 2
      (1) Chronic bronchitis
         (a) Productive cough
         (b) Dyspnea, especially on exertion
         (c) Wheezing and rhonchi
         (d) Cyanosis—"blue bloater"
         (e) Peripheral edema from *cor pulmonale*—right-sided heart failure caused by pulmonary insufficiency from increased pulmonary vascular resistance or pulmonary hypertension; noncardiogenic
         (f) Clubbed fingers
      (2) Emphysema
         (a) Dyspnea with exertion, progressing to dyspnea at rest
         (b) Accessory muscle use

        (c) Increase anterior-posterior diameter of the chest

        (d) Wheezes

        (e) Overall emaciation

        (f) Pink color associated with dyspnea—"pink puffer"

        (g) Peripheral edema from cor pulmonale

        (h) Clubbed fingers

    (3) Asthma

        (a) Dyspnea

        (b) Tight feeling in chest

        (c) Nonproductive cough

        (d) Inspiratory or expiratory wheezes, or both

        (e) Clubbed fingers

    (4) Bronchiectasis

        (a) Dyspnea

        (b) Cough with large amount of sputum production

        (c) Accessory muscle use

        (d) Weight loss

        (e) Emaciation

        (f) Fever

        (g) Clubbed fingers

  c. Abnormal laboratory findings

    (1) ABGs—decreased PaO_2, increased PCO_2 as disease processes progress; commonly PaO_2 is 60 to 80 mm Hg, and $PaCO_2$ is 50 to 60 mm Hg

    (2) CBC—polycythemia when client becomes chronically hypoxemic

    (3) Sputum culture—may indicate chronic bacterial infection

  d. Abnormal diagnostic test results

    (1) CXR—flattened diaphragm, increased lung markings, cardiac enlargement, lung hyperinflation

    (2) Pulmonary function tests—*decreased forced expiratory volume* in one second (FEV_1) (total lung capacity, and residual volumes may be increased due to air trapping)

6. Expected medical interventions

  a. Oxygen when needed to maintain a PaO_2 over 60 mm Hg or during exercise; PaO_2 of 80 mm Hg or less because PaO_2 over 80 mm Hg may result in respiratory depression

  b. Drug therapy—bronchodilators, mucolytics, and expectorants; oral and nebulizer routes

  c. Physical therapy—postural drainage and chest percussion to assist with sputum expectoration

  d. Mechanical ventilation when conservative medical interventions fail

7. Nursing diagnoses

  a. Ineffective airway clearance related to thick, tenacious secretions and fatigue

b. Ineffective breathing pattern related to fatigue and obstruction of the bronchial tree

c. Impaired gas exchange related to changes in the alveolar-capillary membrane and increased sputum production

d. Activity intolerance related to hypoxemia and fatigue

e. Altered nutrition (less than body requirements) related to increased metabolic demands, fatigue, and anorexia

f. Anxiety or fear related to inability to breathe effectively

8. Client goals

a. Client will be able to effectively clear airway as evidenced by stating that airway feels clear and respirations are not labored

b. Client will have an effective breathing pattern as evidenced by a rate within 10% of baseline for the client and use of only abdominal muscles

c. Client will maintain a PaO_2 over 60 mm Hg or within 10% of baseline, and a $PaCO_2$ under 60 mm Hg or within 10% of baseline

d. Client will demonstrate increased activity with decrease in dyspnea or fatigue as stated by client

e. Client will maintain present weight; or if underweight, client will gain 0.5 lb/wk

f. Client will state feeling less anxious or fearful with each episode of dyspnea

9. Nursing interventions

a. Acute care

(1) Assess

(a) Patency of airway; apply suction if cough is ineffective or not present

(b) Respiratory rate, pattern, and depth

(c) Accessory muscle use

(d) Lung sounds for changes, that is, increased or decreased rhonchi, crackles, wheezes. In severe asthma attacks the sudden absence of wheezing is ominous and indicates that the small airways are totally collapsed

(e) Skin color changes

(i) Rubor indicates hypercapnia, which indicates a $PaCO_2$ over 45 mm Hg

(ii) Cyanosis or gray skin color indicates hypoxemia, which indicates a PaO_2 under 60 mm Hg

(f) ABGs as drawn

(g) Effectiveness of bronchodilator therapy

(h) Whether anxiety is increased or diminished; increased anxiety commonly indicates increased respiratory distress

(2) Monitor oxygen administration

b. REMEMBER! Normal drive to breathe is in clients with normal lungs an elevated level of carbon dioxide

> ## ⚠ Warning!
>
> REMEMBER that some clients with COPD have an altered drive to breathe. The drive to breathe is hypoxemia. Increasing the PaO_2 with supplemental oxygen administration may suppress the client's drive to breathe and cause bradypnea or apnea. Note: With any decrease in RR of less than 20% of the client's baseline, oxygen might need to be discontinued. The drive in clients with COPD is usually from PaO_2 less than 80 mm Hg.

   (1) Oxygen administration is usually maintained with a nasal cannula at 1 to 2 L/min (approximately 24% oxygen as opposed to 21% oxygen in room air)

   (2) Monitor fluid intake to ensure appropriate hydration to keep secretions thin

c. Home care regarding client education

   (1) Teach client respiratory maintenance techniques

      (a) Avoid irritants, especially smoking or secondhand smoke; suggest the use of nicotine patch to assist in quitting

      (b) How to use the appropriate technique for pursed lip breathing

         (i) Inhale through nose counting to two and pausing for one count

         (ii) Exhale slowly through pursed lips, as if blowing a kiss or blowing into a straw, while counting to four

      (c) How to cough effectively

         (i) Do not force a cough—may be damaging to the airways

         (ii) Take three deep breaths

         (iii) Bear down against throat—feel pressure against throat

         (iv) Cough will occur as pressure increases in throat and chest area

      (d) How to use the appropriate technique for use of abdominal muscles for breathing

         (i) Abdomen should rise with inspiration

         (ii) Abdomen should fall with exhalation

      (e) How to balance rest and activity at home

         (i) Activities no longer than 20 minutes

         (ii) Rest at least 30 minutes between activities

      (f) How to plan meals. Meals should be small, frequent, and high in calories and carbohydrates. Avoid foods that form gas to prevent gastric bloating, which could put pressure on the diaphragm and impede ventilation. Avoid large, high-carbohydrate meals because when digested, carbohydrates give off more CO_2 than other substances, and result in an increased workload of breathing. Because carbohydrates are needed for adequate energy to breathe, however, they should be consumed frequently in small amounts.

- (g) How to use inhalers correctly
  - (i) Deep breathe and exhale slowly
  - (ii) On second deep breath with inhaler within about 1 inch from the mouth, push down to release medication. Keep the mouth wide open to facilitate aerosol medication movement into lungs instead of the back of the throat. If a spacer is used, lips may be put loosely around the opening.
  - (iii) Hold breath as long as possible, then exhale slowly
- (h) How to determine the amount of medication left in inhaler. Put canister in water. If it floats, it is empty; if it sinks, it is full.
- (i) Avoid known allergens
- (j) Avoid people with upper respiratory illnesses
- (k) Seek treatment for upper respiratory illness within 24 hours of initial onset
- (l) Keep humidity in the home at least at 40% with use of a humidifier
- (2) Check on home care equipment—make sure arrangements have been made for oxygen and for nebulizer equipment in the home if necessary
- (3) Discuss necessary changes in sexual fulfillment, such as changes in positions or the use of bronchodilators before sexual intercourse; suggest and refer to a sexual counselor for further assistance if necessary

10. Evaluation protocol
    a. How do I know that my interventions were effective?
       (1) Does client feel short of breath? Has it improved?
       (2) Was client able to complete bath independently this morning? Did client become short of breath while bathing?
       (3) Is client using oxygen? Is client using it just with activity or all the time?
       (4) Has client been feeling anxious? Has client been feeling less anxious?
    b. Which criteria will I use to change my interventions?
       (1) Increased SOB at rest
       (2) Decreased activity level from increased SOB
       (3) Sputum that is difficult to expectorate

(4) Lung sounds that are deteriorating

(5) ABGs that are deteriorating

c. How will I know that my client teaching has been effective?

(1) Client demonstrates appropriate pursed lip breathing technique

(2) Client demonstrates appropriate abdominal breathing technique

(3) Client demonstrates appropriate use of inhalers or nebulizer equipment

(4) Client is drinking high-calorie supplements, eating small meals, and is avoiding foods that form gas

11. Older adult alert

a. Most clients affected with COPD are in the population classified as older adults

b. In older clients the thoracic muscles have become weaker, meaning they will be unable to tolerate the increased work of breathing required of COPD

c. Older adult clients have fewer alveoli than younger adults, and thus, oxygen exchange will be even more impaired in older adult clients with COPD

d. The weaker thoracic muscles in older adults will also make coughing more difficult, and thus, retained secretions will be a problem in many instances

F. Lung cancer

1. Definition—a malignancy of the lower respiratory tract

2. Pathophysiology—uncontrolled growth of undifferentiated cells that invade surrounding tissues

a. Adenocarcinoma is the most common form—originates in peripheral lung tissue

b. Squamous cell carcinoma—originates in bronchial epithelium

c. Small cell carcinoma (oat cell)—originates in cells of the airways

d. Large cell carcinoma—originates peripherally in the lung; multiple masses occur

3. Etiology—tobacco smoke is the major cause (approximately 80%) of lung cancers; exposure to asbestos and radon also are factors

4. Incidence—has been increasing significantly over the past 10 years

5. Assessment

a. Questions to ask

(1) Do you experience a cough? Do you produce sputum with your cough? How much? How thick is it? What does it look like?

(2) Do you ever feel short of breath?

(3) Do you ever cough up blood?

(4) Do you ever experience hoarseness?

(5) How many pillows do you sleep on at night?

(6) Have you lost a noticeable amount of weight in the past few months?

   b. Clinical manifestations
- (1) Chronic cough, productive or nonproductive
- (2) Dyspnea
- (3) Hoarseness
- (4) Chest tightness or pain
- (5) *Hemoptysis*—blood in sputum
- (6) Shoulder or arm pain
- (7) Frequent occurrences of bronchitis or pneumonia
- (8) *Superior cava syndrome*—edema of the face, neck, arms, and upper torso when the lung tumor presses on the superior vena cava

   c. Abnormal laboratory findings—sputum for cytology: malignant cells identified

   d. Abnormal diagnostic test results
- (1) CXR—nodule or lesion identified
- (2) CT scan—nodule or lesion identified and position pinpointed in chest
- (3) Lung scan—identifies size, shape, and actual position of lesion
- (4) Brain and bone scans—identify metastases

6. Expected medical interventions
   a. Surgery—lobectomy, pneumonectomy, wedge resection, segmental resection if lesion is operable
   b. Radiation therapy—may be sole therapy if client has an inoperable tumor; also can be used preoperatively and postoperatively to decrease lesion size
   c. Antineoplastic therapy—used for small cell carcinoma

7. Nursing diagnoses
   a. Ineffective airway clearance related to thick, tenacious sputum and chest muscle weakness
   b. Ineffective breathing pattern related to chest pain and muscle weakness
   c. Impaired gas exchange related to impaired ventilation secondary to invasive tumor
   d. Altered nutrition (less than body requirements) related to anorexia
   e. Anxiety related to difficulty breathing and fear of death

8. Client goals
   a. Client will maintain a patent airway as evidenced by clear upper airway sounds
   b. Client will maintain RR between 18 and 22 breaths per minute, with appropriate breath sounds in bases
   c. Client will maintain PaO_2 and $PaCO_2$ within 10% of baseline
   d. Client will remain at present weight without any further loss
   e. Client will state that anxiety has reached a manageable level and anxiety does not prevent the maintenance of an active life

9. Nursing interventions
   a. Acute care
      (1) Assess
         (a) Airway patency at least every 1 to 2 hours; suction if cough is ineffective or if client has no secretions with coughing
         (b) RR, effort, and respiratory depth at least every 2 to 4 hours
         (c) Lung sounds for changes, especially wheezing, which may reflect impaired and narrowed lower airways
         (d) ABGs for deterioration
         (e) Accessory muscle use
         (f) Sputum—evaluate consistency, color, and odor; hemoptysis
         (g) Hydration status
      (2) For clients after thoracotomy, assess all of the above
         (a) In addition, assess
            (i) Chest tube patency and drainage. Immediately after surgery expect 150 ml/hr of sanguinous drainage, decreasing in amount and changing from sanguinous to serosanguinous or serous drainage within 48 hours. Bubbling in the water-seal chamber may be seen on exhalation for the first 24 hours, as air escapes from chest; continuous bubbling in the water-seal chamber indicates an air leak from the lung. However, continuous bubbling in the suction-control chamber is normal when it is connected to suction of (usually) 20 cm H_2O. Chest tubes usually are removed 3 to 6 days after surgery.
            (ii) Chest wall for subcutaneous emphysema—air trapped in subcutaneous tissue. Feels like crumpled plastic wrap under the skin. Check around chest tube insertion site first, then shoulder and neck areas.
            (iii) Dressing for bleeding; check behind the client's back for blood
            (iv) Pain—adequate pain medication will allow client to turn, cough, and deep breathe deeply more effectively
         (b) Have client turn, cough, and breathe deeply every 2 hours after pain medication is given. Deep breathing frequently is accomplished through the use of incentive spirometer mechanisms. REMEMBER: When positioning a client on his or her side, the lung facing upward is the one that is ventilated most effectively; in contrast, the lung the client is lying on is compressed and not as effectively ventilated.

      (c) Adhere to specific positioning guidelines

          (i) Pneumonectomy—place client on back and tilt them to the *operative side* ONLY. Remember that the remaining lung is on the side that was not operated on. Placing the client on the side of the remaining lung will prevent adequate expansion of the remaining lung. The remaining lung now receives all the blood from the heart and therefore, adequate **perfusion** is less of a concern. Engorgement of this remaining lung may occur. Right heart failure may also be a problem. There is also an increased risk of mediastinal shift—mediastinum can shift toward remaining lung from a lack of anchoring tissue on the empty cavity side, especially in the first few days after surgery

          (ii) All other thoracotomies—turn client to back and *unoperative side* ONLY; may tilt to the operative side. Lying on the operative side prevents reexpansion of lung tissue that remains on the operative side, may cause compression of the chest tubes, and this is more uncomfortable to client.

      (d) Assist with active and passive **range-of-motion** exercises for the arm on the operative side to prevent tightening of shoulder muscles

      (e) Encourage semi-Fowler's position for optimal ventilation of remaining lung tissue

   b. Home care regarding client education

    (1) Postoperative needs

      (a) Incisional care—frequency, technique, and observations that are normal and those necessary to report to the physician

      (b) Activity limitations—varies with individuals

      (c) Specific assessment factors the client needs to report or discuss with physician

      (d) Continue postoperative coughing and deep-breathing exercises with the use of an incentive spirometer at home

      (e) Continue arm exercises

    (2) Nonsurgical clients

      (a) Take weight weekly

      (b) East small frequent meals

      (c) Use antiemetics before meals

      (d) Balance rest and activity

      (e) Instruct how to have physician-ordered oxygen delivered to the home and used in the home

      (f) Instruct clients and significant others about use of nebulizer therapy

(g) Instruct client as to adequate amount of fluid intake to liquefy secretions

10. Evaluation protocol
    a. How do I know that my interventions were effective?
       (1) Does client feel short of breath? Has the feeling of SOB increased or decreased from 2 hours ago?
       (2) Is client's sputum difficult to cough up?
       (3) Is client having chest or incisional pain?
       (4) Is client feeling anxious? More anxious than yesterday?
    b. Which criteria will I use to change my interventions?
       (1) Client has increased or unresolved SOB
       (2) Client has thick, tenacious sputum that is difficult to expectorate
       (3) Client is experiencing increased or unresolved chest or incisional pain
       (4) Client describes anxiety that prevents activity
    c. How will I know that my client teaching has been effective?
       (1) Client demonstrates correct wound care technique
       (2) Client states conditions that should be reported to physician
       (3) Client demonstrates correct use of oxygen and nebulizer equipment
       (4) Client describes eating small meals and using an antiemetic before meals
       (5) Client shows a chart of weekly weights taken in the home with an evaluation of gain or loss

11. Older adult alert
    a. The cough is weak in older clients owing to a decrease in chest wall muscle strength. These clients are at a greater risk for atelectasis and pneumonia than are younger clients.
    b. After thoracic surgery, older clients are at greater risk for hypoxemia owing to the loss of lung tissue and normal decrease of functioning alveoli as a result of the aging process

G. **Chest and lung trauma**
    1. Definition—injury that occurs to the chest wall or the lung, or both, as a result of a blunt or nonpenetrating impact or penetrating impact to the chest
       a. Rib fracture—break in the integrity of the rib
       b. Flail chest—multiple rib fractures that leave an area of the chest wall unstable, with a need for mechanical ventilation
       c. Pneumothorax—air entering the space between the visceral and parietal pleura. Breath sounds are absent. Pneumothorax can be a consequence of rib fracture and flail chest.
       d. Hemothorax—blood entering the space between visceral and parietal pleura. Breath sounds are absent. Potential signs of shock can be seen. Hemothorax can be a consequence of rib fracture and flail chest.

e. Tension pneumothorax—air entering the pleural space and becoming trapped to the point of causing increased thoracic pressure and a mediastinal content shift. Acute tracheal deviation to the side opposite of the pneumothorax commonly occurs. This is a medical emergency because disruption of cardiac output (CO) and respiratory embarrassment can occur.

2. Pathophysiology—there is normally negative pressure (suction) between the visceral and parietal pleura. Any injury that allows air or positive pressure to enter the pleural space will prevent the lung from remaining inflated.

   a. Injury that allows blood to enter the pleural space may also prevent the lung from remaining inflated

   b. Tension pneumothorax—air enters the pleural space through a hole in the lung, such as when a *bleb* (a fragile thin-walled alveoli) ruptures and then becomes trapped in the thorax, causing an increase in pressure. This pressure pushes the heart, vena cava, and aorta out of position, resulting in poor venous return to the heart, which leads to poor CO (Figure 5-1).

3. Etiology—most common causes of blunt chest trauma are motor vehicle accidents and falls; penetrating traumas are commonly caused by gunshot and knife injuries

4. Assessment

   a. Questions to ask

      (1) Are you having difficulty breathing?

      (2) Do you have pain in your chest? Point to your pain with one finger.

   b. Clinical manifestations

      (1) Some degree of SOB

      (2) Chest pain at point of injury

      (3) Tachycardia

      (4) Anxiety—may be extreme

   c. Abnormal laboratory findings—ABGs. PaO_2 is decreased. Initially $PaCO_2$ is decreased related to tachypnea, followed by increased $PaCO_2$ as the ability to hyperventilate is lost.

   d. Abnormal diagnostic test results—CXR, which indicates the percentage of pneumothorax and amount of space occupied by blood in the pleural space with a hemothorax. CXR also can identify rib fractures and flail chest.

5. Expected medical interventions

   a. Rib fractures—rest, heat to area, and pain relief

   b. Flail chest—chest tube with water-seal drainage if a hemothorax or pneumothorax exists with flail chest. Mechanical ventilation to support ventilation may be required.

   c. Pneumothorax—chest tube insertion and water-seal drainage. Location of the chest tube is usually in the anterior upper thorax to remove air.

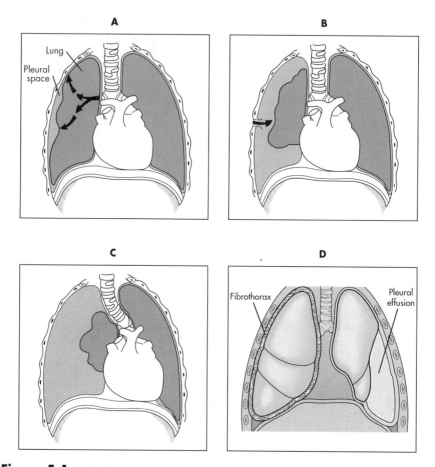

Figure 5-1. **A,** Spontaneous pneumothorax. **B,** Open or traumatic pneumothorax, resulting from collapse of lung owing to disruption of the chest wall and outside air entering. **C,** Tension pneumothorax. As pleural pressure on the affected side increases, mediastinal displacement ensues with resultant respiratory and cardiovascular compromise. **D,** Disorder of the pleura. Fibrothorax resulting from an organization of inflammatory exudates and pleural effusion. (**A–C** from Wilson S, Thompson J: *Respiratory disorders,* St. Louis, 1994, Mosby. **D** *from* Lewis SM, Heitkemper MM, Dirksen SR: *Medical-surgical nursing: assessment and management of clinical problems,* ed 5, St. Louis, 2000, Mosby.)

     d. Hemothorax—chest tube insertion and water-seal drainage. Location of the chest tube is usually in the lower thoracic area to drain blood from the chest. Blood transfusion may be required.
6. Nursing diagnoses
     a. Ineffective breathing pattern related to decreased lung expansion
     b. Impaired gas exchange related to decreased alveolar membrane surface available for gas exchange
     c. Anxiety related to inability to ventilate effectively

7. Client goals
   a. Client will maintain RR between 20 to 24
   b. Client will maintain a PaO_2 between 80 and 100 mm Hg and a $PaCO_2$ between 35 and 45 mm Hg
   c. Client will state feeling less anxious
8. Nursing interventions
   a. Acute care
      (1) Assess
         (a) Airway patency
         (b) Respiratory rate, effort, depth, and character
         (c) Lung sounds for absence
         (d) Chest for rise and fall of chest symmetrically with respirations
         (e) ABGs
         (f) Chest wall for subcutaneous emphysema, especially with rib fractures and flail chest
      (2) Maintain semi-Fowler's position to assist with ventilatory effort
      (3) Medicate for pain
      (4) Provide appropriate care for pleural chest tubes with water-seal drainage (Figures 5-2 and 5-3). Sequence of chambers from client to system are as follows
         (a) Collection chamber—collects drainage from chest and allows measurement of drainage
         (b) Water-seal chamber—seals end of chest tube with 2 cm H_2O so that air cannot enter the chest tube and eventually the thoracic cavity
            (i) Normal function—water will fluctuate with respirations and may bubble on exhalation when air escapes from a significant pneumothorax. Note: This not found with a hemothorax.
            (ii) Abnormal function—continuous bubbling indicates air is leaking into the system
         (c) Suction control chamber—filled to level of ordered suction *with sterile water.* Normal suction is -20 cm H_2O.
            (i) Normal function—should gently bubble continuously when suction is on. Suction source is attached to the chamber or bottle.
            (ii) Abnormal functioning—intermittent or no bubbling occurs. Check that suction is turned on, not disconnected, or tubing is not kinked.
         (d) Taped connections—make certain all connections are taped to prevent air leaks
         (e) Free-draining tubing—tubing should not have kinks
         (f) Drainage system must be below the level of the insertion site on chest wall at all times

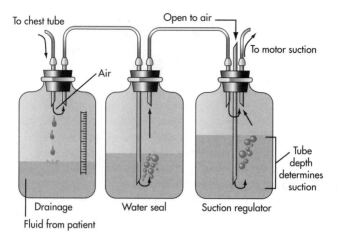

Figure 5-2. Three-bottle disposable water-seal suction. Bottle I is the drainage bottle. A vertical piece of tape should be applied to the outer surface of the drainage bottle. The fluid level and time should be marked hourly on the tape. Bottle II is the water-seal bottle. Bottle III is the suction-control bottle. The length of glass tube below the water surface determines the amount of suction. (From Lewis SM, Heitkemper MM, Dirksen SR: *Medical-surgical nursing: assessment and management of clinical problems,* ed 5, St. Louis, 2000, Mosby.)

     (g) Clamps with rubber tips should be at bedside for emergency situations only. Clamping for extended periods especially with a large leak from a pneumothorax may cause a tension pneumothorax. The chest tube must be clamped during a change of the water-seal drainage collection system.

     (h) Prevention of atelectasis—encourage turning, coughing, and deep breathing

   b. Home care regarding client education

     (1) Care for chest tube insertion site and on signs of infection at site

       (a) If in place, do not remove dressing until physician evaluates the site

       (b) If no dressing, clean site with soap and water. Watch for and report redness, swelling, or any drainage from area.

     (2) Follow-up on evaluation for care for further pulmonary impairment

     (3) Increase activity as able

     (4) Balance rest and activity

 9. Evaluation protocol

   a. How do I know that my interventions were effective?

     (1) Is client having difficulty breathing?

     (2) Has client's chest pain diminished?

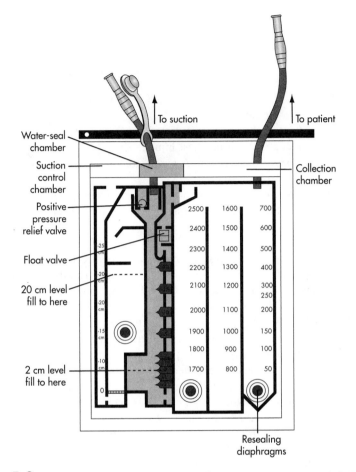

Water-seal chamber

Suction control chamber

Positive pressure relief valve

Float valve

20 cm level fill to here

2 cm level fill to here

To suction

To patient

Collection chamber

Resealing diaphragms

Figure 5-3.   Pleur-evac disposable chest suction system. (From Lewis SM, Heitkemper MM, Dirksen SR: *Medical-surgical nursing: assessment and management of clinical problems,* ed 5, St. Louis, 2000, Mosby.)

   (3) What does an objective evaluation show concerning
     (a) Equal lungs sounds
     (b) Bilateral chest movement
     (c) Decreased chest tube drainage with a change of color from sanguinous to serosanguinous to serous
 b. Which criteria will I use to change my interventions?
   (1) Increased dyspnea with activity or at rest, or dyspnea not improved
   (2) Increased chest pain or unrelieved chest pain with prescribed medications
   (3) Lung sounds remain absent in one area of chest
   (4) Unilateral chest movement
   (5) Significant serosanguinous chest tube drainage, over 50 cc/hr after the first 8 hours

    c. How will I know that my client teaching has been effective?
      (1) Client demonstrates correct care of chest tube site
      (2) Client keeps scheduled follow-up visits with physician
      (3) Client walks half a block or more daily

10. Older adult alert
    a. Older adults are at high risk for infection owing to a decreased immune response. Chest injuries should be evaluated carefully for signs of infection. A temperature of 99° F may indicate an initial infection.
    b. Cough will be impaired owing to decreased muscle strength, and thus, older adults are at a greater risk for atelectasis and pneumonia after a chest injury.

H. Pneumoconiosis

1. Definition—occupational lung disorder related to inhalation of particulate matter during working schedule. The three most common disorders are silicosis, asbestosis, and coal or granite worker's pneumoconiosis.
2. Pathophysiology—when inhaled silicone and asbestos produce an inflammatory and fibrotic type of reaction, resulting in emphysematous type of lung disorder. Coal or granite dust inhaled over many years is deposited in the alveoli, becomes very difficult to clear, and eventually interferes with alveolar membrane function.
3. Etiology—inhalation of silicone from ceramic or building material; asbestos when manufactured into fireproofing products; coal or granite dust from prolonged exposure during mining
4. Assessment, diagnoses, interventions, and evaluations of these clients will be identical to the client with COPD. Please refer to COPD on pp. 161-166, numbers 5 through 11, for discussion of nursing care.

I. Pulmonary embolism

1. Definition—blockage of a branch of the pulmonary artery by a thrombus, piece of fatty tissue, piece of tumor, air, or a particle of amniotic fluid. Blood is prevented from entering the lungs for gas exchange.
2. Pathophysiology—the embolism is freed from the point of origin, travels to the pulmonary artery, and becomes lodged in one of the branches. The larger the embolism the larger the obstruction in the pulmonary artery. Ventilation is greater than perfusion: the lungs are appropriately ventilated but blood is unable to come into contact with oxygen-rich alveoli owing to the embolism. Blood is shunted to the left side of heart unoxygenated, and the client becomes hypoxemic.
3. Incidence—over 6000 cases per year in the United States, with a mortality rate of over 35%

4. Etiology—thrombus formation usually originates in veins of the legs or pelvis
   a. Thrombus follows prolonged bed rest, venous stasis, dehydration, or some other cause of increased coagulability
   b. Fat embolism follows fracture of the long bones—typically the femur
   c. Air embolism may occur from a central venous catheter or during cardiopulmonary bypass
   d. Amniotic embolism follows childbirth
   e. Tumor embolism is associated with a malignancy
5. Assessment
   a. Questions to ask
      (1) Are you having difficulty breathing?
      (2) Do you have chest pain? Point to where it hurts the most with one finger.
      (3) Have you experienced any fever?
   b. Clinical manifestations
      (1) Sudden onset of dyspnea
      (2) Anxiety, fear, and the "feeling of impending doom"
      (3) Sinus tachycardia and dysrhythmias
      (4) Fever over 100° F
      (5) Crackles and pleural friction rub that can be either localized or generalized, depending on the size of embolism
      (6) Pleuritic chest pain
   c. Abnormal laboratory findings—ABGs. PaO_2 is under 80 mm Hg. $PaCO_2$ initially is decreased owing to tachypnea but may increase to over 45 mm Hg as the client tires.
   d. Abnormal diagnostic test results
      (1) Ventilation-perfusion lung scan (definitive for diagnosis)—ventilation with radioactive gas shows normal ventilation. Injection with radioactive dye shows areas of lung not appropriately perfused.
      (2) CXR—may show some decrease in vascular markings on the effected area of the lung
6. Expected medical interventions
   a. Bed rest for 2 to 3 days followed by a slow increase in mobility
   b. Anticoagulation therapy with continuous heparin drip, usually for 7 to 10 days. Therapeutic aPTT of 1.5 to 2 times the normal should be maintained.
   c. Oral anticoagulant therapy begun 3 days before heparin is stopped to allow time for oral anticoagulant to reach therapeutic level. Prothrombin time (PT) of 1.5 to 2 times normal should be maintained for at least 6 months.
   d. Surgical intervention—vena cava umbrella for repeated incidence of pulmonary embolism

e. Thrombolytic therapy—streptokinase or urokinase in the face of massive pulmonary embolism. Medication is directly injected into the pulmonary artery that contains the clot.

7. Nursing diagnoses
   a. Impaired gas exchange related to ventilation-perfusion abnormality
   b. Ineffective breathing pattern related to chest pain, hypoxemia, and anxiety
   c. Chest pain related to inflammatory process initiated by embolism
   d. Anxiety related to difficulty breathing and fear of death

8. Client goals
   a. Client will maintain PaO_2 and $PaCO_2$ within 10% of client baseline
   b. Client will maintain RR within 20 to 24 breaths per minute
   c. Client will state chest pain has diminished
   d. Client will state anxiety has decreased to a manageable level and the feeling of doom is gone

9. Nursing interventions
   a. Acute care
      (1) Immediate care
         (a) Take vital signs every 15 minutes until within 10% of baseline for client; may require vasopressor therapy for support
         (b) Evaluate neurologic status every 1 to 2 hours for changes related to hypoxemia
         (c) Evaluate lung sounds every 1 to 2 hours for changes: increased respiratory effort at rest, increased crackles, onset of wheezing, and rhonchi
         (d) Evaluate SaO_2 and ABGs parameters as ordered for increased hypoxemia
         (e) Administer oxygen as per orders—usually ordered to keep SaO_2 above 90%
         (f) Medicate for pain as vital signs permit. Morphine sulfate relieves feelings of anxiety and promotes bronchial dilation.
         (g) Monitor for indications of right-sided heart failure and acute cor pulmonale
            (i) Distended neck veins with head of bed elevation of 35 degrees or higher
            (ii) CVP is greater than 10 cm H_2O, or greater than 8 mm Hg
            (iii) Right ventricular gallop
            (iv) Peripheral edema; edema of sacrum, ankles, or feet

b. Ongoing care
(1) Monitor for signs of excessive anticoagulation: blood in stool or urine; bleeding gums; bruising; and petechiae, especially over the chest wall
(2) Avoid IM injections owing to anticoagulant therapy
(3) Wean off of oxygen as soon as possible with physician orders and the use of SaO_2 monitoring
c. Home care regarding client education
(1) Instructions regarding anticoagulant therapy
(a) Clients understand any abnormal or excessive bruising or bleeding may be an indication of over-anticoagulation, and they should notify physician immediately
(b) Use a soft toothbrush
(c) Know how often to have PT taken to evaluate maintenance dose of anticoagulant
(d) Notify all caregivers they are taking an anticoagulant; client may want to obtain a medical-alert bracelet
(e) Know which foods should not be eaten, such as green leafy vegetables, because they will interfere with anticoagulants
10. Evaluation protocol
a. How do I know that my interventions were effective?
(1) Is client still having difficulty breathing?
(2) Has client's chest pain gone away or decreased?
(3) Objective assessment
(a) Vital signs are stable
(b) Neurologic status is stable
(c) SaO_2 or ABGs indicate hypoxemia has resolved
(d) APTT is at therapeutic level
b. What criteria will I use to change my interventions?
(1) Unstable vital signs
(2) Deterioration in neurologic status
(3) SaO_2 or ABGs indicate continued hypoxemia
(4) APTT not in therapeutic range
c. How will I know that my client teaching has been effective?
(1) Client indicates that PT must be drawn weekly
(2) Client takes oral anticoagulant at the same time each day
(3) Client uses a soft bristled toothbrush, or if wearing dentures, client checks gums daily for bleeding
(4) Client indicates no excessive bruising or evidence of bleeding
11. Older adult alert
a. Older adults are at great risk for pulmonary embolism as a result of decreased CO experienced with aging. They are also at

risk as a result of proneness to venous stasis from decreased exercise or walking and from decreased tone in venous walls.

b. Older adults can become dehydrated very quickly as a result of diuretic therapy and poor nutritional habits, which also increases the risk of pulmonary embolism.

WEB resources

http://www.lungusa.org/popup6a.html
    American Lung Association

http://www.cancer.org/
    American Cancer Society

http://www.umdnj.edu/~ntbcweb
    NJMS National Tuberculosis Center

REVIEW QUESTIONS

1. When assessing a client, who has had a pulmonary embolism, the nurse would expect to see which type of sudden respiratory findings?
    1. RR over 30 breaths per minute
    2. Cheyne-Stokes pattern
    3. Accessory muscle use
    4. Rapid, shallow breathing

2. A client with newly symptomatic COPD is being started on theophylline. The nurse's understanding of the action of this drug will help the nurse to understand that the expected effect in this client will be
    1. A decreased RR
    2. A decreased work of breathing
    3. To help clear secretions
    4. To help liquefy secretions

3. A client with asthma informs the nurse that he carries cromolyn (Intal) with him wherever he goes in case he has an asthma attack. The best intervention in relation to this statement is to
    1. Praise him for thinking ahead to prevent a problem
    2. Instruct him that this drug works over a long period of time to decrease airway secretions
    3. Instruct him that there is no reason to carry it with him because it is used only for emphysema
    4. Instruct him that this drug is used prophylactically to prevent an asthma attack, not to stop or treat an acute attack

4. A common assessment finding associated with viral pneumonia is
    1. Accessory muscle use during inspiration and expiration
    2. Bronchial breath sounds heard over the area of pneumonia
    3. A dry, hacking cough especially with increased activity
    4. Night sweats with intermittent high temperatures

5. A nurse has placed a purified protein derivative skin test on a client suspected of having TB. The nurse understands a check of this site must be done
    1. Within 24 hours
    2. In 2 to 3 days
    3. In 3 to 4 days
    4. Within 5 to 7 days

6. A client has been diagnosed with adult regulatory distress syndrome (AARDS). In the early stages of the illness expected findings on ABGs are
    1. Low partial pressure of oxygen in arterial blood (PaO_2), low partial pressure of carbon dioxide in arterial blood ($PaCO_2$)
    2. Low PaO_2, high $PaCO_2$

3. High PaO$_2$, low PaCO$_2$
4. Normal PaO$_2$, normal PaCO$_2$

7. Clients with noncardiogenic pulmonary edema would have which of these nursing diagnoses placed on their nursing care plan?
1. Ineffective airway clearance related to thin secretions and fatigue
2. Ineffective breathing pattern related to hypoxia and accessory muscle use
3. Impaired gas exchange related to changes in the alveolar capillary membrane
4. Activity intolerance related to hypervolemia and changes in H&H levels

8. A client with emphysema and an admission diagnosis of respiratory incompetence is complaining to the food service supervisor because he is not being given a choice of cabbage, which he enjoys eating. The nurse's best intervention is to
1. Explain that this is a gas-forming food, and he cannot have those types of food
2. Explain to the food service supervisor that he can have whatever he wants
3. Ask his wife to bring him food from home if the food service group will not give it to him
4. Instruct him that gas-forming foods produce more gas, which then pushes up on his diaphragm to strain it

9. The nurse would expect a client with a tension pneumothorax to display which types of assessment findings?
1. Cyanosis and hypertension
2. Sustained bradypnea and hypotension
3. Boring chest pain and diaphoresis
4. Acute dyspnea and tachycardia over 120

10. When discharging clients, who have been hospitalized for 10 days with the diagnosis of pulmonary embolism, appropriate education must include
1. To eliminate green leafy vegetables from their diet while on medication
2. To eliminate any green vegetables from their diet while on medication
3. That they must have a PT drawn every week throughout the course of therapy
4. They should only take aspirin for fever or pain with avoidance of other NSAIDs

ANSWERS, RATIONALES, AND TEST-TAKING TIPS

Rationales	Test-Taking Tips

1. Correct answer: 4

The best answer in this group is rapid, shallow respirations. The pain of pulmonary embolism causes clients to not want to breathe deeply, and therefore they breathe more rapidly to maintain oxygenation. Option 1 is not the best answer because these clients may have RRs in the 20s or 30s. The Cheyne-Stokes pattern of breathing is associated with diagnoses of CVAs or strokes, increased ICP with head injuries, and the dying process in the terminally ill. Accessory muscle use is more likely to be seen with progressive respiratory distress when the diaphragm as a muscle has become weakened and fatigued.

The key term in the question is "sudden respiratory findings." Option 1 is too restrictive of an answer to be the best choice. Options 2 and 3 are more likely found in situations of progressive or ongoing respiratory difficulties.

2. Correct answer: 2

Bronchodilators enlarge the diameter of the airways to allow for easier passage of air. Thus, clients will have a decrease in their work of breathing. Option 1, a decreased RR, is a secondary benefit of these drugs. Option 3, to help clear secretions, also is a secondary benefit because larger airways allow for better passage of mucus. Also, remember that clearing secretions is best done by a strong cough. Two things liquefy pulmonary secretions, fluid intake and the drug Mucomyst given by inhalation.

The key words in the stem are "expected effect in this client." Avoid adding information to the stem which has no data about a client with secretions. Therefore, options 3 and 4 can be eliminated. To choose between decreased RR and decreased work of breathing, think logically. When the workload is diminished, the rate of respirations tends to decrease. If you decreased the rate of respirations, the workload does not necessarily change. Associate or compare this workload and rate of respirations for respiratory problems to your workload and rate of actions on your nursing unit.

Rationales	Test-Taking Tips

3. Correct answer: 4

Cromolyn has no use in the event of an acute asthma attack. It is used only to prevent asthma attacks. Option 1 is incorrect. The initial part of option 2 is correct but the last part "to decrease airway secretions" is incorrect. Similarly, the initial part of option 3 is correct but the rationale is incorrect.

The approach to select the correct option is to eliminate choices until the only option left is the correct one. An important clue in this stem is the stated client situation, an "asthma attack." In option 1, the word "preventing" contradicts the stated need by the client; also the word "problem" is too general to relate to the situation of an asthma attack. In option 2, the verbiage "over a long period of time" contradicts the given situation of an asthma attack. To eliminate option 3, remember that there is no drug to treat emphysema, only drugs to treat the effects of emphysema. The only option left is 4, the correct option.

4. Correct answer: 2

Bronchial breath sounds, normally heard over the trachea, can be heard over the area of consolidation in clients with pneumonia. These sounds are rough, coarse, and loud. This client typically will not be using accessory muscles, but will be breathing rapidly and shallowly from the pain. A productive cough is a usual finding. Night sweats are seen in clients with TB, AIDS, Hodgkin's disease, or menopause. clients with pneumonia will have a spike in temperature, usually of 102 or higher, rather than intermittent high temperatures.

Use this technique only if you have no educated guess to narrow the options down to two. This technique is to match words in the question and in the option, and it works well here—match "pneumonia" in the question with option 2, which has the word "pneumonia." Another technique is to identify clues in each option to eliminate that option. In option 1, if clients with pneumonia used accessory muscles it would most likely be on inspiration, not expiration, because they need help to pull air into the lung areas that are full of mucus and infection. In option 3, the clue is "dry" cough. Clients with pneumonia have productive coughs. In option 4, the clue is "intermittent high temperatures." Because pneumonia is an acute infection, temperature elevations are most likely to be acute, not intermittent.

5. Correct answer: 2

Skin tests for TB must be checked in 48 to 72 hours for an accurate evaluation. A positive finding is an induration of over 10 mm on clients with no immune problems. Erythema over 10 mm may be a finding but is not considered a positive result. The other options are either too soon or too late for an effective evaluation.

Remember the T in the TB test requires waiting at least Two to Three days to check the site, not Four or Five!

6. Correct answer: 1

The PaO_2 will be low as a result of the hypoxemia of the syndrome; the $PaCO_2$ will be low from the rapid RR associated with hypoxemia. The time "in the early stages" is important to note. The client will be blowing off a lot of CO_2, and because of the congestion there will be little O_2 exchanged at the alveolar level. Hypoxemia occurs when the PaO_2 is under 80 mm Hg.

Use the vertical process of reading to make the options more distinct. Read the first item in each option. As you do this, it is evident that options 1 and 2 are better because there is decreased oxygen in respiratory distress situations. Then, recall that in the "early" period of any type of respiratory distress, the RR is usually fast. Thus, clients have a tendency to blow off CO_2. Select option 1.

7. Correct answer: 3

The primary problem in ARDS or noncardiogenic pulmonary edema is at the alveolar capillary membrane site. In option 1, ineffective airway clearance is related to thick secretions. An ineffective breathing pattern is related to hypoxemia—a laboratory diagnosis with the PaO_2 under 80 mmHg—not hypoxia, which is a clinical diagnosis of decreased tissue oxygenation. Option 3 introduces new information of a different system, hypervolemia, as the cause of activity intolerance in ARDS. Activity intolerance is related to fatigue.

ARDS is a respiratory problem located at the site of the alveolar capillary membrane. Hypoxia is a small word. Think small at the cell level—a lack of oxygen. Hypoxemia is a larger word. Think of a larger area—the blood levels of oxygen.

| Rationales | Test-Taking Tips |

8. Correct answer: 4

Option 4 gives the most thorough explanation. Option 1 reflects rigidity with emphasis on rules as opposed to the client's needs, and thus, it is not the best approach. The other two options, 2 and 3, are obviously incorrect actions.

Options 2 and 3 can be clustered under the approach that the client can eat whatever he wants. The way in which the question is asked gives the clue that this is not a correct approach to a diet problem. Eliminate these options. With options 1 and 4 left, option 1 reflects inflexibility. Option 4 gives an association of the food restriction to breathing difficulty. The client will more easily understand this explanation.

9. Correct answer: 4

Acute changes in heart and lung function occur as a result of movement restriction within the thoracic cavity. Cyanosis, option 1, is a very late sign. Also, cyanosis might be present with hypotension, not hypertension. Sustained bradypnea is not a finding. Neither chest pain nor diaphoresis is a common assessment with this condition.

Terms in three of the options can be clustered to eliminate them: in options 1, 2, and 3, respectively, the key words are "hypertension," "sustained, and "boring." Remember that hypotension occurs more often than does hypertension in acute clinical problems. The word "acute" in option 4 is a clue that this is the correct answer because tension pneumothorax usually is an acute situation.

10. Correct answer: 1

Green leafy vegetables, which contain Vitamin K, may render the coumadin ineffective or less therapeutic. In option 2, not all green vegetables have this effect, only the green leafy ones. Clients must have a PT drawn weekly until the dosage is stabilized and not throughout the course of therapy. Clients must not take aspirin with coumadin because aspirin increases the risk of bleeding. Other NSAIDs may be used as directed by the physician.

The clues that render options 1, 2, and 3 incorrect are the terms "any," "every," and "only," respectively. Options with absolute words such as these usually indicate a wrong answer.

6

The Gastrointestinal System

FAST FACTS

1. Parasympathetic (cholinergic) stimulation increases peristalsis and gland secretion.
2. Sympathetic (adrenergic) stimulation decreases peristalsis and gland secretion.
3. Intrinsic factor, secreted by the parietal cells in the stomach, is required for absorption of vitamin B_{12}.
4. Many of the nutritional problems of the elderly are related to poor dentition or to poorly fitted dentures.
5. Hydrochloric acid in the stomach is increased in the stress response, which results in gastric or duodenal irritation and bleeding, especially in clients on mechanical ventilation. The resulting ulcer is called a *stress ulcer.* In burns, it is called *Curling ulcer.*
6. After gastric surgery, the client's nasogastric (NG) tube should not be repositioned or irrigated without specific instructions by the physician. Because the tube is positioned near the gastric incision, movement may cause the suture line to be disrupted.
7. The normal GI drainage colors are as follows: 'G'astric—'G'reen (G), 'B'ile—'B'rownish-yellow (B), and 'B'M (bowel movement)—brownish from the bile (B).
8. Abnormal findings associated with common bile duct obstructions are the following: (1) BM is clay or gray colored (lack of bilirubin); (2) increased bilirubin: skin is jaundiced, or *icteric;* and (3) urine is brownish or tea colored, and if shaken, is foamy.
9. An abnormal finding associated with small bowel obstruction is that gastric drainage is brownish-yellow mixed with green.

CONTENT REVIEW

I. **The GI system is responsible for the ingestion and *digestion* of food, *absorption* of nutrients, and storage and elimination of waste products**

II. **Structure and function**

   A. Mouth (buccal cavity)—mastication or chewing of food breaks down food into smaller particles to make *digestion* easier. Lubrication of food also occurs in the mouth with introduction of the enzyme ptyalin.

   B. Esophagus—muscular tube responsible for propelling food from the mouth to the stomach through *peristalsis*

   C. Stomach—J-shaped organ found in the upper abdomen responsible for continuation of the digestive process
      1. Four stomach areas
         a. Fundus—left upper stomach
         b. Body—main section
         c. Cardia—base of the esophagus
         d. Antrum—right lower section, just above the pylorus
      2. **Secretions**
         a. Hydrochloric acid
         b. Intrinsic factor
         c. Pepsin
         d. Pepsinogen
         e. Lipase
         f. Bile
         g. Mucous, to protect the walls of the stomach from autodigestion
      3. Endocrine cells of the stomach secrete gastrin, which controls gastric **secretions** and **motility**

   D. Pancreas—called an accessory organ, it is found behind the stomach. The pancreas secretes a liquid rich in sodium bicarbonate to decrease the acidity of gastric contents as well as trypsin, chymotrypsin, lipase, and amylase. These *secretions* enter from the pancreatic duct into the duodenum.

   E. Liver—right side of the upper abdominal cavity, just under the diaphragm. The liver is made up of microscopic lobules, each with a central venule and surrounded by the hepatic artery. It is also called an accessory organ.
      1. Maintains blood glucose and amino acid levels by removing excesses from the portal circulation and secreting glucose if the serum level decreases
      2. Synthesizes blood glucose, proteins, amino acids, and fats
      3. Produces and secretes bile and bile salts necessary for digestion of fat
      4. Bile is delivered and then stored in the gallbladder, which is situated beneath the liver

F. Small intestine
1. Three distinct areas—the duodenum, jejunum, and ileum, which are positioned anatomically as listed
2. Mucosa of the small intestines is covered with millions of fingerlike projections called *villi,* which are responsible for the absorption of food particles after further digestion in the small intestines
3. *Brush border,* made up of microvilli, lines the outer surface of the villi and is responsible for most enzyme or digestive activity in the small intestines
4. Enzymes available at the brush border are peptidase, sucrase, lactase, and maltase
5. Contents of the small intestines are constantly churned by **peristalsis** of the wall of the small intestines, allowing more food particles to come into contact with the villi and thus be further digested and absorbed

G. Large intestine
1. Five distinct areas—ascending colon, transverse colon, descending colon, sigmoid colon, and rectum, which are positioned anatomically as listed. Water, urea, and electrolytes are absorbed by the transverse, descending, and sigmoid colon.
    a. Ascending colon—right side of the abdomen; accepts contents of the ileum and pushes them forward in the colon
    b. Ileocecal valve—between the ileum and cecum, or beginning pouch of the colon; prevents backflow of material into the ileum
    c. Transverse colon—lies horizontally just below the stomach; contents are continuously pushed through the transverse colon
    d. Descending colon—left side of the abdomen; contents are continuously pushed through the descending colon
    e. Sigmoid colon—intestinal contents are then pushed into it, so called because of its S shape
    f. Rectum—contents first enter the rectum and then are expelled through the anus
2. Feces is stored in the distal half of the colon until defecation occurs. Feces are composed of three fourths water and one fourth solid matter, which is food residue, digestive enzymes, bile pigments, and mucus.

III. Targeted concerns
A. Pharmacology—priority drug classifications
1. Antacids—neutralize gastric acid
    a. Expected effects—relief of gastric pain, indigestion, and gastroesophageal reflux
    b. Commonly given drugs
        (1) Aluminum hydroxide (Amphojel)
        (2) Calcium carbonate (Tums)
        (3) Magnesium hydroxide (Milk of Magnesia)

    c. Nursing considerations

        (1) Antacids can alter the absorption of other medications if taken concurrently or within 1 hour of other medications

        (2) Shake preparations well before taking

        (3) Follow with a glass of water to ensure medication has entered the stomach

        (4) Commonly taken 1 hour after eating and at bedtime

2. Combination antacids—a combination of aluminum and magnesium

    a. Expected effects—relief of gastric pain, indigestion, and gastroesophageal reflux

    b. Commonly given drugs

        (1) Magaldrate (Riopan)

        (2) Aluminum and magnesium hydroxide (Maalox Extra Strength)

        (3) Aluminum, magnesium, and simethicone (Mylanta Double Strength)

    c. Nursing considerations—same as above; used by clients who have experienced diarrhea or constipation with single-agent antacids

3. Antidiarrheal agents—slows intestinal **motility** and peristalsis

    a. Expected effect—decreased episodes of diarrhea

    b. Commonly given systemically acting drugs

        (1) Diphenoxlate hydrochloride and atropine sulfate (Lomotil)

        (2) Loperamide hydrochloride (Imodium)

        (3) Camphorated tincture of opium (Paregoric)

    c. Nursing considerations

        (1) Hold drug and call physician if client's abdomen becomes distended and bowel sounds decrease

        (2) Encourage client to ensure that fluid intake is increased to at least 2000 ml/day during this period to prevent dehydration

        (3) Caution client that these medications may cause drowsiness

4. Antiemetics—most agents act on the chemoreceptor trigger zone in the brain to prevent or decrease nausea and vomiting

    a. Expected effects—decreased or inhibited nausea and vomiting

    b. Commonly given drugs

        (1) Prochlorperazine maleate (Compazine)

        (2) Trimethobenzamide hydrochloride (Tigan)

        (3) Metoclopramide hydrochloride (Reglan)—acts by increasing motility of the GI tract; empties the stomach and increases the tone of the esophageal-gastric sphincter

    c. Nursing considerations

        (1) Warn clients that they may feel sleepy and not to drive or use machinery for 6 to 8 hours after taking medication

(2) Instruct clients not to use alcohol while taking these drugs because it enhances the drowsiness effect
5. Inhibitors of gastric acid secretion (H_2 histamine receptor antagonists and proton pump inhibitors)—inhibit the release of hydrochloric acid by occupying the histamine receptor in the gastric mucosa
   a. Expected effect—decreased gastric acid secretion
   b. Commonly given drugs
      (1) Cimetidine (Tagamet)
      (2) Ranitidine (Zantac)
      (3) Famotidine (Pepcid)
      (4) Omeprazole (Prilosec)—proton pump inhibitor
   c. Nursing considerations
      (1) May cause dizziness and headache
      (2) Warn client that medications may cause constipation
      (3) Clients commonly take these medications 30 minutes before or immediately before meals and at bedtime
6. Laxatives—used to treat or prevent constipation or to prepare the bowel for examination
   a. Expected effects—bowel evacuation and bowel normalization
   b. Commonly given drugs
      (1) Bulk-forming agents
         (a) Psyllium hydrophilic mucilloid (Metamucil)
         (b) Methylcellulose (Citrucel)
         (c) Bran
      (2) Emollients—provides additional fluid and fat, thus softening the stool
         (a) Docusate sodium (Colace)
         (b) Docusate calcium (Surfak)
      (3) Irritants—increase peristalsis
         (a) Cascara (Cas-Evac)
         (b) Senna (Senokot)
         (c) Bisacodyl (Dulcolax)
      (4) Lubricants—lubricate the intestines, such as mineral oil
      (5) Saline osmotics—increase water in the stool, distend the bowel, and increase peristalsis
         (a) Milk of Magnesia
         (b) Magnesium sulfate
         (c) Magnesium citrate—commonly used as a preparation before lower GI X-ray films
         (d) Lactulose (Cephulac)—commonly used in liver disease when serum ammonia levels are elevated
   c. Nursing considerations
      (1) Assess client's abdomen for bowel sounds, distension, and tenderness before administration; evaluate for intestinal obstruction

(2) Encourage client to increase fluid intake, roughage, and bulk in diet to normalize bowel elimination

(3) Educate client about the impact of adequate exercise, fluid, and dietary fiber

7. Anticholinergics—inhibit the action of acetylcholine
   a. Expected effects—decreased GI secretions and decreased colon spasms
   b. Commonly given drugs
      (1) Propantheline (Pro-Banthine)
      (2) Dicylcomine hydrochloride (Bentyl)
   c. Nursing interventions
      (1) Warn client that drugs may cause drowsiness and blurred vision; caution against driving or using machinery until effects have subsided
      (2) Encourage client to increase fluid, bulk, and roughage in diet to counteract constipating effect of these drugs

8. Mucosal healing agents—adhere to ulcer to protect it from acid; stimulate release of prostaglandins, which increase protection of mucosal layer; absorbs pepsin
   a. Expected effect—protects inflamed mucosa from acid
   b. Commonly given drug—sulcralfate (Carafate)
   c. Nursing interventions
      (1) Educate client to take on an empty stomach, usually 45 to 60 minutes before eating
      (2) Inform client to avoid antacids within 30 minutes of taking drug
      (3) Inform client that medication works best if dissolved in a small amount of liquid and then taken, rather than swallowing the pill whole

B. Procedures

1. Abdominal X-ray films—show intestinal gas, fluid, masses, and size and position of organs

2. Ultrasonography—sound waves are used to produce images of the abdominal contents; usually used for gallbladder or liver visualization

3. CT scan—X-ray images are taken at several angles, then synthesized by a computer to produce an accurate picture of the structure being assessed; contrast material may be used orally, rectally, or intravenously

4. MRI scan—a magnetic field is used to produce images of areas being assessed

5. Endoscopy—a fiberoptic scope is used for direct visualization of an area of the GI tract; the prefix denotes the area being visualized
   a. Esophagogastroduodenoscopy (EGD)—esophagus, stomach, and duodenum
   b. Proctosigmoidoscopy—rectum and sigmoid colon
   c. Colonoscopy—entire length of large colon

    d. Endoscopic retrograde cholangiopancreatography (ERCP)—esophagus, stomach, and duodenum; dye is injected into the pancreatic and bile ducts, and x-ray films are taken

6. Barium swallow with an upper GI series—thickened barium is administered orally, and serial X-ray films are taken while the client assumes several positions on the X-ray table; films are taken as the client swallows and then at 30 minute to 1 hour intervals
7. Barium enema—barium is introduced into the large intestines through an enema, and x-rays films are taken with the client in several different positions
    a. Water-soluble contrast study—meglumine diatrizoate (Gastrografin)—is used in the same way as barium but is safer for clients who may be suffering from a perforation
8. Oral cholecystography—radiopaque dye is administered to the client orally, and X-rays are taken of the gallbladder
9. Stool analysis—abnormal constituents, such as blood, pathogens, and fats, are identified from a stool sample
10. Schilling test—small bowel absorption of vitamin B_{12} and possible lack of intrinsic factor are evaluated

C. Psychosocial concerns
1. Anxiety—an uncomfortable feeling associated with an unknown direct cause; common in this client as a result of sometimes vague symptoms with unknown causes
2. Social isolation—common in the client with a chronic illness of the GI tract as a result of the sometimes unpredictable nature of the symptoms and the inability to tolerate many foods
3. Fear—an uncomfortable feeling associated with a known cause; in these clients the causes range from abdominal pain to nausea and rectal bleeding
4. Lifestyle changes—apparent especially in the client who must learn to cope with an ostomy
5. Body-image disturbances—may be seen in the client who must learn to cope with an ostomy
6. Substance abuse—ingestion of alcohol may be more common in patients with GI dysfunction and may result in lifestyle or work problems

D. Health history—questions and sequence
1. What is your height and weight?
2. What specifically about your eating, stomach, or bowels has been bothering you lately?
3. Do you have any pain or sores in your mouth? Do you have any difficulty chewing?
4. When did the problem first occur?
5. How often do you have this problem? Does it occur in relation to eating, activity, or having a bowel movement?
6. If the problem is pain, can you point to the pain?

7. Can you describe the pain? Is it sharp, burning, or dull? When does it occur in relation to your daily activities such as work, rest, and meals?
8. On a scale of 0 to 10 where would you rate your pain?
9. Is there anything you do or eat that makes the pain worse or better?
10. What relieves the pain?
11. Do you notice any other symptoms when you are having discomfort?
12. Are you following a special diet?
13. Are you being treated by a physician for any other medical problems?
14. Are you presently taking any medications that the physician has prescribed?
15. Are you presently taking any medications that you buy without a prescription?
16. Have you ever had surgery of the GI tract?
17. Do you have any allergies to foods or medications?

E. Physical examination—appropriate sequence
1. ABCs—vital signs
2. Height and weight
3. Inspection of oral cavity
4. Inspection of abdomen
5. Auscultation of abdomen—bowel sounds in all four abdominal quadrants; normal frequency of 5 to 35 sounds per minute in an irregular manner
   a. Listen for at least 5 minutes in each quadrant to determine absence of bowel sounds
   b. Auscultate for bruits—none should be heard
6. Abdominal percussion—each quadrant
7. Abdominal palpation—each quadrant

IV. Pathophysiologic disorders
A. Oral candidiasis (thrush)
1. Definition—overgrowth of the normal oral flora with *Candida albicans,* a fungus
2. Pathophysiology—disruption of the normal balance of oral flora allows *Candida albicans* to become overgrown
3. Etiology—immunosuppression or the use of antibiotics
4. Incidence—common in the client who is immunosuppressed, has diabetes, or is on extended use of antibiotics
5. Assessment
   a. Questions to ask
      (1) Do you have any pain in your mouth?
      (2) Have you noticed any bleeding in your mouth?
      (3) Are you presently taking an antibiotic?
      (4) Do you have any strange sensations in your mouth?

    b. Clinical manifestations

       (1) Patchy white areas on tongue and oral mucous membranes, resembling milk curds

       (2) Patches adhere to mucous membranes; not easily removed

  6. Expected medical intervention—oral nystatin (Mycostatin); swish medication in mouth then swallow

  7. Nursing diagnosis—pain related to impaired oral mucous membranes

  8. Client goal

    a. Client will state mouth pain has decreased or been relieved

  9. Nursing interventions

    a. Acute care

       (1) Analgesics as needed for pain relief

       (2) Warm saline mouth washes with small amounts of hydrogen peroxide

       (3) Decrease diet to liquids or pureed foods

    b. Home care regarding client education

       (1) Explain dental hygiene to be followed at home

       (2) Instruct client on how to continue administration of medication at home correctly

       (3) Teach client how to identify a new onset of infection

 10. Evaluation protocol

    a. How do I know that the interventions were effective?

       (1) Is client's mouth pain relieved or decreased?

       (2) Is client able to tolerate meals without excess pain?

    b. Which criteria will I use to change my interventions?

       (1) Client has increased or unrelieved mouth pain

       (2) Client is unable to tolerate food that is served

    c. How will I know that client teaching has been effective?

       (1) Client demonstrates correct oral hygiene technique

       (2) Client demonstrates correct technique for medication administration

       (3) Client identifies changes in oral mucosa to be brought to physician's attention

 11. Older adult alert

    a. This problem is common in older adults owing to normal changes in the oral flora

    b. The use of dentures may aggravate any alteration in gum integrity

B. Gastroesophageal reflux disease (GERD)

  1. Definition—regurgitation of stomach contents into lower esophagus

  2. Pathophysiology—lower esophageal sphincter does not close appropriately in between swallowing. Reflux of gastric contents very often leads to esophagitis. Eventually, the basal epithelial layer of the esophagus will thicken and lead to esophageal strictures. In severe cases, may cause inflamed larynx with a change in voice to that of a whisper tone.

3. Etiology—alcohol, anticholinergic drugs, caffeine, increased estrogen levels
4. Assessment
   a. Questions to ask
      (1) Do you ever feel a burning behind your breastbone?
      (2) When do you experience this burning?
      (3) Do certain foods aggravate this burning?
      (4) Do you ever notice a pain behind your breastbone?
      (5) How long does it last?
      (6) Does anything relieve this pain?
   b. Clinical manifestations
      (1) Heartburn—midsternal area
      (2) Heartburn or pain radiation into the back, neck, jaw, or both arms
      (3) Discomfort to an aching feeling
      (4) Usually relieved within 3 to 5 minutes
      (5) Relieved with liquid antacids
   c. Abnormal diagnostic test results
      (1) Barium swallow—shows evidence of reflux and changes in esophageal wall
      (2) Continuous ambulatory 24-hour esophageal pH monitoring—identifies acid reflux into the esophagus and the amount
      (3) Esophagoscopy—identifies presence of hiatal hernia and esophagitis
5. Expected medical interventions
   a. Antacids to neutralize stomach acid
   b. H_2 histamine receptor antagonists to decrease acid production
   c. Metoclopramide hydrochloride (Reglan) to increase lower esophageal sphincter tone and decrease reflux
6. Nursing diagnoses
   a. Pain related to reflux of stomach contents into the esophagus
   b. Diarrhea or constipation related to administration of antacids
7. Client goals
   a. Client will state pain had decreased or subsided
   b. Client will state diarrhea or constipation is controlled with a return to normal bowel habits
8. Nursing interventions—client education
   a. Teach client the medication administration regimen
   b. Instruct client on diet modifications—restrict foods that are spicy, acidic, fatty, contain caffeine or garlic, or cause an increase in symptoms
   c. Instruct client to eat slowly—chew each mouthful 20 to 30 times before swallowing

d. Encourage client to eat small meals every 2 hours

e. Encourage client to prevent stomach distention when eating by not overeating and by avoidance of swallowing air

f. Instruct client to sit erectly for at least 2 hours after meals

g. Teach client to avoid wearing tight clothing around the abdomen

9. Evaluation protocol

a. How will I know that client teaching has been effective?

(1) Client reports appropriate medication administration

(2) Client produces a food diary, indicating that appropriate foods are being eaten

(3) Client identifies specific foods and drinks that aggravate the symptoms

(4) Client reports fewer episodes of heartburn or pain

(5) Client reports a change in wardrobe to decrease tight-fitting abdominal clothing

10. Older adult alert—older clients will have aggressive medical treatment for the prevention of surgery and the complications of impaction or perforation, which occur more commonly in this population

C. Hiatal hernia

1. Definition—protrusion of a portion of the stomach up into the thoracic cavity through an enlarged opening of the diaphragm near the lower esophagus

2. Pathophysiology—muscle support is decreased around the opening in the diaphragm for the esophageal protrusion, and the stomach is permitted to move up through this weakness and into the thoracic cavity. There are two types of hiatal hernia:

a. Type I—sliding hiatal hernia: a portion of the upper stomach and the gastroesophageal junction are displaced upward into the thorax

b. Type II—rolling hiatal hernia: a portion or all of the stomach is displaced upward into the thorax

3. Etiology—aging, congenital muscle weakness, trauma or surgery at the level of the esophageal opening in the diaphragm

4. Incidence—more common in the female population, and the incidence increases with age

5. The remainder of the information about hiatal hernia would be identical to the client with gastroesophageal reflux (refer to pp. 195-197)

D. Peptic ulcer disease

1. Definition—a term used to depict the disorders known as gastric ulcer and duodenal ulcer

a. Gastric ulcer—a break in the mucosa of the stomach

b. Duodenal ulcer—a break in the mucosa of the duodenum

TABLE 6-1	Assessment of Peptic Ulcer Disease	

Assessment Concerns	Gastric	Duodenal
Type of pain	Aching, burning, gnawing	Same
Placement of pain	Epigastric, slightly left	Epigastric, slightly right
Cause of pain	Food may cause pain	Empty stomach may cause pain
What relieves pain	Vomiting may help	Food or antacids
Eating effects	Anorexia and weight loss	Normal appetite
Belching	Occurs	More common
Vomiting	Occurs	Uncommon

2. Pathophysiology
   a. Gastric
      (1) Most found in the distal half of stomach or in area of lower curvature
      (2) Failure of the mucosal defense mechanisms from gastric acid
         (a) Inhibition of prostaglandin production such as that caused by NSAIDs
         (b) Prostaglandins are thought to be responsible for mediating a protective mechanism
   b. Duodenal
      (1) Increased parietal cell mass causes increased acid release
      (2) Increased gastrin stimulates histamine, a powerful secretory mechanism for acid
      (3) Increased emptying time of the stomach increases the acid load in the duodenum and lowers the duodenal pH, leading to an insufficient buffer in the duodenum to protect it
3. Etiology
   a. Gastric—NSAIDs, alcohol, and cigarette smoking inhibit prostaglandin production and thus alter mucosal defense
   b. Duodenal—hypersecretion of hydrochloric acid, secondary to increased gastrin release and a decrease in duodenal pH, which allows pepsin to become more active and damage the mucosa
4. Assessment
   a. Questions to ask (Table 6-1)
      (1) Where is your pain? Point to it.
      (2) Do you have your pain before or after you ingest food?
      (3) Is there anything you can take or do to relieve the pain?
      (4) Have you lost your appetite?
   b. Clinical manifestations are listed in Table 6-2

TABLE 6-2	Symptoms of Gastric and Duodenal Ulcers	
Symptom	**Gastric Ulcers (%)**	**Duodenal Ulcers (%)**
Anorexia	46-57	25-36
Belching*	48	59
Bloating*	55	49
Fatty food intolerance	−	14-72
Heartburn	19	27-59
Nausea	54-70	49-59
Pain		
Epigastric*	67	61-86
Radiation to back*	34	20-31
Frequently severe	68	53
Gnawing*	13	16
Episodic	16	56
At night	32-43	50-88
Increased by food	24	10-40
Food relief	2-48	20-63
Not related to food*	22-53	21-49
Relief with antacids*	36-87	39-86
Vomiting	38-73	25-57
Weight loss	24-61	19-45

Modified from Soll AH, Isenberg JI: Duodenal ulcer disease. In Sleisenger MH, Fordtran JS, editors: *Gastrointestinal Diseases,* ed 3, Philadelphia, 1983, WB Saunders.
*Symptoms are similar for both types of ulcers.

  c. Complications
    (1) Bleeding
      (a) Gastric—manifested as hematemasis: vomiting blood
      (b) Duodenal—seen as melena or tarry stools
    (2) Perforation—penetration of an ulcer through a wall; severe abdominal pain, a boardlike abdomen, emesis, and fever are the most common findings
    (3) Gastric outlet obstruction—ulceration and healing repeatedly cause scar tissue, which obstructs the outlet; more common in ulcers in the pyloric region
  d. Abnormal diagnostic tests
    (1) Esophagogastroduodenoscopy—visualization of an ulcer
    (2) Barium swallow for UGI series—identification of an ulcer on x-ray films
5. Expected medical interventions
  a. Antacids—neutralize acids; 1 hour after meals and at bedtime; up to seven doses daily if meals are eaten frequently
  b. H_2 histamine receptor antagonist

    c. Mucosal healing agents—adhere to ulcer to protect from acid; stimulate release of prostaglandins which increase protection of the mucosal layer

    d. Diet—remove from diet those foods that cause discomfort; frequent small feedings; milk stimulates gastric acid production

    e. Surgery

       (1) Billroth I and Billroth II (Figure 6-1)

       (2) Vagotomy and pyloroplasty—severing parasympathetic stimulation and opening of pylorus to compensate for resultant decrease in gastric emptying (Figures 6-2 and 6-3)

6. Nursing diagnoses

    a. Pain related to action of gastric acid against a gastric or duodenal ulcer

    b. Anxiety related to unknown cause of pain or unknown outcome or chronicity of illness

    c. Alteration in nutrition related to anorexia and nausea as evidenced by weight loss

7. Client goals

    a. Client will state pain has decreased or has been relieved

    b. Client will state anxiety has decreased

    c. Client will demonstrate a weight within 2 pounds of baseline or normal range

8. Nursing interventions

    a. Acute care

       (1) Client with GI bleeding

          (a) Monitor client's vital signs every 15 to 60 minutes until within 10% of baseline and stable

          (b) Evaluate client for postural hypotension and sustained sinus tachycardia

          (c) Prepare client for blood or blood product administration

          (d) Maintain a large-bore IV needle, 16 or 18 gauge

          (e) Monitor I&O

          (f) Monitor urine output every 1 to 2 hours

          (g) Insert NG tube—gastric lavage usually if active bleeding

             (i) Use tap water—best at room temperature

             (ii) Instill 50 to 100 ml, leave in the stomach for several minutes, then allow drainage by gravity or low suction; repeat every 30 to 45 minutes as necessary

             (iii) Measure amount inserted and amount returned for accurate I&O, especially if not equal; that is, 1200 ml returned in 8 hours minus 1000 ml inserted by lavage equals 200 ml of actual gastric output

       (2) Client who has undergone gastric surgery

          (a) Normal postoperative regimen as described in Chapter 9, pp. 311-312

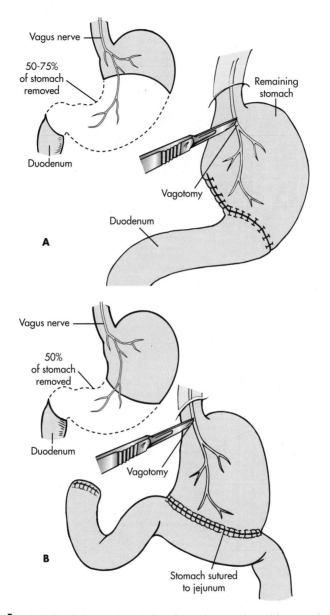

Figure 6-1   **A,** Billroth I procedure (subtotal gastric resection with gastroduodenostomy anastomosis). **B,** Billroth II procedure (subtotal gastric resection with gastrojejunostomy anastomosis). (From Lewis SM, Heitkemper MM, Dirksen SR: *Medical-surgical nursing: assessment and management of clinical problems,* ed 5, St. Louis, 2000, Mosby.)

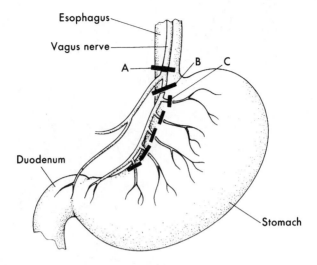

Figure 6-2 Vagotomy procedures. **A,** Truncal. **B,** Selective. **C,** Parietal cell vagotomy. (From Beare PG, Myers JL: *Adult health nursing,* ed 3, St. Louis, 1998, Mosby.)

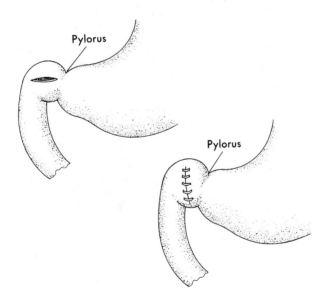

Figure 6-3 Pyloroplasty (Heinke-Mikulicz procedure). The pyloric outlet is widened and a vagotomy done to allow emptying of gastric contents. (From Beare PG, Myers JL: *Adult health nursing,* ed 3, St. Louis, 1998, Mosby.)

Warning!

Flush NG tube **only** as per physician's order—commonly every 4 hours with 30 ml of sterile normal saline. **Do not reposition NG tube.** It sits near the anastomosis, and repositioning it may push through the suture line.

     (b) Evaluate NG drainage—should change from bright red to coffee brown, to bile, to a greenish characteristic over 24 to 48 hours

  b. Home care regarding client education

    (1) *Dumping syndrome*—a complex reaction thought to be secondary to excessively rapid emptying of the gastric contents into the jejunum

      (a) Follows gastric surgeries

      (b) Food in duodenum and jejunum is hypertonic—pulls extravascular fluid toward it, further distending duodenum or jejunum. A *diet high in carbohydrates aggravates the condition.*

      (c) Client has nausea, epigastric pain, vomiting, diarrhea, dizziness, and tachycardia; orthostatic hypotension within 30 to 45 minutes after eating

      (d) Several hours after a meal the client experiences hypoglycemia owing to increased insulin released in response to rapid gastric emptying

      (e) Can be prevented by

        (i) Eating six small meals per day

        (ii) Having meals low in carbohydrates, high in proteins and fats

        (iii) Eating slowly and chewing each bite 20 to 30 times

        (iv) Not drinking fluids with meals because doing so increases gastric emptying

        (v) Lying on the left side for 30 to 60 minutes after a meal to inhibit emptying time

    (2) Specific medication regimen

      (a) Sulcralfate (Carafate)—take on an empty stomach 1 hour before meals and at bedtime

      (b) Antacids inactivate Carafate; therefore do not take them with and 30 minutes before or after taking Carafate

9. Evaluation protocol

  a. How do I know that my interventions were effective?

    (1) Vital signs are stable, plus or minus 10% of baseline

    (2) Urine output is acceptable, at least 30 ml/hr

        (3) Gastric lavage has been effective as indicated by decreased bloody drainage

        (4) Client's NG drainage after surgery returns to greenish drainage within 48 hours

        (5) No bleeding episodes have occurred

    b. Which criteria will I use to change my interventions?

        (1) Vital signs not within plus or minus 10% of baseline

        (2) Urine output less than 30 ml/hr

        (3) The client experiences bloody drainage for over 24 hours after surgery

    c. How will I know that my client teaching has been effective?

        (1) Client reports no episodes of dumping syndrome

        (2) Client reports medication administration is appropriate and effective

  10. Older adult alert

    a. Many drugs prescribed for older adults, such as NSAIDs, can predispose them to peptic ulcers

    b. Older clients may not have early manifestations of peptic ulcer disease and therefore may present only when life-threatening manifestations occur, such as GI hemorrhage

E. Cholecystitis and cholelithiasis

  1. Definition—inflammation of the gallbladder; presence of calculi in the gallbladder

  2. Pathophysiology—stone blocks bile drainage from gallbladder. Gallbladder becomes inflamed and bile, being an irritant, causes inflammatory changes in the walls of the gallbladder.

  3. Etiology—most cases of cholecystitis are caused by gallstones of which there are two types

    a. Cholesterol stones—occur when bile becomes supersaturated with cholesterol

    b. Pigment stones—of unknown origin

  4. Incidence—more common in females. More common in pregnant women or within a few months of delivery. Female sex hormones may play a role in the formation of gallstones. Increased incidence after menopause.

  5. Assessment

    a. Questions to ask

        (1) Are you experiencing pain? Point to your pain.

        (2) Does your pain coincide with food intake? If yes, any specific foods or types of food?

        (3) Have you been running a fever?

        (4) Have you experienced nausea, vomiting, or diarrhea?

    b. Clinical manifestations

        (1) Right upper quadrant pain—may radiate to right scapular area or shoulder

        (2) Pain follows ingestion of a high-fat meal

        (3) Pain may be accompanied by anorexia, nausea, vomiting, and flatulence

        (4) If there is a stone lodged in the common bile duct, there may be mild jaundice, clay-colored stools, and tea-colored urine

    c. Abnormal laboratory findings

        (1) CBC—elevated WBC count

        (2) Serum bilirubin—may be elevated if there is an obstruction of common bile duct

    d. Abnormal diagnostic test results

        (1) Ultrasonography of the gallbladder—identifies gallstones and thickened wall of gallbladder

        (2) Oral cholecystogram—identifies gallstones

        (3) Intravenous cholangiography—identifies stones in the bile duct

6. Expected medical interventions

    a. Fat reduction in the diet

    b. Dissolution of gallstones with medication—chenodeoxycholic acid (CDCA)

    c. Lithotripsy—done as outpatient

    d. Cholecystectomy—if stones are removed from the common bile duct or if the common bile duct is explored, a T-tube must be inserted (Figure 6-4). Hospitalization usually is required for 3 to 5 days.

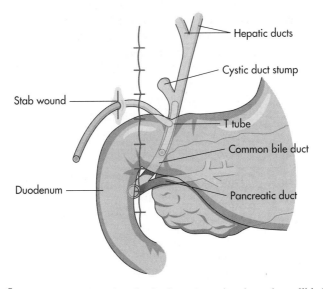

Figure 6-4 Placement of T-tube. Cystic duct stump is where the gallbladder was removed. (From Beare PG, Myers JL: *Adult health nursing,* ed 3, St. Louis, 1998, Mosby.)

    e. Laparoscopic cholecystectomy—done either on an outpatient basis or in the hospital; if in the hospital, the stay is from 24 to 48 hours

7. Nursing diagnoses

    a. Pain related to inflammation of the gallbladder or to the effects of surgery

    b. Ineffective breathing pattern related to pain associated with cholecystectomy incision

    c. Risk for fluid volume deficit related to nausea and vomiting

8. Client goals

    a. Client will state pain has decreased or has been relieved

    b. Client will take 10 deep breaths every 1 to 2 hours and have clear breath sounds

    c. Client will have appropriate fluid volume as evidenced by input equal to output within plus or minus 300 ml

9. Nursing interventions

    a. Acute care

        (1) Acute cholecystitis

            (a) Frequent vital signs as indicated by status

            (b) Analgesics are given for pain

            (c) NPO status is maintained

            (d) If present, NG patency is maintained

            (e) IV line is maintained and fluid administered as ordered to replace lost fluids

            (f) Preoperative teaching is done if surgery is planned

            (g) I&O are monitored

        (2) Postoperative cholecystectomy—open cholecystectomy

            (a) Same interventions as listed above

            (b) If present, T-tube care required as follows

                (i) Prevent kinking

                (ii) Keep bile drainage bag below the level of the insertion site

                (iii) Change dressing as needed—bile, having a very high pH, is irritating to the skin

                (iv) Never irrigate the tube

                (v) Do not allow traction on the tube

                (vi) Measure drainage every shift

                (vii) Clamp tube when ordered during meals to determine patency of common bile duct. If the client has nausea or vomiting, unclamp the tube. This means that some edema is probably still present.

            (c) Drain and recharge continuous suction device such as a Jackson Pratt drainage tube—empty when half full or every shift; measure drainage; recharge after emptying

            (d) Have client turn, cough, and breathe deeply every two hours, which is best achieved with adequate pain relief and use of an incentive spirometer. Atelectasis is a common problem postoperatively owing to the close proximity of the incision to the rib cage.

(e) Administer meperidine hydrochloride (Demerol), which is the drug of choice. Morphine can cause spasm of the sphincter of the common bile duct and result in increased pain.

b. Home care regarding client education

(1) Postoperative diet—clients have no dietary restrictions after discharge unless something they eat bothers them

(2) Instructions about how to care for incision if traditional surgery and for puncture wounds if laparoscopic surgery

(3) Instruct client on the findings that are indicative of wound infection and when to call physician

10. Evaluation protocol

a. How do I know that my interventions were effective?

(1) Vital signs are within plus or minus 10% of baseline

(2) Client states pain is relieved

(3) NG is patent with minimal drainage

(4) I&O is balanced; input equals output within plus or minus 300 ml

(5) T-tube is patent and draining approximately 200 ml/day of yellow-brown drainage

(6) Skin around T-tube is intact, without breakdown

(7) Client is turning, coughing, and deep breathing every 2 hours using incentive spirometer; lung sounds are clear

b. Which criteria will I use to change my interventions?

(1) Client's vital signs are not within plus or minus 10% of baseline

(2) Client states pain is unrelieved

(3) NG drainage has decreased or stopped

(4) I&O is not within plus or minus 300 ml

(5) Skin around the T-tube is red and edematous

(6) No drainage from the T-tube is observed, or the drainage is a color other than yellowish-brown

(7) Basilar breath sounds are diminished

c. How will I know that my client teaching has been effective?

(1) Client states a regular diet is being followed without gastric upset

(2) Client states the changes in the wound that should be called to physician's attention

(3) Client demonstrates a wound that is clean and dry without evidence of infection

11. Older adult alert

a. The incidence of gallbladder disease increases with age and should be suspected with new onset of right upper quadrant pain

   b. Cancer of the gallbladder is a disorder of older adults. Clients must be carefully evaluated.
F. **Pancreatitis**
   1. Definition—inflammation of the pancreas
      a. Acute—sudden onset
      b. Chronic—long-term process with a continuous course of symptoms
   2. Pathophysiology
      a. Inflammation of the pancreas causes the pancreatic ducts to close off
      b. Eating stimulates the pancreas to release enzymes
      c. Enzymes become trapped in the pancreatic duct, and the duct eventually ruptures
      d. Rupture of the duct causes release of pancreatic enzymes into the pancreas
      e. Enzymes begin to autodigest the pancreas; hemorrhage can result
      f. Necrosis of the pancreas can occur
      g. Walls are formed around this cystic fluid and debris, and pseudocysts are formed, which may lead to abscess formation
   3. Etiology—biliary disease, alcohol abuse, trauma, obstruction of the pancreatic duct or duodenum
   4. Assessment
      a. Questions to ask
         (1) Are you having pain? Point to where your pain is located.
         (2) On a scale of 0 to 10 where would you rate your pain?
         (3) Have you had any nausea or vomiting?
         (4) Have you noticed that your abdomen is swollen?
         (5) Have you been running a fever?
      b. Clinical manifestations
         (1) Epigastric pain—may be severe
         (2) Hypotension and sinus tachycardia
         (3) Intractable vomiting
         (4) Abdominal distention
         (5) Low-grade fever
         (6) Steatorrhea—fatty, foul smelling stools; more with chronic type
      c. Abnormal laboratory findings
         (1) Serum amylase elevated
         (2) Serum lipase elevated
         (3) Calcium—low
         (4) CBC—elevated WBC
         (5) Serum glucose elevated if endocrine function is affected
      d. Abnormal diagnostic test results
         (1) Abdominal ultrasonography—pancreatic edema and pancreatic fluid collection
         (2) CT scan—pancreatic edema, necrosis, fluid collections, abscesses, and pseudocysts

5. Expected medical interventions
   a. Vital signs are stabilized by use of monitoring lines, with instillation of fluids commonly at high rates of 150 to 250 ml/hr and blood or blood products such as plasmanate
   b. Pain relief is provided—meperidine hydrochloride (Demerol) is the drug of choice. Current controversy whether morphine causes complications such as spasm of the sphincter of Oddi (Banks, 1998).
   c. Insulin is provided for hyperglycemia
   d. Sodium bicarbonate is given for metabolic acidosis of pH less than 7.10
   e. NPO status is maintained; NG tube to decrease stimulation of pancreatic enzyme release
   f. Hyperalimentation if NPO is maintained for long periods
   g. Surgery is performed for ruptured pseudocysts or hemorrhage
   h. Antibiotics are not used to treat pancreatic inflammation. Antibiotics are usually given to treat secondary infections.
6. Nursing diagnoses
   a. Pain related to inflammatory process of the pancreas
   b. Fluid volume deficit related to blood loss and fluid shifts
   c. Decreased CO related to blood loss and fluid shifts
   d. Altered nutrition (less than body requirements) related to nausea and vomiting
7. Client goals
   a. Client will state pain is relieved or decreased
   b. Client will maintain vital signs within plus or minus 10% of baseline and appropriate I&O
   c. Client will demonstrate appropriate CO as evidenced by BP and HR within plus or minus 10% of normal baseline
   d. Client will maintain weight within 10% of normal baseline
8. Nursing interventions
   a. Acute care
      (1) Vital signs are taken at least every 2 hours until within plus or minus 10% of normal, or more often if not within set parameters
      (2) Pain medication is administered as needed
      (3) IV access is maintained, and IV fluid administration is monitored
      (4) Electrolyte balance and acid-base balance are monitored
      (5) NPO status is maintained. NG tube patency is maintained, and drainage is evaluated. pH is tested, and antacids are administered as per physician orders.
      (6) Total parenteral nutrition (TPN) is maintained as ordered (Box 6-1)
      (7) If in place drainage tubes or sump tubes are monitored; drainage and sites are evaluated

Box 6-1
Total Parenteral Nutrition (TPN)

Definition

TPN is a method for nutritionally sustaining clients who cannot or should not ingest, digest, or absorb nutrients. TPN solutions consist of an individually calculated combination of amino acids, glucose, minerals, vitamins, and trace elements. Lipid emulsions are frequently given daily by IV piggyback to make the feedings complete.

Administration

TPN may be delivered through either a peripheral or central vein. Peripheral delivery necessitates excellent venous access, and glucose concentrations are limited to 10%. Solutions of 15% to 35% glucose may be administered centrally. TPN is associated with significant potential risks of infection and metabolic imbalance and necessitates careful monitoring.

Nursing Interventions

Monitor insertion site; provide site care and dressing changes according to institution policy.

Administer TPN solutions through inline filters; *lipids do not require filters.*

Weigh client daily and maintain records.

Assess for fluid overload.

Monitor laboratory values daily.

Avoid drawing blood or administering other fluids and medications through TPN catheter.

Monitor blood glucose levels throughout therapy; provide sliding-scale regular insulin coverage as needed.

Encourage active exercise as tolerated to support the production of muscle rather than fat cells.

Monitor respiratory rate; excess carbohydrates increase carbon dioxide production and may cause tachypnea.

Instruct client to use Valsalva maneuver and clamp tube during central line tubing changes to prevent air emboli.

Carefully monitor infusion times and do not increase drip rate more than 10% of ordered rate to catch up if behind.

Adapted from *AJN/Mosby nursing board review,* ed 9, St Louis, 1994, Mosby.

b. Home care regarding client education
  (1) Low-fat, high-calorie, high-carbohydrate diet
  (2) No alcohol and no caffeine

⚠ Warning!

If hyperalimentation drip rate is stopped suddenly, that is, if the IV comes out, observe for a severe decrease in serum glucose level within 1 to 2 hours. If the rate is increased too quickly, observe for severe increase in serum glucose level within 1 to 2 hours with a possible hyperosmolar diuresis effect for a significantly increased urine output.

   (3) Alcohol rehabilitation if alcohol consumption is the source of pancreatitis
   (4) Pancreatic enzyme administration if needed
   (5) Insulin administration if continued endocrine function is impaired
   (6) Medical follow-up
9. Evaluation protocol
   a. How do I know that my interventions were effective?
      (1) Vital signs are within set parameters
      (2) Pain is controlled
      (3) I&O is balanced, with input equal to output within plus or minus 300 ml
      (4) Amylase and calcium levels are within acceptable ranges
      (5) NG is patent with appropriate drainage; pH is maintained with antacid administration
      (6) TPN is administered without complications
   b. Which criteria will I use to change my interventions?
      (1) Client's vital signs are not within plus or minus 10% of baseline
      (2) Client's pain is unrelieved or increased
      (3) Client's I&O, enzyme levels, and electrolytes are out of balance
      (4) Client is experiencing complications of TPN—central line infection, hyperglycemia, or fluid overload
   c. How will I know that my client teaching has been effective?
      (1) Client produces a diet diary with documentation of appropriate food intake
      (2) Client discusses alcohol rehabilitation process positively
      (3) Client demonstrates appropriate insulin administration
      (4) Client demonstrates appropriate pancreatic enzyme administration
10. Older adult alert
    a. Older clients may not have the physical stamina to survive the life-threatening nature of pancreatitis
    b. Older clients have decreased production of pancreatic enzymes, which may be valuable in decreasing the occurrence of the complications of pancreatitis

G. Cirrhosis

1. Definition—a disorder that results in widespread fibrosis of the liver and subsequent dysfunction
2. Pathophysiology—cirrhosis is the outcome of a liver insult
   a. The liver insult leaves it with scar tissue and destroyed hepatocytes, which are responsible for bile formation. This function will be decreased and eventually lost.
   b. Blood flow through the liver is impeded by massive scar tissue. Blood backs up into the portal vein and then eventually into the

veins that empty into the portal vein (mesenteric veins, pancreatic and splenic veins), leading to portal hypertension.

c. Through the process of inflammation and injury, the liver becomes inflamed and enlarged in the early stages of insult

d. In the later stages the liver becomes hard and nodular

e. Through these changes the liver loses its ability to perform necessary functions, and the client suffers the consequences of hepatic insufficiency

f. When blood cannot enter the portal vein because of high pressure, collateral circulation develops around the liver to return blood flow to the superior vena cava. The vessels that comprise the collateral circulation have thin walls that are unable to withstand the high pressures exerted on them by the portal hypertension, and they rupture—esophageal bleeding.

g. High pressure from portal vein causes increased pressure in the veins dumping blood into the portal vein. These veins dilate, and venous pressure pushes plasma out of the vascular space and into the extravascular space. The most common manifestation of this is ascites.

h. The liver no longer is able to detoxify ammonia. The ammonia levels increase and become toxic to the brain, which is called *hepatic encephalopathy.*

i. Damaged hepatocytes are unable to produce albumin. Vascular fluid is normally held in the vascular space by the osmotic pull of albumin. Without albumin, vascular fluid will leave the vascular space, causing generalized interstitial edema, *anasarca.*

3. Etiology—alcohol ingestion, hepatitis, chemical or drug ingestion
4. Incidence—more common in the male population
5. Assessment
   a. Questions to ask
      (1) Have you been feeling tired lately?
      (2) Have you experienced loss of appetite or nausea and vomiting?
      (3) Have you experienced any discomfort in the right upper side of your abdomen?
      (4) Have you noticed a change in your skin color?
   b. Clinical manifestations
      (1) Early findings—may not seek medical attention
         (a) Fatigue
         (b) Weakness
         (c) Anorexia
         (d) Nausea, vomiting, and diarrhea
         (e) Epigastric or right upper quadrant abdominal discomfort
         (f) Flatulence
      (2) Progressive findings
         (a) Jaundice
         (b) Bleeding tendencies—bruising and bleeding from gums

        (c) GI bleeding

        (d) Frequent infections

        (e) Menstrual irregularities in females

        (f) Gynomastia and impotence in males

        (g) *Spider angioma* on the skin, which is an elevated red dot from which thin blood vessels radiate in a starlike pattern

        (h) Ascites

    (3) Hepatic encephalopathy

        (a) *Asterixis*—flapping tremor of the hands

        (b) Drowsiness, stupor, and hepatic coma

  c. Abnormal laboratory findings

    (1) ALT elevated

    (2) AST elevated

    (3) LDH elevated

    (4) PT elevated

    (5) PTT elevated

    (6) Bilirubin (total and direct) elevated

    (7) Serum albumin decreased

    (8) Sodium, potassium, and chloride decreased

    (9) H&H decreased

  d. Abnormal diagnostic tests

    (1) Paracentesis—done to confirm presence of ascites; also used for evacuation of fluid to ease breathing effort

    (2) Abdominal ultrasonography—presence of ascites

    (3) EGD—presence of esophageal varices

    (4) EEG—abnormal tracing in the event of encephalopathy

6. Expected medical interventions

  a. Elimination of cause—alcohol, drugs, or chemicals

  b. High-protein, high-calorie diet. Note: Decrease protein in the event of encephalopathy.

  c. Sodium and fluid restriction for ascites

  d. LeVeen peritoneovenous shunt for reinfusion of ascites (Figure 6-5)

  e. For bleeding esophageal varices

    (1) NPO, NG intubation

    (2) Room temperature saline lavage of NG tube

    (3) IV fluid and blood replacement

    (4) Balloon tamponade of bleeding varices with a Sengstaken-Blakemore tube (Figure 6-6)

    (5) IV vasopressin to vasoconstrict arteries and decrease bleeding

    (6) Endoscopic injection of sclerotherapy—injection of sclerosing agent into varices to cause inflammation followed by fibrosis. This procedure prevents and controls bleeding.

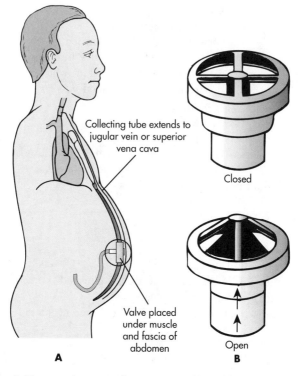

Figure 6-5 LaVeen continuous peritoneovenous shunt. **A,** Collecting tube. **B,** Valve in closed and open positions. (From Lewis SM, Heitkemper MM, Dirksen SR: *Medical-surgical nursing: assessment and management of clinical problems,* ed 5, St. Louis, 2000, Mosby.)

    f. Portacaval shunt—decreases portal hypertension; diversion of blood from portal vein to inferior vena cava

    g. Bowel cleansing with lactulose and neomycin sulfate (Neo-Diloderm) to prevent or minimize ammonia production in the bowel and thus decrease or prevent hepatic encephalopathy

7. Nursing diagnoses

    a. Ineffective breathing pattern related to pressure on the diaphragm from enlarged liver and the presence of ascites

    b. Pain related to enlarged, inflamed liver and spasms of the bile ducts

    c. Altered nutrition (less than body requirements) related to nausea, anorexia, and vomiting

    d. Activity intolerance related to fatigue that is secondary to anemia

    e. Risk for injury (hemorrhage) related to decreased clotting factors

8. Client goals

    a. Client will maintain RR of 20 to 24 per minute without use of accessory muscles

    b. Client will state pain is decreased or improved

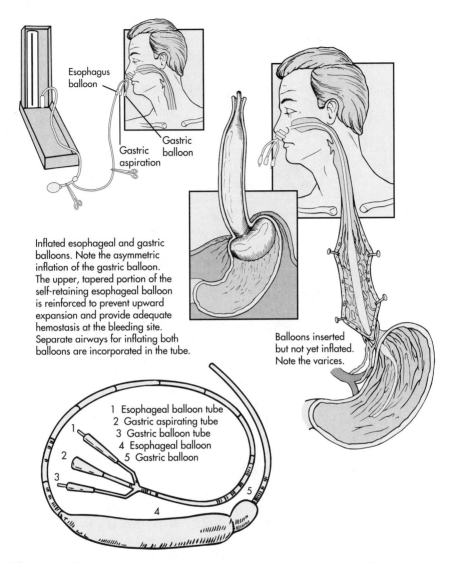

Esophagus
balloon

Gastric
balloon

Gastric
aspiration

Inflated esophageal and gastric
balloons. Note the asymmetric
inflation of the gastric balloon.
The upper, tapered portion of the
self-retaining esophageal balloon
is reinforced to prevent upward
expansion and provide adequate
hemostasis at the bleeding site.
Separate airways for inflating both
balloons are incorporated in the tube.

Balloons inserted
but not yet inflated.
Note the varices.

1 Esophageal balloon tube
2 Gastric aspirating tube
3 Gastric balloon tube
4 Esophageal balloon
5 Gastric balloon

Figure 6-6   Esophageal tamponade accomplished with Sengstaken-Blakemore tube.
(From Lewis SM, Heitkemper MM, Dirksen SR: *Medical-surgical nursing: assessment and management
of clinical problems,* ed 5, St. Louis, 2000, Mosby.)

    c. Client will maintain baseline weight plus or minus 1 kg
    d. Client will increase activity by 10% each day without increased
       fatigue as stated by client
    e. Client will show no evidence of bleeding or bruising
  9. Nursing interventions
    a. Acute care—client regimen
      (1) Rest with elimination of substances toxic to the liver such
         as sedatives and acetaminophen

(2) Nutritional support for weight and energy maintenance

(3) An increase in activity by 10% each day (e.g., each day, 10 more feet walked, 5 more steps climbed, and so on)

(4) Avoidance of infections and contact with others who have an infection

(5) Evaluation of all stools and urine for blood as well as any other bodily excrement

(6) Prevention of any trauma that could cause bruising or bleeding; avoid IM injection

(7) Care of the client with bleeding esophageal varices

   (a) Monitoring of vital signs every 5 to 15 minutes until within plus or minus 10% of normal; temperature taken every 4 hours and PRN

   (b) Large-bore IVs for fluid and blood administration

   (c) NG lavage with room temperature saline to clear stomach of clots and slow bleeding

   (d) Comparison of amount of lavage inserted to amount drained to evaluate fluid loss

(8) Monitoring of the Sengstaken-Blakemore tube

   (a) Awareness of the pressure in each balloon, and use of the correct amount of traction if ordered

   (b) Insurance that only the ordered balloons are inflated. Many physicians will attempt to control bleeding with only the gastric balloon inflated owing to the risk of airway obstruction with the esophageal balloon inflated.

> ⚠️ **Warning!**
>
> When caring for a client with a Sengstaken-Blakemore tube with the esophageal balloon inflated, **evaluate the client's airway frequently.** The upward displacement of the tube could cause airway obstruction. Have scissors at the bedside to quickly deflate the balloon by cutting the airport of the esophageal balloon in the event of airway obstruction. Remember that clients are unable to swallow their saliva when either of the balloons is inflated.

(9) Accurate I&O, daily weight

(10) Monitor abdominal girth; measure at least every 8 hours

(11) Evaluate electrolyte balances

(12) Monitor intake of dietary protein

b. Home care regarding client education

   (1) Teach the client to avoid precipitating factors, that is, substances that could be toxic to the liver or require detoxification by the liver

    (2) Instruct the client to meet dietary requirements: enough protein to build tissue but not so much as to cause encephalopathy, low sodium, and fluid restriction

    (3) Teach the client which changes should be brought to attention of physician

10. Evaluation protocol

  a. How do I know that my interventions were effective?

    (1) Airway is patent and unobstructed

    (2) Vital signs are within plus or minus 10% of baseline

    (3) Fluid balance is adequate with input equal to output within plus or minus 300 ml

    (4) Urine output is at least 30 ml/hr

    (5) Abdominal girth is within 1 inch of baseline

    (6) No evidence exists of trauma or bruising to skin or extremities

    (7) Urine, stool, and excrement are free of blood

    (8) No evidence exists of infection—WBC within acceptable parameters

    (9) Rest and activity are balanced; ambulatory activity is increasing by 30 minutes per day

    (10) No substance has been ingested that is toxic to the liver

  b. Which criteria will I use to change my interventions?

    (1) Obstructed airway

    (2) Vital signs not within plus or minus 10% of baseline

    (3) Findings indicative of infection

    (4) Findings indicative of bleeding, bruising, or trauma to the tissues

    (5) I&O out of balance

    (6) Abdominal girth increasing in size by half an inch each time it is measured

  c. How will I know that my client teaching has been effective?

    (1) Diet diary indicative of correct food choices

    (2) Client indicates which substances to avoid

    (3) Client is able to identify the changes in health status that would necessitate calling physician

11. Older adult alert

  a. Older adults have a higher occurrence of CHF and ingestion of multiple hepatotoxic drugs

  b. Concerns with clients over the age of 50 are a decrease in liver size, decrease in storage capacity, decreased ability to synthesize protein, and potential decreased hepatic blood flow from a decrease in CO

H. Hepatitis

1. Definition—an inflammation of the liver; may be acute or chronic

2. Pathophysiology—virus invades the liver through the portal tracts and causes inflammation of the liver

  a. Liver parenchyma cells are destroyed

  b. Hepatocytes are destroyed

TABLE 6-3	Hepatitis Etiology, Transmission, and Incubation	
Hepatitis	**Transmission**	**Incubation period**
A	Feces, contaminated water and food	2-6 wk
B	Parenteral, sexual, perinatal	2 wk-6 mo
C	Same as hepatitis B	5-10 wk
D	Complication of hepatitis B	2-26 wk
E	Fecal, oral	2-9 wk

    c. Leukocytes invade the liver
    d. Liver enzymes are released, and liver function is decreased
    e. Hepatocytes are removed and replaced with scar tissue
    f. Cirrhosis or chronic hepatitis can be the result
3. Etiology—can be caused by virus, bacteria, hepatotoxins, or drugs (Table 6-3)
4. Incidence—over 70,000 cases per year
5. Assessment
    a. Questions to ask
        (1) Have you had symptoms that have made you feel as if you have the flu?
        (2) Have you been feeling tired and weak?
        (3) Have you been noticing a loss of appetite?
        (4) Have you noticed a change in your skin color?
        (5) Has your urine become dark in color?
        (6) Are your bowel movements a gray color?
    b. Clinical manifestations
        (1) Preicteric stage (prodromal stage)—lasts 1 week
            (a) Flu-like symptoms
            (b) Malaise
            (c) Weakness
            (d) Low-grade fever
            (e) Cough, chills, and rhinitis
            (f) Anorexia
            (g) Nausea, vomiting, and diarrhea
            (h) Dyspepsia
            (i) Dull pain over right upper abdominal quadrant
            (j) Hepatomegaly
            (k) Lymphadenopathy
            (l) Urticaria
            (m) Weight loss
        (2) Icteric stage—lasts 2 to 6 weeks; most contagious stage
            (a) Jaundice—liver cannot metabolize bilirubin
            (b) Dark-amber-colored urine—bilirubin excreted by the kidneys instead of the stool

    (c) Clay-colored stools—no bilirubin in the stool to induce a brown color

    (d) Pruritus

    (e) Fatigue and weakness continue

    (f) Abdominal pain continues

    (g) Abnormal laboratory results are found

   (3) Posticteric stage—lasts 2 to 6 weeks

    (a) Client remains quite fatigued

    (b) Liver size decreases as do liver enzymes

    (c) Symptoms slowly recede

  c. Abnormal laboratory findings

   (1) Direct bilirubin elevated

   (2) ALT and AST elevated

   (3) Blood glucose may be decreased

   (4) PT may be elevated

   (5) LDH elevated

   (6) Stool tests positive for hepatitis A

6. Expected medical interventions

  a. Vaccination against hepatitis B in high-risk clients or health care personnel

  b. Hepatitis B immune globulin for clients who have been in transmission contact with another person

  c. Immune globulin for clients traveling to areas of high levels for hepatitis A or for clients who have been exposed to hepatitis A

  d. Bed rest

  e. No substances are to be administered that are toxic to the liver such as acetaminophen or alcohol

  f. Findings that occur are treated

7. Nursing diagnoses

  a. Pain related to inflammation of the liver

  b. Fatigue related to increased metabolic demands of the body

  c. Fluid volume deficit related to vomiting and diarrhea

  d. Diarrhea related to inability of the liver to metabolize food appropriately

8. Client goals

  a. Client will state pain has decreased or is relieved

  b. Client will tolerate longer periods of activity without increased fatigue

  c. Client will have input equal to output within plus or minus 300 ml

  d. Client will have decreased episodes of diarrhea within 24 hours of initial therapy

9. Nursing interventions

  a. Acute care

   (1) Maintain universal precautions

   (2) Balance rest and activity to meet client needs

(3) Turn, cough, and deep breathing along with leg exercises to prevent the complications of bed rest

(4) Encourage the use of electric razors and soft toothbrushes to decrease risk of bleeding

(5) Monitor nutrition—high-carbohydrate low-fat diet

(6) Give antiemetic agents before meals to decrease nausea and increase nutrition

(7) Increase fluid intake to 3000 ml/day

(8) Avoid soap and harsh linens if client suffers from pruritus

(9) Administer antihistamines if pruritus is severe

b. Home care regarding client education

(1) Instruct client not to share personal items or meal items

(2) Instruct client that sexual intercourse should be avoided during infectious period

(3) Teach client to launder clothes separately

(4) Instruct client to use separate bathroom facilities or cleanse shared bathrooms with chlorine solution daily

(5) Instruct client to abstain from alcohol for at least 1 year

(6) Teach client that checkups with physician must be scheduled every 2 to 3 months for at least 1 year

(7) Inform health care persons of illness for up to 1 year after treatment

10. Evaluation protocol

a. How do I know that my interventions were effective?

(1) Is client feeling more rested or less fatigued?

(2) Is client having any difficulty breathing? Is client taking deep breaths every 2 hours? Is client flexing ankles at least 3 times an hour?

(3) Has client noticed any blood in urine or stool, or blood when brushing teeth?

(4) Has client's feeling of nausea diminished?

(5) Is client's itchy skin feeling better?

b. Which criteria will I use to change my interventions?

(1) Fatigue is more pronounced

(2) Atelectasis, pneumonia, or phlebitis has developed

(3) Bruising or bleeding of gums is evident

(4) Nausea is preventing maintenance of nutritional intake

(5) Pruritus is intractable

c. How will I know that my client teaching has been effective?

(1) Client states the use of separate bathroom and eating utensils and is washing clothes separately

(2) Client states the avoidance of all alcohol products

(3) Client indicates the avoidance of sexual intercourse at present

(4) Client indicates scheduling of a monthly appointment with physician

(5) Client indicates the conveyance of the fact that he or she has this illness to health care providers

11. Older adult alert

    a. Older adult clients are at great risk for complications related to their illness and must be monitored carefully

    b. Older adults have a decreased CO as well as decreased respiratory efficiency. These factors open older adults to many complications during times of illness, such as hepatitis.

I. Inflammatory bowel disease

1. Definition—chronic inflammatory disorder of the small or large bowel, or both

    a. Two disorders

        (1) Ulcerative colitis—chronic inflammatory process of the mucosa of the colon, usually the descending colon, and the rectum

        (2) Crohn's disease or regional enteritis—chronic inflammatory disorder of any area of the GI tract from the mouth to the anus

2. Pathophysiology (Table 6-4)

    a. Ulcerative colitis—affects only the large bowel and only the mucosa. It begins at the rectosigmoid area, moves up the descending to the transverse colon, and then moves over to the right side of the colon, the ascending colon. Small abscesses form in the walls of the colon and progress to large purulent ulcerations. Stools eventually will be liquid and full of pus and blood from the ulcerated areas.

    b. Crohn's disease—affects any area of the bowel and all layers. It usually starts in the ileum and moves toward the left colon. Granulomas found initially in the lymph follicles of the mucosa eventually ulcerate. The lymphatics are destroyed, and edema and inflammation result. Fibrosis and serositis occur as well as the development of fistulas from the bowel to other areas of the bowel or adjacent structures.

    c. Toxic megacolon—life-threatening complication of both disorders, though more often a complication of ulcerative colitis. Destruction of circular and longitudinal muscles causes the colon to dilate. The walls become thin, and rupture is imminent.

3. Etiology—genetic, environmental, microbial, and immunologic as well as psychological factors have been implicated in these disorders

4. Incidence—more common in the 20- to 30-year-old age group, and more common in the higher socioeconomic level

    5. Assessment

       a. Questions to ask

          (1) Do you ever have rectal bleeding or bloody diarrhea?

          (2) Do you ever experience abdominal cramping?

          (3) Have you been losing weight?

          (4) Do you ever feel as if you must strain to have a bowel movement? *(intestinal tenesmus)*

       b. Clinical manifestations—dependent on pathologic findings

          (1) Ulcerative colitis—(see Table 6-4)

          (2) Crohn's disease—(see Table 6-4)

TABLE 6-4   Comparison of Ulcerative Colitis and Crohn's Disease

	Ulcerative Colitis	Crohn's Disease
Usual area affected	Left colon, rectum	Distal ileum, right colon
Extent of involvement	Diffuse areas, contiguous	Segmental areas, noncontiguous
Inflammation	Mostly mucosal	Transmural
Mucosal appearance	Ulcerations	Cobblestone effect, granulomas
Character of stools	Blood present	No blood present
	No fat	Steatorrhea
	Frequent liquid stools	3-5 semisoft stools daily
Abdominal pain	May occur, mild	Right lower quadrant pain, cramping
Abdominal mass	No	Common in right lower quadrant
Complications	Toxic megacolon	Fistulas
	Pseudopolyps	Perianal disease
	Hemorrhoids	Strictures
	Hemorrhage	Abscesses
		Perforation
Extraintestinal	Anemia	Anemia
manifestations	Erythema nodosum	Malabsorption of fat and
	Pyoderma gangrenosum	fat-soluble vitamins
	Arthritis	Arthritis
	Liver disease	Hepatobiliary disease
	Iritis, conjunctivitis	Iritis, conjunctivitis
	Stomatitis	Renal stones, obstructive
	Thrombophlebitis	uropathy
Reasons for surgery	Poor response to medical therapy	Presence of complications
	Complications	
Response to surgery	Curative	Noncurative, high recurrence rate

Modified from Phipps WJ, Sands JK, Marek JR: *Medical-surgical nursing: concepts and clinical practice,* ed 6, St Louis, 1999, Mosby.

(3) Toxic megacolon
    (a) Severe abdominal pain
    (b) Abdominal distention
    (c) Fever
    (d) Leukocytosis
    (e) Tachycardia

c. Abnormal laboratory findings
    (1) CBC—H&H may be low as well as RBCs
    (2) Stool for blood—positive during period of active bleeding

d. Abnormal diagnostic test results
    (1) Upper GI series with barium (in Crohn's disease)—shows ulcerations and fistula formations, "cobblestoning" of mucosa, and narrowing
    (2) Barium enema—shows ulcerations and mucosal irregularities in both disorders
    (3) Endoscopy—shows inflamed mucosa; cobblestone appearance of mucosa in Crohn's disease, and granular appearance in ulcerative colitis
    (4) CT scan—shows mesenteric abnormalities and thickening of the colon wall
    (5) Biopsy—shows diffuse inflammation and rules out malignancy

6. Expected medical interventions
  a. Administration of IV fluids and possibly TPN during acute exacerbations
  b. Blood administration as needed
  c. Maintenance of regular diet. Client should eliminate foods that exacerbate symptoms; high residue foods may cause exacerbated symptoms.
  d. Take the four A's approach to medication—anti-inflammatory, antibacterial, antidiarrheal, antianxiety, along with immunosuppressive drugs are utilized
  e. Surgical intervention as necessary, that is, when all medical regimens have failed or a life-threatening illness has occurred

7. Nursing diagnoses
  a. Altered nutrition (less than body requirements) related to increased peristalsis and poor absorption
  b. Diarrhea related to inflammatory process of the bowel
  c. Risk for fluid volume deficit related to frequent diarrhea

8. Client goals
  a. Client will maintain baseline weight within 1 to 2 kg
  b. Client will have decreased episodes of diarrhea by two bowel movements per day
  c. Client will demonstrate input equal to output within plus or minus 300 ml

9. Nursing interventions
    a. Postoperative care
       See routine postoperative care in Chapter 9, pp. 311-312
       (1) Maintain NG suction—irrigate as per orders
       (2) Begin ostomy care—ileostomy drainage may begin almost immediately after surgery
       (3) Protect skin from the alkaline effluent from the ileostomy, which is corrosive, by using an appliance with a protective barrier such as stoma adhesive
       (4) Evaluate stoma
           (a) Immediately after surgery the stoma may be pale
           (b) When the client's body temperature warms, the stoma may be red, ruddy, and slightly edematous
           (c) Within several weeks the stoma should be pink with no edema
           (d) Any change should be reported to the physician immediately
    b. Home care regarding client education
       (1) Self-care of the stoma
       (2) Changes in the stoma that must be reported to physician
           (a) Gray, blue, or bright red stoma
           (b) Bleeding spots on the stoma
           (c) Swollen stoma
       (3) Diet—no special diet is required but have the client remove food items he or she finds irritating
       (4) Fluids—encourage the client to drink fluids. Findings associated with fluid and electrolyte imbalances are a major issue in clients with an ileostomy.
10. Evaluation protocol
    a. How do I know that my interventions were effective?
       (1) NG drainage decreases as bowel sounds return
       (2) Stoma remains pink and above the level of the skin
       (3) Skin surrounding the stoma remains free of breakdown
    b. Which criteria will I use to change my interventions?
       (1) NG drainage continues in large amounts, more than 600 ml/day
       (2) Peristalsis does not return within 24 to 48 hours
       (3) Stoma color changes to a dusky pink, blue, or black
       (4) Skin ulcerates around the stoma
    c. How will I know that my client teaching has been effective?
       (1) Client demonstrates all aspects of ileostomy care, including care of the appliance
       (2) Client states changes in the stoma that should be reported to physician

        (3) Client states assessment findings associated with fluid and electrolyte imbalance that should be reported to physician

        (4) Client indicates which foods have been removed from the diet and why

  11. Older adult alert

    a. These disorders are uncommon in the older adult population

    b. If the client is an older adult and requires surgery, care of the ostomy may require more time than in a younger adult

    c. Older clients may not be able to care for the ileostomy, and thus care may have to be assumed by family members

J. Diverticular disease

  1. Definition

    a. Diverticulosis—outpouching of the wall of the colon (diverticulum)

    b. Diverticulitis—inflammation and obstruction of a diverticula

  2. Pathophysiology—fiber in the diet assists in passing feces through the colon more quickly and more efficiently. Owing to decreased fiber content, passage time is decreased, lumen pressure increases, and pressure on the wall increases. Blood supply to the area also is impaired, resulting in outpouching of the wall.

  3. Etiology—diet low in fiber and roughage

  4. Incidence—over 30 million people in the United States are affected, with the largest percentage over the age of 60

  5. Assessment

    a. Questions to ask

      (1) Have you ever experienced an unusual pain in the left lower side of your abdomen?

      (2) Do you ever have alternating diarrhea and constipation?

      (3) Have you ever noticed rectal bleeding?

    b. Clinical manifestations

      (1) The client may be asymptomatic until diverticulitis occurs

      (2) Unusual pain in left lower quadrant of the abdomen

      (3) Alternating diarrhea and constipation

      (4) Rectal bleeding

      (5) Diverticulitis

        (a) Crampy, left lower quadrant pain

        (b) Abdominal distention

        (c) Nausea and vomiting

        (d) Low-grade fever

    c. Abnormal laboratory findings

      (1) WBC—elevated

      (2) CBC—H&H may be low

    d. Abnormal diagnostic test results

      (1) Flat-plate x-ray film of the abdomen—evaluates for free air under the diaphragm with perforation of the bowel

(2) Barium enema—identifies diverticular sacs with decreased lumen size

(3) Sigmoidoscopy or colonoscopy—visualize openings to the diverticula; rule out carcinoma

6. Expected medical interventions
   a. High-fiber diet, omitting seeds and kernels that can lodge in diverticula
   b. Bran therapy, Metamucil, or a similar agent taken daily
   c. During acute diverticulitis—NPO, or low-residue diet, IV fluids, and antibiotics
   d. Colon resection with end-to-end anastomosis if episodes of diverticulitis are more frequent
   e. Colon resection with diverting or loop colostomy if bowel perforation has occurred—repeat anastomosis at a later date
   f. Peritonitis as a result of bowel perforation—correction of the rupture with irrigation of the peritoneum and IV antibiotic therapy

7. Nursing diagnoses
   a. Alteration in bowel elimination—constipation and diarrhea related to bowel inflammation
   b. Pain related to bowel inflammation

8. Client goals
   a. Client will state bowel movements have become soft and formed and occur once or twice a day
   b. Client will state pain is decreased or relieved

9. Nursing interventions
   a. Acute care
      (1) Diverticulitis
         (a) Maintain IV access
         (b) Maintain hydration with oral or IV fluids
         (c) Administer pain medication as needed by client, which may take the form of antispasmodic agents
      (2) Postoperative care
         (a) See routine postoperative care in Chapter 9, pp. 311-312
         (b) Maintain NG patency if present, irrigating as per orders
         (c) Evaluate stoma for color and size if present (see stoma assessment p. 224)
         (d) Begin stoma care—dressings may be used initially; apply appliance when appropriate, usually within 48 hours
   b. Home care regarding client education
      (1) Diet—high in fiber, Metamucil, or similar agent daily with adequate fluid intake
      (2) Stool softeners if needed

        (3) Assessment findings that must be called to attention of physician: abdominal distention and sudden onset of severe abdominal pain, which may be indicative of a perforation

        (4) Stoma care if stoma is present

10. Evaluation protocol

    a. How do I know that my interventions were effective?

        (1) Client states pain is relieved or decreased

        (2) I&O is adequate, that is, input is equal to output within plus or minus 300 ml; 30 ml/hr of urine output

        (3) Stoma remains pink or reddish in color

        (4) Stoma output begins in 2 to 3 days

    b. Which criteria will I use to change my interventions?

        (1) Pain unrelieved

        (2) I&O not balanced within plus or minus 300 ml

        (3) Stoma changes color to dusky pink, blue, or black

        (4) Stoma output does not begin within 3 days

    c. How will I know that my client teaching has been effective?

        (1) Client produces a food diary indicative of a high-fiber content

        (2) Client reports taking Metamucil or a similar agent every day

        (3) Client states no need for stool softeners

        (4) Client demonstrates care of the stoma and appliance

11. Older adult alert

    a. This is a disorder of older adults and may require frequent teaching periods regarding dietary changes. Eating habits are difficult to change.

    b. The ability to care for a stoma requires evaluation for minimal vision and manual dexterity. If the client is unable to do the care because of arthritis or vision problems, another person may have to assume the responsibility.

K. Colorectal cancer

1. Definition—malignancy of the colon or the rectum

2. Pathophysiology—tumors are graded according to cell differentiation. When the cells of a tumor are well differentiated, the outcome is more favorable. The tumor spreads through the walls of the colon, through the lymphatics, by way of the bloodstream, across the peritoneum, or by way of incision lines or the drain. Intestinal obstruction can result, as well as wall ulceration and hemorrhage, abscess, or fistula formation.

3. Etiology—risk factors

    a. Ulcerative colitis or Crohn's disease for many years

    b. High-fat, low-fiber diet

    c. Family history

    d. Polyposis—presence of polyps in the colon

4. Incidence—second most common type of cancer with over 150,000 new cases per year in the United States. Most cancers are found in the rectum, with the next most common being found in the sigmoid colon.

5. Assessment
   a. Questions to ask
      (1) Have you noticed any rectal bleeding?
      (2) Have you had a change in your bowel movements lately?
      (3) Have you lost any weight over the past year? Were you trying to lose weight?
   b. Clinical manifestations
      (1) Rectal bleeding
      (2) Vague abdominal pain
      (3) Alternating constipation and diarrhea
      (4) Spastic pain of the colon or sphincters
      (5) Abdominal distention
      (6) Weight loss
   c. Abnormal laboratory findings
      (1) Stool for occult blood or guiac—positive
      (2) H&H—low
      (3) Carcinoembryonic antigen (CEA)—elevated indicative of intestinal tumor
   d. Abnormal diagnostic test results
      (1) Digital rectal examination—feel the presence of a tumor
      (2) Barium enema—depicts a constriction in the colon and tumor location
      (3) Sigmoidoscopy or colonoscopy—presence of lesion; biopsy confirms malignancy
      (4) Endorectal ultrasonography—identifies involved lymph nodes

6. Expected medical interventions
   a. Surgical resection of the tumor; end-to-end anastomosis if possible; anterior-posterior resection if necessary, with permanent colostomy
   b. Removal of involved lymph nodes
   c. Radiation therapy as an adjunct to surgery
   d. Chemotherapy if surgery is not advised or to reduce the tumor before surgery

7. Nursing diagnoses
   a. Altered nutrition (less than body requirements) related to anorexia
   b. Fatigue related to tumor growth and decreased nutrition
   c. Body-image disturbance related to presence of colostomy

8. Client goals
   a. Client will maintain present weight or gain 0.5 kg/week
   b. Client will state fatigue is reduced

    c. Client will state feeling comfortable with the presence of the colostomy

9. Nursing interventions
   a. Acute care—will be identical to the client with inflammatory bowel disease and diverticular disease (pp. 221-227)
   b. Home care regarding client education
     (1) Stoma care, appliance care, and where to purchase equipment
     (2) Normal diet with plenty of fluids
     (3) Colonoscopy may be repeated 6 to 12 months after surgery and then yearly
     (4) Stool for occult blood done yearly
     (5) CEA levels are drawn at regular intervals, every 3 to 6 months for the next 5 years
     (6) Technique for colostomy irrigation if necessary (Figure 6-7)
       (a) Remove appliance and apply an irrigating sleeve
       (b) Use 1000 ml of warm water; hang the bag 18 to 24 inches above stoma
       (c) Insert cone into the stoma until it forms a seal to prevent irrigation fluid from coming out
       (d) Let water run in stoma
       (e) Remove cone and allow solution to drain
       (f) Remove irrigating sleeve and apply clean appliance

10. Evaluation protocol
   a. How will I know that my client teaching has been effective?
     (1) Client demonstrates effective care and irrigation of the colostomy

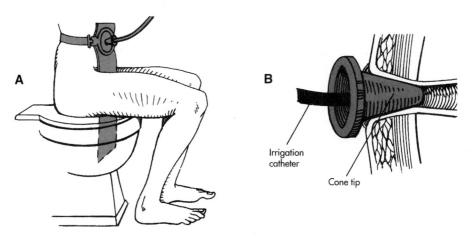

Figure 6-7 Colostomy irrigation. **A,** Colostomy irrigation with person sitting on toilet: irrigating sleeve drains into toilet. **B,** Cone irrigating tip inserted into stoma. (From Phipps WJ, Sands JK, Marek JF: *Medical-surgical nursing: concepts and clinical practice,* ed 6, St. Louis, 1999, Mosby.)

(2) Client indicates following of a regular diet without difficulty

(3) Client exhibits an understanding of the postoperative laboratory and diagnostic regimen

11. Older adult alert—these will be the same as for the client with inflammatory bowel disease and diverticular disease (pp. 225, 227)

WEB resources

http://www.ccfa.org/
   CCFA: Crohn's & Colitis Foundation of America

http://www.niddk.nih.gov/health/digest/digest.htm
   NIDDK Health Information: Digestive Diseases

http://www.iffgd.org/
   Functional Gastrointestinal Disorders (IFFGD)

REVIEW QUESTIONS

1. Clients with gastroesophageal reflux should be counseled to remove which of the following items from their diet?
   1. Pizza
   2. Alcohol
   3. Whatever results in the return of discomfort
   4. Coffee and soda

2. When lavaging a client's stomach tube, the nurse must calculate the correct gastric output from fluid intake. This is accomplished by
   1. Subtracting the output from the intake
   2. Subtracting the intake from the output
   3. Irrigating the gastric tube, and removing the irrigation immediately
   4. Irrigating the gastric tube, and allowing the gastric suction to pull the fluid out into the collection container

3. When evaluating the abdomen of a client who has just had open cholecystectomy surgery, the nurse notices that the continuous portable suction device is half full. It is only 4 hours into the shift. The best intervention at this time is to
   1. Empty the device now, record the output, and recharge the system
   2. Wait until 8 hours have passed to empty the device, record the total output, and reset the vacuum in the system
   3. Wait another hour until calculating the output and resolving the lost vacuum
   4. Squeeze the air out of the device but do not empty it at this time

4. A client with pancreatitis has asked the nurse why the insulin shot is needed. The best response would be
   1. "You are producing more glucose because of your illness, so we must give you insulin."
   2. "Your pancreas usually makes insulin, but because it is inflamed the insulin is not made in the amounts you need."
   3. "We are giving you more glucose in your IV feeding today, so you need a little extra insulin."
   4. "You ate a little more today, so you need some extra insulin."

5. A priority assessment for clients with ascites is
   1. Abdominal girth measurement every 8 hours
   2. Blood pressure checks every 4 hours
   3. Daily weight in the morning
   4. Respiratory effort continuously

6. Understanding of the pathophysiology of cirrhosis of the liver allows the nurse to explain to the client's family why their family member is having bleeding episodes. The nurse explains that
   1. The bleeding is because of the inability to eat; it has left the client's body in a weakened state.
   2. The liver is responsible for making substances that produce clotting of the blood. A liver that is affected by cirrhosis will not make those substances, and the blood will not clot.
   3. Something in the medication we are giving him to help the liver is affecting the clotting of the blood.
   4. This is a temporary problem caused by inflammation of the client's liver. It will subside with appropriate therapy.

7. A client with hepatitis B is complaining of severe nausea that is interfering with his eating meals. The best nursing intervention is to
   1. Offer antiemetics at least 2 hours before meals
   2. Give antiemetics with complaints of any degree of nausea
   3. Routinely give an antiemetic injection 30 minutes before meals
   4. Administer antiemetics immediately before the client eats

8. During the assessment of a client who *has just returned* from surgery into the post-anesthesia unit after a total colectomy and placement of an ileostomy, the nurse expects the ileostomy stoma to be which color?
   1. Pale
   2. Deep purple
   3. Ruddy red
   4. Dusky blue-gray

9. Which of these statements by a client would alert the nurse to encourage the client to see a physician?
   1. "I have diarrhea when I drink milk."
   2. "I have a crampy right lower abdominal pain just before a bowel movement."
   3. "I keep changing back and forth between diarrhea and constipation."
   4. "I use laxatives several times a month."

10. A classic finding associated with a perforated diverticulum is
   1. Rectal bleeding
   2. Abdominal distention
   3. Severe abdominal pain
   4. Fever

ANSWERS, RATIONALES, AND TEST-TAKING TIPS

Rationales	Test-Taking Tips

1. Correct answer: 3

Clients can eat whatever does not cause the return of the reflux symptoms. The items in the other three options are known to cause problems of reflux and are correct answers. However, they are not the best answer because option 3 is most specific to the individual client's needs.

If you have no idea of the correct answer, cluster options 1, 2, and 4 with specific food items. These options do not consider individual needs. Select option 3.

2. Correct answer: 2

The output should be higher than the amount instilled into the gastric tube; that is: 1000 ml instilled—intake from 1300 drained out—output. 1300 minus 1000 equals plus 300 ml for gastric drainage. If you subtracted the output from the intake you would have 1000 minus 1300 equals minus 300 ml, or a deficit of 300 ml, which is not the case. More came out than what was put in. Option 3 is an incorrect action for the given situation. Option 4 is a correct action but it does not answer the question about calculating the fluid volumes.

The best approach to these types of questions is to write a sample on the provided scratch paper as shown in the rationale above. After you calculate it both ways as stated in options 1 and 2, reread the question to make sure you understand it. Select option 2. This is an example of a question about an action that you do often. Yet in print the question may result in confusion in your mind. Go to the basics and write it down for the calculation. Avoid doing such calculations mentally, which increases your chances of selecting an incorrect answer.

3. Correct answer: 1

Drainage collection devices should be emptied when half full or at the end of 8 hours, whichever comes first. The other options are incorrect actions at this time.

Read the options carefully. Avoid allowing the distractor "now" in option 1 push you to select option 4. The question asks for a best action "at this time." Option 1 best answers the question. A second warning regarding this question is to "know" that option 1 is correct

Rationales	Test-Taking Tips

and not read the other options. Remember that this type of approach to test questions will increase your chances of failure. Correct such bad actions by first identifying that you have the problem. In the future, for all questions for which you select option 1 as the answer, go immediately to option 4. Read options 4, 3, and 2, and then reread option 1. Select option 1 only after you have given equal consideration to all of the options.

4. Correct answer: 2

An inflamed pancreas cannot appropriately manufacture or release insulin, so it must be administered subcutaneously. The initial part of option 1 is correct in that with illness the glucose levels may be elevated. However, that is not the reason for the insulin. Options 3 and 4 are obviously incorrect rationales.

If you have no idea of the correct answer, simply match words—the patient has "pancreatitis"—select option 2, which has the word "pancreas" in it. Another approach, if the answer is unknown to you, is to select the longest answer for explanations to clients because they most likely give more details.

5. Correct answer: 4

Respiratory effort always has top priority over other assessments, especially in clients who have ascites. Ascites of the abdomen pushes up on the diaphragm and impedes ventilation. Note that all of the options are correct actions. Use the clue of the timeframe in each option to select the priority action. Option 1 is every 8 hours, option 2 is every 4 hours, option 3 is in the morning, and option 4 is continuously.

This question falls into the harder category because all of the options are correct as suggested by the clue in the question when it asks for a "priority" assessment. If you have no idea of the correct answer, use the ABCs to guide the selection of option 4, respiratory before circulation and safety factors.

6. Correct answer: 2

In cirrhosis, the liver is no longer able to produce clotting factors at a normal pace or even at all. Options 1 and 3 obviously are incorrect statements. Option 4 may have been considered as a possible answer. The first sentence in this option is acceptable. However, the second sentence is incorrect information. No "appropriate therapy" is directly associated with accessory organ malfunctions such as the pancreas, liver, and gallbladder. The primary action taken is to rest the involved organ. In fact, antibiotics are contraindicated in pancreatitis because their use may cause abscesses to develop.

If you have no idea of the correct answer, an approach is to select the most complete statement, which is usually the longest one. This is option 2.

7. Correct answer: 3

Removal of nausea before a meal increases the chance that the client will eat some of the meal. Option 1 is too far in advance of the meal, and option 4 is too close to mealtime. When given 2 hours before or right before the meals, the effects to decrease nausea will be minimal. Option 2 may be an approach in some situations. It is not the best answer in this situation of severe nausea that interferes with the consumption of meals. If the information about the meals were not included in the stem, then option 2 would be the best answer.

The clues in the stem are the key words "severe nausea" and the fact of problems eating meals. It follows that medication would be given before meals. Note that option 3 also states the route as an injection, whereas the other options do not specify the route of administration. Thus, you are confident that an injection of an antiemetic given 30 minutes before a meal will minimize or eliminate nausea.

8. Correct answer: 1

The stoma is initially pale, as is the client's skin and other mucous membranes on just

The key words in the stem are "who has just returned." Recall that in the operating and recovery rooms the

Rationales	Test-Taking Tips

returning from surgery. As the client warms, the stoma becomes red to a ruddy red. Deep purple, cyanotic, or a dusky blue-gray color indicates vascular compromise of the stoma.

temperature is cooler than on a surgical unit. Therefore, the client's skin usually is cool and pale.

9. Correct answer: 3

Alternating constipation and diarrhea may be indicative of colon cancer. This problem needs further assessment. Options 1 and 2 may be normal findings in many clients. Option 4 is considered within the normal usage of laxatives.

The approach to this situation is to use common sense. Option 1 indicates the situation of lactose intolerance. In option 2, this type of pain on the right or left side before bowel movements may indicate the accumulation of gas in the large intestine. Thus, you may have narrowed the options to 3 and 4. Option 4 could be selected because of a need for further assessment. However, because you must decide between options 3 and 4 in the given situation, option 3 is the better answer. Cancer risk is a more serious problem than the possibility of dehydration or electrolyte imbalance from the use of laxatives.

10. Correct answer: 3

Severe abdominal pain is more indicative of a ruptured diverticulum. Rectal bleeding is indicative of an internal or external hemorrhoid problem or rectal fistula. Abdominal distention could be indicative of many problems such as an intestinal obstruction, paralytic ileus, or stool impaction. Fever is present in many pathologic conditions. A spike in temperature to at least 102° F is classic in conditions such as pneumonia, urinary tract infections, and ear infections.

If you have no idea of the correct answer, try an approach to match the level of severity in the question and option. "Perforated diverticulum" can be matched with "severe abdominal pain"—both are intense findings.

7

The Renal System

FAST FACTS

1. The kidney maintains a homeostasis in the body only with an adequate perfusion of blood volume, approximately 20% of cardiac output (CO).
2. A mean arterial pressure (MAP) of greater than 70 mm Hg is needed to sustain the glomerular filtration rate (GFR).
3. Renal glomerular filtration is driven by hydrostatic pressure, which is generated by BP. Decreased BP results in a decreased renal filtration rate.
4. A MAP of less than 70 mm Hg for more than 40 minutes significantly increases the risk of acute tubular necrosis (ATN) or acute renal failure (ARF).
5. Acute renal failure has one finding—a decreased urine output of less than 30 ml/hr or 400 ml/day. This is documented as *oliguria,* the first stage of renal failure.
6. A serum creatinine level greater than 1.2 indicates impaired renal function.
7. The creatinine clearance test for glomerular filtration evaluation requires serum creatinine levels and a 24-hour urine collection.
8. The kidney is the essential channel for excretion of water-soluble drugs and drug metabolites.
9. The kidneys regulate water, electrolytes, nitrogenous wastes, acids, and bases.
10. When homeostasis is lost, the kidneys depend on the nervous and endocrine systems to adjust the renal mechanisms by hormonal activity.
11. Chronic renal failure results in the problem of anemia when Epogen, synthetic erythropoietin, is not given regularly.

CONTENT REVIEW

I. The renal system—excretes water-soluble wastes, stimulates RBC production, and maintains the balance of pH, plasma water, and electrolytes

II. Structure and function

A. **Definition—a pair of organs each weighing approximately 6 ounces, situated at the level of the costovertebral angle (CVA) in the retroperitoneum**

B. **Structure—the kidney has three distinct structural areas (Figure 7-1)**
   1. Cortex—outer layer; glomeruli, proximal and distal tubules
   2. Medulla—middle layer; 6 to 10 renal pyramids comprised of collecting ducts and tubules
   3. Pelvis—interior layer or collection area
   4. Calyces separate the pyramids of the medulla from the renal pelvis

C. **Nephron—functional unit of the kidney; approximately 1 million per kidney (Figure 7-2)**
   1. Structure and blood flow sequence
      a. Renal corpuscle—glomerulus of the renal capillaries situated in Bowman's capsule; filtration
      b. Proximal convoluted tubule—reabsorption and secretion (Figure 7-3, Table 7-1)
      c. Loop of Henle—reabsorption
      d. Distal convoluted tubule—acid-base balance and secretion
      e. Collecting ducts—concentration

D. **Functions of the kidney**
   1. Fluid and electrolyte balance
      a. Sodium—filtered by the glomeruli and reabsorbed in the tubules
      b. Chloride—follows sodium
      c. Potassium—filtered by the glomeruli and reabsorbed in the proximal tubules

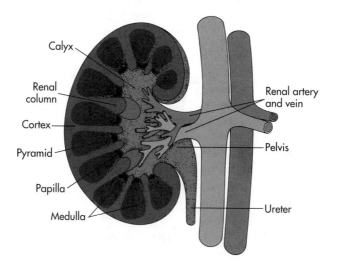

Figure 7-1   Frontal section of kidney. (From Beare PG, Myers JL: *Adult health nursing,* ed 3, St. Louis, 1998, Mosby.)

d. Water—ADH concentration in the collecting duct controls reabsorption

2. Acid-base balance
   a. Excretes organic acids
   b. Releases free hydrogen ions
   c. Conserves bicarbonate

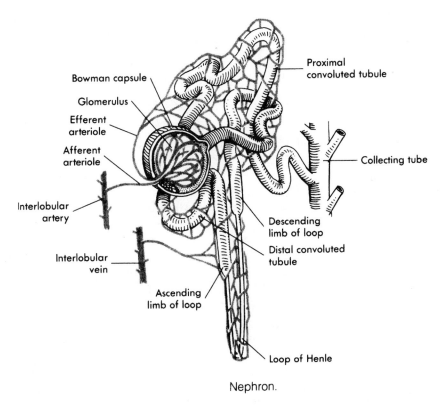

Nephron.

Part of Nephron	Function	Substance
Glomeruli	Filtration	H_2O and solute, electrolytes (Na, K, PO_4, Ca, Cl, Mg), urea, creatinine, uric acid, glucose, amino acids
Proximal tubules	Reabsorption, secretion	H_2O, electrolytes (Na, K, Mg, Ca, Cl, HCO_3), glucose, amino acids
Loop of Henle	Reabsorption	H_2O, electrolytes (Na, K)
Distal tubule	Acid-base balance, secretion	Hydrogen ions (H), Na
Collecting tubule	Concentration	H_2O

Figure 7-2 The nephron. (From Phipps WJ, Sands JK, Marek JF: *Medical-surgical nursing: concepts and clinical practice,* ed 6, St. Louis, 1999, Mosby.)

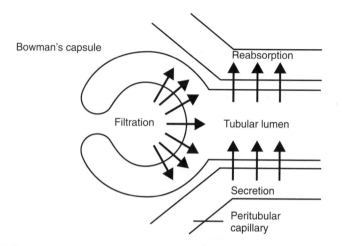

Figure 7-3 Processes of filtration, secretion, and reabsorption in urine formation. (From Richard C: *Comprehensive nephrology nursing,* Boston, 1987, Little, Brown.)

TABLE 7-1	Tubular Reabsorption and Secretion	
Region of Tubule	**Reabsorption**	**Secretion**
Proximal convoluted tubule	• Water • Glucose • Vitamins • Amino acids and protein • Urea • Ions: sodium, potassium, chloride, phosphate • Bicarbonate (regulated by acid-base balance)	• Hydrogen ions (regulated by acid-base balance) • Bicarbonate (regulated by acid-base balance) • Creatinine • Ammonia • Urea • Drugs (e.g., penicillin, digoxin)
Loop of Henle	• Descending limb: water • Ascending limb: sodium, chloride, calcium, potassium, magnesium	
Distal convoluted tubule	• Sodium (regulated by aldosterone) • Calcium and phosphorus (regulated by parathormone) • Water (regulated by ADH) • Bicarbonate (regulated by acid-base balance)	• Sodium and potassium (regulated by aldosterone) • Calcium and phosphorus (regulated by parathormone) • Water (regulated by ADH) • Hydrogen ions (regulated by acid-base balance) • Potassium • Ammonia • Potassium
Collecting tubules	• Water (regulated by ADH) • Sodium	• Hydrogen • Ammonia

From Dennison RD: *Pass CCRN,* ed 2, St. Louis, 2000, Mosby.

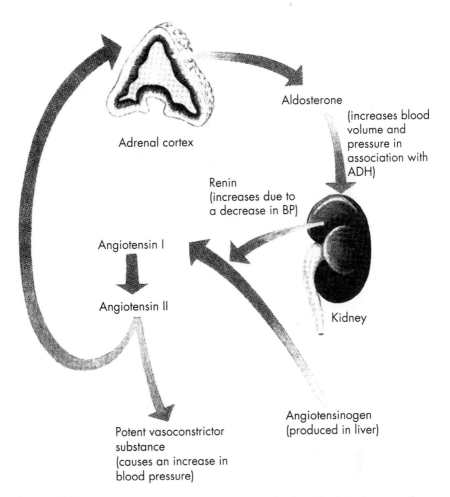

Figure 7-4   The renin-angiotensin-aldosterone mechanism. Angiotensin-converting enzyme made in the lung converts angiotensin I to angiotensin II. The vasoconstriction then leads to increased blood volume, resulting in an increased blood pressure. (From Brundage DJ: *Renal disorders,* St. Louis, 1994, Mosby.)

3. Excretion of waste products—urea and creatinine, bacterial toxins, and drugs and drug metabolites
4. Production and secretion of erythropoietin, which stimulates the bone marrow to manufacture hemoglobin
5. Facilitation of the production and activation of vitamin D, which is necessary for calcium metabolism
6. Regulation of arterial BP by releasing renin and activating the renin-angiotensin-aldosterone system (Figure 7-4)

III. **Targeted concerns**

A. **Pharmacology—priority drug classifications**

1. Diuretic agents—induce the renal excretion of water, sodium, potassium, or any combination of these from the body

   a. Expected effect—reduction in circulating blood volume

   b. Commonly given drugs

      (1) Loop diuretics—act on the ascending loop of Henle; furosemide (Lasix), bumetanide (Bumex)

      (2) Thiazide diuretics—inhibit sodium and chloride reabsorption in the distal tubule; chlorothiazide (Diuril)

      (3) Potassium-sparing diuretics—action is in the collecting tubule; spironolactone (Aldactone)

      (4) Osmotic diuretics—pulls water from extravascular space into vascular space; mannitol (Osmitrol)

   c. Nursing considerations

      (1) Hydration level and electrolyte balance must be monitored carefully in clients who receive diuretic drugs

      (2) Potassium supplements may be required with loop and thiazide diuretics

      (3) With potassium-sparing diuretics, life-threatening hyperkalemia can occur if clients are not instructed that they do not require potassium supplements or foods high in potassium in the diet

2. Phosphate-binding agents—bind with phosphate in the treatment of hyperphosphatemia

   a. Expected effect—ingested phosphates bind with aluminum in the intestine forming a complex that can be excreted in feces

   b. Commonly given drugs

      (1) Aluminum carbonate gel (Basaljel)

      (2) Aluminum hydroxide gel (Amphojel)

      (3) Calcium acetate (Phos-Ex)

   c. Nursing considerations

      (1) Aluminum preparations are constipating and should be given with a stool softener

      (2) Phos-Ex should not be given in the client with high calcium levels

3. Erythrocyte-stimulating hormone—treats anemia caused by a lack of erythropoietin in chronic renal failure; promotes the production of erythrocytes

   a. Expected effect—increase in hematocrit is seen approximately 2 weeks after initiation of therapy

   b. Commonly given drug—recombinant human erythropoietin (Epogen)

   c. Nursing considerations

      (1) May elevate BP

(2) Do not shake the vial because doing so will inactivate the drug

(3) Clinical response will not be seen for several weeks; not for immediate correction of anemia

B. Procedures

1. Urinalysis—identifies normal and abnormal constituents; can indicate abnormalities in the kidney function or structure; *requires a clean specimen*

2. Urine culture and sensitivity—identifies bacterial organisms and the antibiotics to which the organisms are sensitive; *requires a sterile specimen*

3. Creatinine clearance—most useful test of kidney function; 24-hour specimen
   a. Measures amount of creatinine filtered by the glomeruli
   b. A decrease in creatinine cleared indicates a decrease in GFR

4. Kidney-ureter-bladder (KUB) x-ray film—abdominal x-ray film without contrast dye; standing or supine; renal structures may be seen; calculi may be visualized

5. Renal sonogram—sound waves are used to project an image of the kidney and structures; calculi and renal tumors can be identified

6. Radionuclide imaging—following injection of radionuclide tracer substances, kidney is scanned and evaluated for obstruction or insufficiency

7. Intravenous pyelography (IVP) or excretory urography—contrast dye is used in conjunction with radiographic X-rays, allowing visualization of the kidney structures and their function through sequencing X-ray films

8. Nephrotomography—X-ray films are taken at several angles to distinguish abnormalities in the kidneys

9. Retrograde pyelography—catheter is passed up into one or both of the ureters and contrast medium injected up into the kidney, allowing visualization of kidney structures and function when clients are not capable of concentrating or excreting urine

10. Renal arteriography—catheter is inserted into the renal artery through the femoral artery, and dye is injected into the renal vasculature; used to evaluate patency of renal vascular structures

11. Renal CT—computer-generated plane images of the kidney used to identify masses or tumors

12. MRI—computer generated images that are created by changes in the magnetic field of the body; very useful for visualization of the kidney and abnormalities

13. Renal biopsy—a needle is inserted percutaneously into the kidney to obtain a sample of kidney tissue; used to evaluate hematuria, proteinuria, or nephrotic syndrome

14. Nephroscopy—endoscopic examination of the kidney; renal pelvis and calyces can be visualized; percutaneous tract established followed by an endoscope into the kidney

C. Psychosocial concerns

1. Anxiety—the uncomfortable feeling associated with an unknown direct cause; clients may display this when symptoms begin but the cause has not yet been identified; also seen when clients are unsure of the outcome of their acute or chronic illness
2. Fear—an uncomfortable feeling associated with a real danger; the real danger may be death in many of these clients owing to irreversible kidney failure
3. Social isolation—may be identified in clients who are confined owing to hemodialysis or physical impairment from chronic renal impairment
4. Depression—in response to a long-standing incurable illness
5. Hopelessness—commonly seen in clients who are waiting for renal transplantation
6. Dependency—may be observed in the client who is in need of renal dialysis; physical limitations may require that the client enlist aid from significant others to complete activities of daily living

D. Health history—question sequence

1. Please describe the problem that you have been experiencing
2. Do you have any other conditions for which you are receiving care?
3. Have you ever suffered any injury to or a problem with your kidneys?
4. Which prescription and nonprescription medications are you currently taking?
5. What is your current height and weight?
6. Has there been any change in your weight? Over what period of time?
7. Is there any history of renal disease in your family?
8. Have you experienced any pain over your sides?
9. Have you noticed any change in your pattern of urinating?
10. Have you experienced any urgency, frequency, or burning?
11. Have you noticed blood or any other particles in your urine?
12. Does your urine have a strange odor or color?
13. Have you experienced any loss of appetite, nausea, vomiting, or diarrhea?
14. Have you experienced frequent urinary tract infections (UTIs)?

E. Physical examination—appropriate sequence

1. ABCs—vital signs
2. Skin color, temperature, turgor, and moisture
3. Inspection of upper abdomen and flank areas
4. Deep palpation of the kidneys bilaterally
5. Percussion of the kidneys posteriorly and anteriorly to outline them
6. Auscultation of the kidneys for bruits—indication of stenosis or aneurysm of the renal artery

IV. Pathophysiologic disorders
A. Acute renal failure (ARF)
1. Definition—a sudden loss of kidney function, which may be reversible
2. Pathophysiology—many theories persist as to what occurs in the kidney experiencing acute renal failure. There is no one accepted theory. The clinical course is
   a. Oliguric phase—client produces less than 400 ml/day of urine for an average time of 1 to 2 weeks. Although this condition may last as long as several months, it rarely lasts longer than 4 weeks. The longer it lasts, the poorer the prognosis.
   b. Diuretic phase—client produces over 3000 ml/day of urine; lasts several days to 3 weeks
   c. Recovery phase—gradual return to function before renal failure; lasts 3 to 12 months. Creatinine levels gradually return to normal.
3. Etiology—three categories of similar origination
   a. Pre-renal—poor circulating blood volume; poor CO
   b. Renal—injury or destruction to renal structures
   c. Post-renal—obstruction of urinary tract distal to kidney
4. Assessment
   a. Questions to ask
      (1) Have you noticed that you have been urinating less?
      (2) Has your weight increased? By how much?
      (3) Have you noticed swelling in any part of your body?
      (4) Have you felt weak or tired?
      (5) Have you noticed a change in the way your urine looks or smells?
   b. Clinical manifestations
      (1) Neurologic—altered sensorium, weakness, and headache
      (2) Respiratory—Kussmaul's respiration (deep and rapid) and pneumonia
      (3) Cardiovascular—anemia, hypertension, and dysrhythmias
      (4) GI—nausea, vomiting, and GI bleeding
      (5) Integumentary—generalized edema and bruising
   c. Abnormal laboratory findings (Table 7-2)
   d. Abnormal diagnostic test results
      (1) EKG—dysrhythmias; T-wave abnormality related to hyper- or hypokalemia
      (2) Renal ultrasonography—may indicate abnormally shaped kidney
      (3) Renal scan—may show impaired perfusion
      (4) Renal biopsy—indicates extent of damage to renal structures
5. Expected medical interventions
   a. Prevention of further injury—increased fluids and osmotic diuretics to increase renal filtration
   b. Maintenance of homeostasis with peritoneal dialysis or hemodialysis until renal function returns (Figure 7-5)

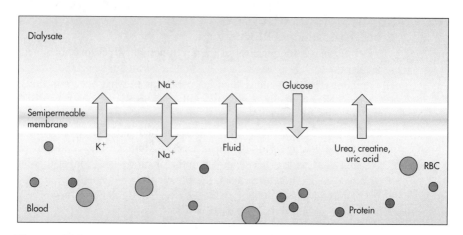

Figure 7-5 Dialysis: net movement of fluid and particles by osmosis and diffusion. (From Lewis SM, Heitkemper MM, Dirksen SR: *Medical-surgical nursing: assessment and management of clinical problems,* ed 5, St. Louis, 2000, Mosby.)

TABLE 7-2	**Abnormal Laboratory Findings of Acute Renal Failure**

Laboratory Tests	Oliguric Phase	Diuretic Phase	Recovery Phase
Serum sodium	Decreased	Elevated, normal, or decreased	Normal
Serum potassium	Increased	Elevated, normal, or decreased	Normal
BUN, creatinine ratio	Increased— ratio >10:1	Increased— ratio >20:1	Normal— ratio <20:1
Specific gravity	Increased	Decreased	Normal
Blood volume	Hypervolemia	Hypovolemia	Normal
Blood pressure	Hypertensive	Hypotensive	Normotensive
Serum phosphorus	High	Same	Resolving
Serum calcium	Low	Same	Resolving
Hemoglobin and hematocrit	Anemia	Anemia	Anemia
	Hemodiluted— low	Hemoconcentrated— high	Resolving
Serum creatinine	Elevated	Elevated	Resolving

   c. Initiation of Continuous Renal Replacement Therapy
      (CRRT)—method to remove excess fluid and wastes slowly.
      CRRT can be utilized in a hemodynamically stable client.
      Vascular access required. Several variations are available
      (Figure 7-6).

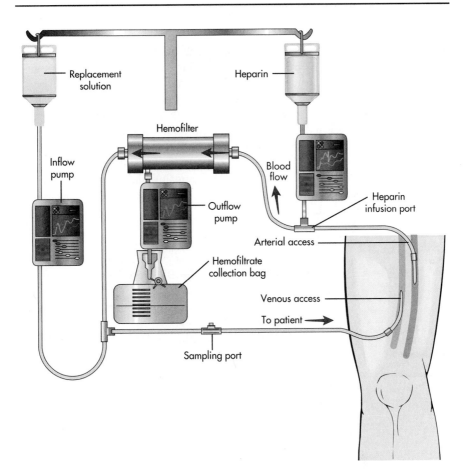

Figure 7-6   Continuous arteriovenous hemofiltration. (From Lewis SM, Heitkemper MM, Dirksen SR: *Medical-surgical nursing: assessment and management of clinical problems,* ed 5, St. Louis, 2000, Mosby.)

   d. Maintain electrolyte balance
   e. Treat infections or anemia as they become apparent
  6. Nursing diagnoses
   a. Fluid volume excess (vascular space) related to failed renal regulatory mechanisms (oliguric phase)
   b. Fluid volume deficit (vascular space) related to failed renal regulatory mechanisms (diuretic phase)
   c. Altered nutrition (less than bodily requirements) related to anorexia
   d. Potential for infection related to depressed immune response
   e. Potential for sensory-perceptual alterations related to abnormal blood chemistry
   f. Potential for impaired skin integrity related to peripheral edema

7. Client goals
   a. Client will maintain fluid volume at appropriate levels as evidenced by CVP reading of 5 to 15 mm Hg. (CVP readings may be at the higher end of normal owing to fluid retention that is expected until resolution of the illness.)
   b. Client will have adequate daily caloric and protein intake
   c. Client will not have an infectious process as evidenced by a normal temperature and WBC count
   d. Client will be oriented to person, time, event, and place
   e. Client will have skin integrity remain intact as evidenced by no skin tears or open areas
8. Nursing interventions
   a. Acute care
      (1) Assess
         (a) Neurologic status at least every 2 hours
         (b) Vital signs with postural BP every 2 to 4 hours
         (c) CVP readings with vital signs
         (d) Lung sounds for fluid accumulation, and heart sounds for gallops with vital signs
         (e) Daily weights—same time, same scale, and same amount of clothing
         (f) Accurate measurements of I&O
         (g) Blood chemistries as ordered for desired changes
      (2) Care of the client receiving in-hospital peritoneal dialysis
         (a) Use meticulous aseptic technique during procedure and dressing changes of peritoneal catheter
         (b) Client maintained in supine position with head of bed up as needed to promote ventilation
         (c) Warm dialysate to body temperature before installation
         (d) Instill 2 L into abdomen (inflow)
         (e) Allow dwell time of 20 to 30 minutes
         (f) Drain fluid from peritoneum; document loss or gain of fluid during procedure (outflow)
         (g) Outflow should be greater than inflow by 100 to 200 ml with each exchange
         (h) Turn client to ensure appropriate drainage
         (i) Check outflow for
            (i) Cloudiness—sign of infection
            (ii) Red tinge—sign of bleeding
            (iii) Brown tinge—sign of bowel perforation
         (j) Repeat cycles for the number ordered by physician; usually 24 in 24 hours
      (3) Evaluate nutritional likes and dislikes to encourage an appropriate nutritional status; consider the use of antiemetics before meals to ensure adequate intake

(4) Meticulous skin care with turning every 2 hours and **range-of-motion** exercises. Consider the use of a special mattress or bed to decrease the risk of skin breakdown. Use a draw sheet for repositioning to prevent skin shearing.

b. Home care regarding client education
   (1) The importance of recording client's weight daily
   (2) The importance of keeping an accurate daily record of I&O
   (3) Special dietary needs of the client with preparation suggestions
   (4) Desired effects, side effects, and effects to report to physician of the medications prescribed on discharge

9. Evaluation protocol
   a. How do I know that my interventions were effective?
      (1) Does client know who and where he or she is? What day or year it is? The situation he or she is in? Neurologic status should improve slowly.
      (2) Have headaches improved?
      (3) Does client feel strength returning?
      (4) Assess for improvement
         (a) Vital signs and CVP readings
         (b) Blood chemistries
         (c) Edema
         (d) Daily weight
         (e) I&Os
   b. Which criteria will I use to change my interventions?
      (1) Neurologic status shows decreased LOC
      (2) Vital signs not within plus or minus 10% of baseline
      (3) CVP readings greater than 15 mm Hg
      (4) Peripheral edema has increased or not decreased
      (5) Weight gain of over 2 lb/wk
   c. How will I know that my client teaching has been effective?
      (1) Client or family member shows a chart of daily weights
      (2) Client tells amount of fluid taken in and urinated each day
      (3) Client shows types of food eaten each day

10. Older adult alert
    a. Older adult clients are at increased risk for developing ARF as a result of unstable cardiovascular status. They have declining COs.
    b. Fluid balance is extremely precarious in older adult clients and difficult to maintain
    c. Older adult clients have less reserve nephrons than do younger adults, and thus there will be less to compensate with in the event of nephron damage
    d. The GFR begins to decline with age and is significantly decreased after the age of 50

B. Chronic Renal Failure (CRF)
1. Definition—irreversible failure of the kidneys. This condition is fatal unless the client receives dialysis or kidney transplantation.

2. Pathophysiology—the affecting etiology causes a destruction of the nephrons, leading to a progressive loss of renal function. A normal GFR is 125 ml/min; **uremia** is present when the GFR decreases to 10 to 20 ml/min
3. Etiology—many causes: injuries, disease processes, drug toxicities, and infectious processes are just a few
4. Incidence—most common in the middle-aged adult; incidence is increasing
5. Assessment
    a. Questions to ask
        (1) Do you urinate frequently? How much urine do you void when you urinate?
        (2) Do you ever have difficulty breathing?
        (3) How is your appetite?
        (4) Do you ever feel as if you cannot think clearly?
        (5) Do you ever feel a burning or tingling sensation in your hands or feet?
        (6) Is your hair and skin dry?
        (7) Has there been a change in your menstrual pattern?
    b. Clinical manifestations (Table 7-3)
    c. Abnormal laboratory finding (see Table 7-2)
    d. Abnormal diagnostic test results
        (1) KUB X-ray film—small, dense kidneys
        (2) Renal ultrasonography—small, dense kidneys
6. Expected medical interventions
    a. Dialysis—continuous ambulatory peritoneal dialysis (CAPD) or hemodialysis
    b. Maintenance of acceptable electrolyte levels
    c. Restriction of fluids
    d. Diet—Controlled protein, carbohydrate, fat, sodium, potassium, and phosphate if on hemodialysis; if on CAPD, usually unrestricted diet with higher protein intake to replace loss of albumin
    e. Administration of supportive drug therapy
    f. Transplantation of kidney—live or cadaveric
7. Nursing diagnoses
    a. Fluid volume excess related to inability of kidney to excrete water
    b. Altered nutrition (less than bodily requirements) related to anorexia and inability of the body to tolerate certain foods
    c. Impaired skin integrity related to tissue edema and structural changes of the skin
    d. Sensory-perceptual alterations related to blood chemistry abnormalities
    e. Potential for infection related to altered immune response
    f. Potential for injury related to altered sensorium, seizure activity, or both

| TABLE 7-3 | Clinical Manifestations of Chronic Renal Failure |

Focus	Assessment Findings
Urine output	Oliguria, <400 ml/day; anuria, <100 ml/day
Metabolic	BUN and creatinine increased, no ratio; phosphorus increased; calcium decreased; potassium increased, metabolic acidosis; sodium increase or decrease, depending on body water
Neurologic, central	Decreased level of consciousness, decreased motor function, decreased cognition
Cardiovascular	Hypertension, CHF, pericarditis
Hematologic	Erythropoietin decreased (anemia); platelet function decreased (bleeding); leukocyte function decreased (infection risk increased); if on CAPD, hypoalbuminemia
Respiratory	Kussmaul's respiration owing to metabolic acidosis, pulmonary edema, pleural effusions, apnea, uremic breath from ammonia (uremic fetor)
GI	Anorexia, nausea, vomiting, mucosal irritation in GI tract, hematemasis, melena, diarrhea, or constipation
Neurologic, peripheral	Peripheral neuropathy, parathesias—numbness, tingling
Musculoskeletal	Soft tissue calcifications, osteodystrophy—bone defect, bone and joint pain
Dermatologic	Pruritus, dry skin (sweat gland atrophy), pallor or sallow skin color, bruising, dry-brittle hair, uremic frost (urea on skin—late sign)
Endocrine	Hypothyroidism
Reproductive	Decreased fertility, decreased libido, amenorrhea, impotence, decreased sperm and testosterone

     g. Potential for body image disturbance related to need for altered elimination of nitrogenous wastes (dialysis)

8. Client goals

     a. Client will maintain an appropriate fluid balance as evidenced by a stable weight within 1 to 2 pounds

     b. Client will demonstrate an appropriate dietary intake as evidenced by a food diary indicating appropriate food choices

     c. Client will maintain skin integrity as evidenced by no new skin tears and skin tears that are no longer weeping fluid

     d. Client will maintain LOC: indicate name, location, situation, and date

     e. Client will have no indication of infection as evidenced by normal temperature and normal WBC count

     f. Client will be free of injury as evidenced by no bruising, fractures, or lacerations

     g. Client will talk about own perception of body image

9. Nursing interventions
   a. Acute care
      (1) Assess all body systems for alterations; changes in any body system are likely
      (2) Care of client—hemodialysis
          (a) Assess access site (Figure 7-7)
              (i) Palpate for thrills; vibrations felt at site mean patency
              (ii) Listen for bruits—turbulent sounds indicate patency
              (iii) Do not use affected extremity for BP or venipuncture; prevents bruising, bleeding, and risk of infection

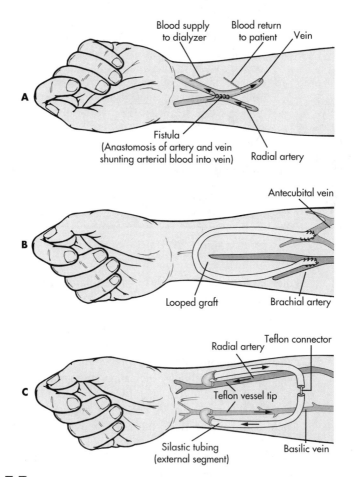

Figure 7-7 Methods of vascular access for hemodialysis. **A,** Internal arteriovensous fistula. Requires 4 to 6 weeks to mature. **B,** Looped graft in forearm. **C,** External canula or shunt can be used immediately. (From Lewis SM, Heitkemper MM, Dirksen SR: *Medical-surgical nursing: assessment and management of clinical problems,* ed 5, St. Louis, 2000, Mosby.)

(iv) If external shunt, have clamps or tourniquets available for accidental bleeding from site

(v) Do not allow constrictive clothing over site

(vi) Keep site and extremity warm

(vii) Check site for infection; wash site daily with antibacterial soap and water; any deodorant soap is acceptable

(b) Prepare Client for dialysis as many as 3 times per week; 4 to 6 hr/dialysis session

(c) Evaluate temperature and BP before dialysis

(d) Monitor BP throughout dialysis

(3) Monitor vital signs for a change of more than plus or minus 10% of baseline

(4) Take daily weights

(5) Record accurate I&Os

(6) Use antiemetics to control nausea and improve nutrition

(7) Encourage eating protein of high biologic value—meat, milk, and eggs

(8) Institute seizure precautions if necessary

(9) Monitor blood chemistries—compare levels versus physical findings

(10) Avoid soap for bathing to prevent drying of skin; use oil in bath water

b. Home care regarding client education

(1) Continuous Ambulatory Peritoneal Dialysis (CAPD)

(a) Prepare client and significant others for CAPD. Instruct how to

(i) Record daily weight and blood pressures

(ii) Use strict sterile technique during procedure

(iii) Instill 2 L of room-temperature dialysate using strict sterile technique

(iv) Keep dwell time: 4 hours during day, 8 hours at night

(v) Continue with usual daily activities

(vi) Allow outflow of fluid and discard into commode

(vii) Repeat with fresh solution at least 4 times daily

(viii) Have dialysate dwell overnight

(ix) Maintain dietary changes: increase protein to 1.5 g/kg/day; increase potassium, salt, and water intake

(x) Follow-up for laboratory studies and their needed frequency

(xi) Follow medication schedule, and report pertinent side effects to physician

(xii) Report problems of which physician should be made aware

    (2) Hemodialysis

        (a) Teach client and significant others

            (i) How to check for infection at access site—fever, redness, swelling, and pain

            (ii) That the client will require dialysis three times per week; 4 to 6 hr/dialysis session

            (iii) How to use clamps or tourniquets—if the client has an external AV shunt in place, have clamps or tourniquets available at all times in case of dislodgement

            (iv) That the physician needs to be notified immediately if the access site bleeds or catheter becomes dislodged

            (v) Not to allow the access site extremity to be used for BPs or venipunctures

            (vi) Not to wear constrictive clothing over the access site

10. Evaluation protocol

    a. How will I know that my client interventions have been effective?

        (1) Vital signs and neurologic status are stable

        (2) Weight is stable

        (3) I&Os are within normal limits for client

        (4) Electrolytes studies are within normal limits for client

        (5) Access site is free of infection and is patent for dialysis use

        (6) Nutritional status is appropriate—client indicates eating suggested diet

        (7) Skin is clean and moist without tears or breakdown

        (8) Client is free of any injury

    b. Which criteria will I use to change my interventions?

        (1) Vital signs are not within plus or minus 10% of baseline

        (2) Neurologic status is decreased

        (3) Weight gain

        (4) Abnormal electrolyte balance

        (5) Skin breakdown is evident

        (6) Bruising, lacerations, or fractures are apparent

    c. How will I know my client teaching has been effective?

        (1) Client is able to demonstrate CAPD using appropriate actions and strict sterile technique

        (2) Client selects correct food choices as indicated in a food diary

        (3) Client maintains stable weight and BP as indicated on weight and BP records

        (4) Client has appointments made for laboratory studies and catheter change

(5) Client has a list of adverse reactions that if experienced should be reported to physician

(6) Client identifies protective measures that should be taken for the extremity with the access site

11. Older adult alert

    a. Older adult clients may have limited options for access sites for hemodialysis as a result of having long-standing cardiovascular disease

    b. Renal transplantation may not be an option for older adult clients because of their age. Clients over the age of 60 must be evaluated on an individual basis to identify if transplantation is a viable option.

    c. Peritoneal dialysis may not be an option for older adult clients who have had several abdominal surgeries and have adhesions from the surgeries

C. Renal calculi

1. Definition—a stone formed and possibly lodged in the kidney; may cause obstruction of urine flow out of the kidney

2. Pathophysiology—stone components are calcium oxalate and carbonate, uric acid, cystine, and struvite. Three factors lead to the production of renal calculi

    a. Urine saturation with a stone element

    b. Inhibitor deficiency or substances that would prevent stone formation

    c. A matrix formation, or the presence of a basis for the stone

3. Etiology—ingestion of calcium carbonate, vitamin D, vitamin C in large doses, and several drug therapies can predispose a client to renal calculi. Abnormalities in the kidney and environmental factors also can predispose a client to stone formation.

4. Incidence—seen in men more than women aged 30 to 50 years, and is more common in the southeastern United States

5. Assessment

    a. Ask the following questions

        (1) Do you have pain? Point to location with one finger.

        (2) Is your pain sharp or dull?

        (3) On a scale of 0 to 10 where would you rate your pain?

        (4) Did your pain come on suddenly or over a period of time?

        (5) Does your pain radiate to anywhere else in your body?

        (6) Have you experienced any nausea, vomiting, or sweating associated with this episode?

        (7) Did you try anything to make your pain better? Did it work?

        (8) Did anything make your pain worse?

    b. Clinical manifestations

        (1) Sharp, severe pain, sudden onset, deep in the lumbar region and radiating into the testicle of the male or bladder of the female if a stone is lodged in the renal

pelvis. In contrast, stones lodged in the ureter cause radiation down into the genitalia and the thigh.

    (2) Pallor

    (3) Nausea and vomiting

    (4) Diaphoresis

    (5) Pain may be intermittent as the stone moves or passes

  c. Abnormal laboratory findings—stone analysis—identifies constituents of stone

  d. Abnormal diagnostic test results

    (1) KUB X-ray film—identification of stone and location

    (2) IVP—identification of obstruction and *hydronephrosis,* which is dilation of the pelvis and calyces of kidney by urine unable to drain

6. Expected medical interventions

  a. Hydration—increased fluids to flush out stone; 3000 to 4000 ml/day

  b. Ambulation—use of gravity to assist removal of stone

  c. Surgery

    (1) Cystoscopy with basket to remove stone

    (2) Transcutaneous shock wave lithotripsy—as client lies in a tub of water, sonic shock waves are fired at the calculi, resulting in disintegration; similar technique for gallstones

    (3) Percutaneous lithotripsy—endoscope is passed through the nephrostomy tract, and lithotripsy is used to disintegrate the stone

    (4) Pyelolithotomy—stone removed through a flank incision (Figure 7-8)

    (5) Nephrolithotomy—stone removed from the renal parenchyma through a flank incision (see Figure 7-8)

    (6) Ureterolithotomy—stone removed from the ureter through a flank incision (see Figure 7-8)

7. Nursing diagnoses

  a. Pain related to irritation from a stone

  b. Anxiety related to pain and unknown cause

  c. Deficit in knowledge regarding dietary restrictions related to new onset; need for education

8. Client goals

  a. Client will state pain is relieved after pain medication or passage of stone

  b. Client will state feeling less anxious

  c. Client will discuss postacute care

    (1) Indicate foods to avoid for the prevention of stone formation, commonly calcium-based foods

    (2) Indicate the need to drink 2 to 3 L/day of water

    (3) Indicate need to void at least every 2 hours to prevent urinary stasis and stone formation

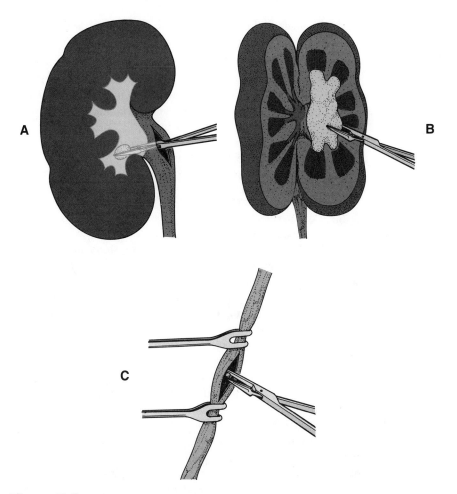

Figure 7-8 Location and methods of removing renal calculi from upper urinary tract. **A,** Pyelolithotomy, removal of stone through renal pelvis. **B,** Nephrolithotomy, removal of staghorn calculus from renal parenchyma (kidney split). **C,** Ureterolithotomy, removal of stone from ureter. (From Beare PG, Myers JL: *Adult health nursing,* ed 3, St. Louis, 1998, Mosby.)

    9. Nursing interventions
       a. Acute care
          (1) Administer pain medication to control pain; narcotics are usually required; assess effectiveness
          (2) Strain all urine for stones
          (3) Maintain IV access
          (4) Increase oral intake if tolerated
          (5) Monitor I&O
          (6) Instruct client to void every 2 hours to prevent stasis of urine
          (7) Monitor incision for signs of infection

(8) Evaluate drainage from penrose drains or ureteral or nephrostomy tubes

> ⚠️ **Warning!**
>
> **Do not irrigate urinary tract tubes** unless specifically directed by physician. Strict sterile technique must be used to prevent infection. If an irrigation is ordered, usually only 5 ml of sterile saline should be used to prevent distention of the kidney pelvis.

   b. Home care regarding client education
     (1) Prevent reoccurrence
       (a) Increase fluid intake to 3000 ml/day; water is preferable
       (b) Limit dietary intake dependent on stone analysis
       (c) Void every 2 hours or when urge to void occurs to prevent urine stasis
       (d) Follow-up with physician for urinalysis and laboratory studies as ordered
     (2) Postoperative care
       (a) Keep incision clean and dry
       (b) Notify physician if incision becomes red, swollen, or drainage occurs
       (c) Notify physician if experiencing urgency, frequency, or burning on urination

10. Evaluation protocol
   a. How do I know that my interventions were effective?
     (1) Has client's pain decreased or been relieved?
     (2) Has a stone been retrieved when straining urine?
     (3) Has client been ingesting and urinating 3000 ml/day?
     (4) Is incision clean, dry, and free of infection?
   b. Which criteria will I use to change my interventions?
     (1) Unrelieved pain
     (2) Stone has not passed
     (3) Client is urinating only 1000 ml/day with ingestion of 3000/day
     (4) Incision is red and swollen
   c. How will I know that my client teaching has been effective?
     (1) Client is drinking 3000 ml/day
     (2) Client has eliminated appropriate foods from the diet
     (3) Client voids as soon as the urge occurs or at least every 2 hours
     (4) Client has an appointment to see the physician for a follow-up visit
11. Older adult alert—take extreme care in hydrating older adult clients with renal stones. These clients have a greater risk of

fluid overload in the event of a compromised heart, diminished vascular tone, and diminished renal function. The essential evaluation during hydration is for the finding of pulmonary edema, indicated by frothy sputum with acute respiratory distress.

D. **Pyelonephritis**
   1. Definition—bacterial infection of the renal pelvis, calyces, and parenchyma; can be acute or chronic
   2. Etiology—usually a result of an ascending urinary tract infection (UTI)
   3. Pathophysiology—usually originates as lower UTI that travels up the urinary tract and infects the kidney. Exudate accumulates in the interstitium of the kidney, and abscesses develop.
   4. Assessment
      a. Questions to ask
         (1) Do you have a fever? Do you have chills?
         (2) Do you have pain in your back?
         (3) Do you have blood in your urine?
         (4) Do you have any particles in your urine?
         (5) Do you have pain when you urinate?
         (6) Do you have frequency or urgency?
      b. Clinical manifestations
         (1) Flank pain; pain at the costovertebral angle; may be described as an aching back or a kink in the back
         (2) Fever and chills
         (3) Nausea and vomiting
         (4) Hematuria and pyuria
         (5) Foul-smelling urine
         (6) May be accompanied by symptoms of cystitis—burning, frequency, and urgency
      c. Abnormal laboratory findings
         (1) Urinalysis—bacteria, pus, WBC, and casts in the urine
         (2) CBC—elevated WBC
         (3) Urine culture and sensitivity—identifies bacteria responsible for infection and which antibiotic(s) would be effective
   5. Expected medical interventions
      a. Anti-infective agents, initially IV, followed by PO administration
      b. IV and oral fluids as tolerated
   6. Nursing diagnoses
      a. Pain related to acute inflammatory process of the kidney
      b. Altered body temperature related to inflammatory process of the kidney
   7. Client goals
      a. Client will state pain is relieved
      b. Client will maintain body temperature at normal level for client or between 37° C and 37.5° C

8. Nursing interventions
   a. Acute care
      (1) Administer antibiotics as ordered
      (2) Monitor culture and sensitivity results
      (3) Administer analgesics, antiemetics, and antipyretics as required by exhibited findings
      (4) Assess hydration status; maintain appropriate hydration
   b. Home care regarding client education
      (1) Necessity of completing the entire course of antibiotics
      (2) Need to make arrangements for repeat urine cultures after antibiotic therapy is completed
      (3) Instruction about the need to seek medical advice as soon as symptoms of a UTI are apparent
      (4) How to prevent further episodes
         (a) Drink at least eight glasses of water daily
         (b) Void at least every 2 hours or as soon as urge is felt
         (c) For females, wiping from front to back after voiding or bowel movements
         (d) Wear cotton underwear especially for females who use pantyhose
9. Evaluation protocol
   a. How do I know that my interventions were effective?
      (1) Has client pain decreased or been relieved?
      (2) Does client feel hot?
      (3) Does client feel nauseated?
   b. Which criteria will I use to change my interventions?
      (1) Flank pain persists
      (2) Fever persists
      (3) Nausea and vomiting persist
   c. How will I know that my client teaching has been effective?
      (1) Client states that antibiotic therapy has been completed
      (2) Client states a repeat urine culture was completed in physician's office
      (3) Client states an intake of at least eight glasses of water daily
      (4) Client states voiding at least every 2 hours
10. Older adult alert
   a. In response to the normally decreased CO and cardiac perfusion seen in older adult clients, blood levels of antibiotics may vary. Thus, antibiotic therapy must be closely evaluated for effectiveness in older adult clients.
   b. The kidneys of older adult clients may be slower to respond to therapy because of the decreased perfusion
E. **Renal cancer**
   1. Definition—malignancy of the kidney
   2. Etiology—unknown

3. Incidence—more common in the male population; represents approximately 3% of all malignancies

4. Pathophysiology—adenocarcinoma is most common. Malignancy begins in the cortex and progresses slowly until the parenchyma is compressed. The lungs are the most common site of metastases.

5. Assessment
   a. Questions to ask
      (1) Do you ever have blood in your urine?
      (2) Do you ever have pain in your back?
      (3) Have you noticed a weight loss?
      (4) Do you ever feel very tired?
   b. Clinical manifestations
      (1) Intermittent gross hematuria
      (2) Flank pain
      (3) Palpable abdominal or flank mass
      (4) Weight loss
      (5) Fatigue
   c. Abnormal laboratory findings
      (1) CBC—anemia if diminished renal function, or polycythemia if erythropoietin is increased
      (2) Erythrocyte sedimentation rate (ESR) elevated
      (3) Urinalysis—hematuria
   d. Abnormal diagnostic tests
      (1) KUB X-ray films—lesion identified
      (2) Renal ultrasonography—identifies solid mass versus a cyst
      (3) Renal biopsy—identifies the type of malignancy

6. Expected medical interventions
   a. Nephrectomy if lymph nodes are not believed to be involved
   b. Radical nephrectomy if lymph nodes are believed to be involved

7. Nursing diagnoses—postoperative
   a. Pain related to effects of surgery
   b. Ineffective breathing pattern related to incisional pain
   c. Anxiety related to unknown prognosis

8. Client goals
   a. Client will state pain has been relieved or is at a tolerable level
   b. Client will maintain a RR of 16 to 20 and will take 10 deep breaths every 2 hours
   c. Client will state anxiety has been reduced

9. Nursing interventions
   a. Acute care
      (1) Monitor vital signs every 2 to 4 hours, evaluating for within plus or minus 10% of baseline

    (2) Make sure client is deep breathing and coughing every 2 hours and using incentive spirometer every hour, with 3 to 5 breaths per session. Breathing is difficult owing to close proximity of incision to the diaphragm. Pain medication must be effective and liberal.

    (3) Splint incision—helpful when coughing and deep breathing

    (4) Assess lung sounds at least every 1 to 2 hours for atelectasis and possible pneumothorax induced by surgery

    (5) Monitor urine output for less than 30 ml/hr and serum creatinine carefully for postoperative ARF

    (6) Assess bowel sounds at least every 2 to 4 hours for postoperative paralytic ileus, a common complication after renal surgery

    (7) Change dressings as needed to protect skin from drainage

  b. Home care regarding client education

    (1) How to care for incision; indications of infection to report to physician

    (2) Need to continue coughing, deep breathing, and performing incentive spirometer exercises

    (3) Have client make appointment for follow-up care with physician

10. Evaluation protocol

  a. How do I know that my interventions were effective?

    (1) Vital signs are within plus or minus 10% of baseline

    (2) Client's pain is decreased or has been relieved

    (3) Client is not having difficulty breathing

    (4) Client is not having abdominal pain or bloating

  b. Which criteria will I use to change my interventions?

    (1) Vital signs over 10% plus or minus that of baseline

    (2) Unrelieved pain

    (3) SOB

    (4) Ineffective coughing and deep breathing or respiratory effort during incentive spirometer exercises

    (5) Decreased urine output

    (6) Absent bowel sounds

    (7) Skin excoriation from drainage

  c. How will I know that my client teaching has been effective?

    (1) Client demonstrates proper incision care

    (2) Client demonstrates coughing, deep breathing, and incentive spirometer exercises, with indications of how often to do the exercises

    (3) Client states when physician follow-up visit has been scheduled and which abnormal findings to report

11. Older adult alert
    a. Renal surgery is a major surgical procedure that may require long anesthesia time. Older adult clients must be medically cleared for this surgery, with cardiovascular status closely monitored.
    b. The renal status of older clients must be evaluated carefully pre- and postoperatively, keeping in mind that one kidney is now completing all the functions of two. Renal excretion is decreased as a normal course of aging.

WEB Resources

http://www.kidney.org/
    National Kidney Foundation - Making Lives Better

http://www.nephroworld.com/
    NephroWorld - The whole world of Nephrology

REVIEW QUESTIONS

1. When monitoring a client who is in the diuretic phase of acute renal failure, a central venous pressure (CVP) line would help to evaluate the
   1. Blood plasma volume
   2. Fluid volume
   3. Renal perfusion capability
   4. Cardiac output (CO)

2. Hypertension in the client with chronic renal failure (CRF) is expected as a result of
   1. Decreased urine output
   2. Decreased H&H
   3. Increased electrolyte retention
   4. Overall increased fluid volume

3. One of the best indicators of peritonitis in the client undergoing a peritoneal dialysis is
   1. Fever of sudden onset
   2. Bloody returned dialysate
   3. Brown returned dialysate
   4. Cloudy returned dialysate

4. A concern in the older adult client diagnosed with kidney stones that are managed conservatively is
   1. Risk for infection
   2. Risk for an MI
   3. Fluid overload while attempting to flush out the stone
   4. Electrolyte imbalance from frequent urination

5. When caring for a client with an internal access site for hemodialysis, an important assessment to make initially would be
   1. Site color being pink
   2. Site temperature having normal warmth
   3. A bruit over the site
   4. A pulse below the site

6. Near the end of the completion of an intermittent peritoneal dialysis sequence for a client in acute renal failure, the nurse observes that the return from the last two runs was less than that inserted. The best intervention to employ at this time is
   1. Call the physician
   2. Turn client carefully from side to side to allow drainage of all areas of the abdomen
   3. Place the catheter to suction for 10 minutes
   4. Irrigate the catheter with sterile saline

7. The peripheral parasthesias seen in clients with CRF are most often a result of
1. High potassium
2. High phosphorus
3. Low H&H
4. Low calcium

8. The client with continuous ambulatory peritoneal dialysis (CAPD) is permitted more protein intake than the client having peritoneal dialysis for acute problems. This would be related to the fact that
1. More protein is lost through CAPD owing to extended contact with the dialysate
2. Protein levels are preserved with CAPD
3. Protein levels are preserved with acute peritoneal dialysis
4. There is some urine formation with CAPD

9. Suggestions given to the nursing assistant for bathing a client with CRF would include using
1. A deodorant soap to minimize skin odors from the uremic frost
2. Bath oil only—soap is drying and the skin is already dry from skin changes
3. Soap to clean and bath oil to counteract the dryness of the skin
4. Only a bubble bath owing to the cleansing nature of the bath with no skin friction

10. A client with CRF has a blood study returned. The nurse reviews it before placing it on the chart. The hemoglobin is 7 and the hematocrit is 24. The next action would be to
1. Call the physician immediately
2. Initiate the standing order for blood from the blood bank
3. Do nothing because this is within the normal range for a client with CRF
4. Ask the doctor to get a type and crossmatch for a blood transfusion, which might be needed within the next 24 hours

ANSWERS, RATIONALES, AND TEST-TAKING TIPS

Rationales	Test-Taking Tips

1. Correct answer: 2

Central venous pressure, measured in the right atrium, is an accurate assessment of fluid volume balance in the body. It reflects if the *preload,* the volume of blood returned from the venous system, is normal, diminished, or increased for different clinical situations. Option 1, blood plasma volume, the straw-colored fluid portion of the total blood volume, is too narrow of an answer to be correct. Plasma, which is water and solutes, contains proteins, lipids, glucose, electrolytes, vitamins, and hormones. Options 3 and 4 have no association with CVP.

Think venous—volume—preload. Arterial—afterload—resistance to pump against. Cluster options 1, 3, and 4 under the focus of specific, and option 2 is more general. Thus, the correct option is 2. Use this approach if you do not know the correct answer.

2. Correct answer: 4

The kidneys of a client in CRF are unable to remove fluid from the body. Thus, the fluid volume rises to result in hypertension. Option 1 is incorrect since a *decrease* in urine output does not directly result in fluid retention and hypertension. Other factors such as fluid intake can also impact the degree of urine output and fluid retention. In option 2, H&H has no impact on the presence of hypertension. Electrolyte retention has many effects on the functions of the body. However, it is not a primary cause of hypertension.

Use the general versus the specific clustering of the options. Options 1, 2, and 3 are specific, and option 4 is the most general. Or, note that the key word in the stem is "hypertension" and of the options an "increased fluid volume" would most likely increase the blood pressure.

3. Correct answer: 4

As with other fluids from the body orifices or parts, any cloudy fluid typically indicates infection. A fever of sudden onset is more typical of pneumonia, or a urinary tract, a sinus, or an ear infection. Bloody dialysate is indicative of a bleeding incident in the abdomen. A brown dialysate is indicative of a ruptured bowel.

Recall your basic terminology, that is, "-itis" typically means an inflammation from trauma or infection.

4. Correct answer: 3

In the conservative approach to managing kidney stones, fluids usually are increased to 3000 to 4000 ml/day. This provides an effort to flush the stones out of the urinary tract system. This extra fluid load could easily cause acute heart failure in older adult clients. The risk of infection with kidney stones is greatest when they are immovable from the urinary tract. This is similar to gallstones in the gallbladder that do not move and result in an infected gallbladder. The risk of MI is more likely if the client has a history of coronary artery problems. Option 4 is an incorrect statement. Frequent urination with normal functioning kidneys does not result in electrolyte imbalances.

Match the key word in the stem "stone" with the option that has this word—option 3. For the selection of option 3, remember that the urine is strained for stones after each voiding, which results from the extra hydration of the body with water.

5. Correct answer: 3

A bruit that is felt over the access site indicates a turbulent blood flow and patency of the site. Options 1, 2, and 4 are correct actions to take but none is as important as the "initial"

This question falls into the harder category because all of the options are correct answers. To get the question correct you need to note the clue in the question—"to make initially." If you read too quickly

Rationales	Test-Taking Tips

assessment. The flow or circulation of blood is a priority. Therefore, option 3 is the best answer.

and missed this clue, you probably had a difficult time making a decision. Remember to reread the question. Within it lies the clue to the selection of the correct answer.

6. Correct answer: 2

Turning the client from side to side would allow pooled fluid to exit the abdomen. The catheter should never be placed to suction, nor should it be irrigated. The physician would be called if the action in option 2 was ineffective to produce more drainage of dialysate.

Noninvasive interventions are typically more appropriate than invasive actions when drainage tubes are involved. Thus, eliminate options 3 and 4. The choice between options 1 or 2 is decided based on the principle that further nursing assessments or interventions are commonly indicated in situations before the physician is called.

7. Correct answer: 4

Serum calcium runs low in the client with CRF because phosphorus is high. A low calcium level is exhibited by numbness or tingling around the mouth or fingers, or dizziness. The other options are not commonly associated with parasthesias.

This question falls into the harder category because all these options are commonly found in CRF. Go with what you know. High potassium results in cardiac problems. Low H&H results in complaints as in anemic clients—fatigue, pallor, SOB at rest or on exertion. Eliminate options 1 and 3. If you cannot remember about high phosphorus just remember the seesaw. If phosphorus is up, calcium is down. Now associate low calcium with low potassium and think of the client on the diuretic Lasix. Recall that a frequent complaint is leg cramps from these clients. Thus, low calcium affects the muscles like low potassium. Thus, option 4 is the correct answer. Remember the low calcium train: tingling, twitching, and tetany—all of which are associated with muscle function.

8. Correct answer: 1

More protein is lost through CAPD than through peritoneal dialysis. Options 2, 3, and 4 are incorrect statements.

Use common sense—with a continuous procedure such as CAPD, clients are more likely to lose protein than with an intermittent procedure.

9. Correct answer: 2

The best answer is one that avoids the use of soap. Any type of soap would be drying to the skin. The skin of these clients is dry from the atrophy of the sebaceous glands, which results from the disease process.

Use your common sense. Cluster the three options 1, 3, and 4 that have soap in them. Select option 2.

10. Correct answer: 3

From a lack of erythropoietin, which is produced by the kidney, the client with CRF will have chronically low H&H. Erythropoietin is one major stimulus to the bone marrow for the production of RBCs, WBCs, and platelets. Without this substance these clients commonly have low serum levels of H&H, WBCs, and platelets. However, sometimes clients with CRF routinely get injections of Epogen, the synthetic erythropoietin, and have fewer problems in these areas.

Look for the clue of a key word: "immediately" eliminates option 1—more physical assessment data would be needed before calling the physician. Initiation of giving blood in option 2 is usually done if the client has other findings associated with a low H&H and not just on the result of one laboratory test. Option 4 is inappropriate for the nurse to do because no other problems or findings are given to support a situation for the administration of blood.

8

The Urinary System

FAST FACTS

1. Provide for privacy. During assessment for urinary dysfunction, clients often feel embarrassed and have difficulty answering questions.
2. Many clients delay seeking treatment for urinary tract dysfunctions until they have severe discomfort. Urinary problems often include problems with sexual dysfunction.
3. Urinary drainage bags must always be positioned below the level of the bladder to prevent reflux of urine, which introduces microorganisms into the bladder and increases the risk of infection.
4. Clients with acute or chronic UTIs must increase their fluid intake to 2500 to 3500 ml/day.
5. Water is the preferred fluid, with the avoidance of caffeinated products.
6. Clients with cardiac and renal dysfunctions must use caution with high fluid intake and ask the physician for strict guidelines.

CONTENT REVIEW

I. **The urinary system is responsible for the transportation, storage, and elimination of urine**

II. **Structure and function**
   A. **Ureters—originate at the renal pelvis and enter the bladder on the dorsal surface. Their purpose is to propel urine from the kidneys to the bladder. Urine is actively propelled by peristalsis.**
   B. **Bladder—situated in the pelvis; comprised of four layers**
      1. Transitional epithelium—innermost layer
      2. Submucosal—supports the inner layer
      3. Layer of smooth muscle bundles referred to as the detrusor muscle. Urination occurs when the detrusor muscle contracts and the internal sphincter relaxes.

4. Serous layer of peritoneum—only in the upper surface of the bladder

C. **Urethra—allows passage of urine from the bladder to the meatus so that urine can exit the body. The male urethra is 18 to 20 cm long, and the female urethra is 3 to 4 cm long. The male urethra is surrounded by the prostate gland at the proximal end and also serves to carry semen during ejaculation.**

III. Targeted concerns

A. **Pharmacology—priority drug classifications**
  1. Anti-infective agents (Table 8-1)
  2. Urinary analgesic agent (see Table 8-1)
  3. Anticholinergics, antispasmodics, and spasmolytics—relax smooth muscle in the bladder
    a. Expected effects—increase bladder capacity; used to treat **incontinence**
    b. Commonly given drugs
      (1) Flavoxate hydrochloride (Urispas)
      (2) Oxybutynin chloride (Ditropan)
      (3) Propantheline bromide (Pro-Banthine)
    c. Adverse reactions—commonly occur with anticholinergic agents: drowsiness, dry mouth, and blurred vision. Medication usually is continued unless findings are severe.
    d. Nursing considerations
      (1) Administer 1 hour before meals
      (2) Instruct client about the possibility of orthostatic hypotension
      (3) Warn client of possible drowsiness, and to avoid driving or using machinery until accustomed to the response
  4. Cholinergic agent—increases esophageal and ureteral peristalsis, and detrusor contraction
    a. Expected effects—increases voiding pressure and decreases bladder capacity
    b. Common agent—bethanechol chloride (Urecholine)
    c. Nursing considerations
      (1) Instruct client that oral doses should be taken on an empty stomach
      (2) Warn clients about orthostatic hypotension and how to intervene by dangling feet for 3 to 5 minutes before standing from a lying position
      (3) Warn clients that until they feel comfortable with the dizziness that may occur, they should not use machinery or drive
      (4) Bladder spasms might occur and must be reported to physician

| **TABLE 8-1** | **Drugs Used to Treat Urinary Tract Infection** |

Generic Name (Trade Name)	Action and Use	Side Effects	Nursing Implications
Urinary Analgesic			
Phenazopyridine hydrochloride (Pyridium)	Exerts an anesthetic effect on the mucosa of the urinary tract as it is excreted in the urine Used for relief of urinary tract pain	Red-orange or rust discoloration of urine	Inform that urine will be orange-colored Take drug with food Use Clinitest for urine testing
Urinary Antiseptics			
Cinoxacin (Cinobac) Methenamine hippurate (Hiprex) Nitrofurantoin (Furadantin, Macrodantin)	Act as disinfectants within the urinary tract Concentrated by the kidneys and reach therapeutic levels only within the urinary tract Used to treat UTIs	Nausea, vomiting, GI upset, diarrhea, hypersensitivity reaction, and dizziness Brown or rust discoloration of urine	Keep urine acidic; give vitamin C (6-12 g/day) or cranberry, plum, prune, or apple juice Give after meals to minimize GI upset Warn that urine may be brown- or rust-colored Monitor I&O; maintain fluid intake of 1500-2000 ml/day
Sulfonamides			
Trimethoprim/ Sulfamethoxazole (Bactrim, Septra) Sulfasalazine (Azulfidine) Sulfisoxazole (Gantrisin)	Bacteriostatic against gram-positive and gram-negative organisms Excreted unchanged and dissolves well in urine Used to treat UTIs, acute otitis media, inflammatory bowel disease, chronic bronchitis, parasitic infections, and for preoperative bowel sterilization	GI disorders, hypersensitivity reactions, headache, peripheral hearing loss, cystaluria, and hypoglycemia	Force fluids to 3000-4000 ml/day *Keep urine alkaline* Give with at least 8 oz water 1 hr before or 2 hr after meals for maximum absorption Monitor I&O Monitor clients with potential renal or hepatic impairment closely Advise clients to complete drug course

Continued

TABLE 8-1	Drugs Used to Treat Urinary Tract Infection—cont'd

Generic Name (Trade Name)	Action and Use	Side Effects	Nursing Implications
Sulfonamides—cont'd			
			Warn about potential increased effect of oral hypoglycemics and false-positive Clinitest results when appropriate
Other Antiinfectives			
Ciprofloxacin hydrochloride (Cipro)	Broad-spectrum antibiotic used for mild to moderate UTIs	GI disturbances, headache, and rash	Give 2 hr before or after administration of antacids containing magnesium Give 2 hr after meals Drink plenty of fluids

Modified from AJN *Mosby Nursing boards review,* ed 9, St. Louis, 1994, Mosby.

B. **Procedures**
1. Urinalysis—see Chapter 7, p. 243
2. Urine culture and sensitivity—see Chapter 7, p. 243
3. KUB x-ray films—see Chapter 7, p. 243
4. IVP—see Chapter 7, p. 243
5. Retrograde pyelography—using an endoscope, the bladder and ureters are directly visualized with the assistance of contrast dye that can be gently injected into the upper urinary tract
6. Voiding cystography—client is catheterized and contrast material instilled into the bladder; x-ray films are then taken of the bladder during filling and during voiding; used to evaluate the bladder for trauma, anomalies, or **reflux**
7. Retrograde urethrography—contrast material is injected into the tip of the male urethra while X-ray films are taken; used to evaluate urethra for strictures or structural changes
8. CT scan—provides axial images of the urinary system; helpful in locating tumors, abscesses, or masses
9. MRI—use of a magnetic field to give an excellent image of the structures of the pelvis but not particularly useful for urinary calculi
10. Endoscopy
    a. Ureteroscopy—visualization of the ureters using a fiberoptic scope

      b. Cystourethroscopy—visualization of the urethra, bladder, and ureters using a fiberoptic scope; any abnormalities of the structures visualized can be identified

11. Urodynamic testing—a series of tests used to measure the transportation, storage, and elimination of urine

      a. Cystometrography (CMG)—most commonly used technique to evaluate bladder filling, bladder capacity, and detrusor stability

12. Ultrasonography—ureters, bladder, and prostate can be visualized using high-**frequency** sound waves; tumors, urinary calculi, or masses can be identified

13. Biopsy—anticipate some bright red blood afterward for about 24 to 48 hours

      a. Ureter biopsy specimen is taken during endoscopy using a nylon brush to retrieve tissue for study

      b. Bladder and urethra biopsy specimens are taken during endoscopy; small forceps are used to pull away pieces of tissue from several areas for study

      c. Prostate biopsy is taken using a transrectal approach, with the assistance of an ultrasonic probe; several pieces of tissue are retrieved for study

C. Psychosocial concerns

1. Anxiety—uncomfortable feeling associated with an unknown direct cause; common in the client with any alteration to urinary elimination as a result of the private nature of the matter

2. Fear—an uncomfortable feeling associated with real danger; common in the client facing any type of malignancy

3. Anger—common response when the client is facing a malignancy

4. Altered body image—a concern for the client who must face a change in bodily functions, such as surgery that will change urinary elimination

5. Social isolation—may occur if the client has incontinence or is uncomfortable with a new body image, such as urinary diversion

6. Depression—not uncommon in the client facing changes in lifestyle or body image

7. Embarrassment—seen in the client with a condition that is difficult to control, such as incontinence

D. Health history—questions and sequence

1. Describe the problem you are experiencing
2. How often do you urinate?
3. Do you urinate in large or small amounts each time?
4. Do you wake up at night to urinate?
5. Do you use any method to stimulate voiding?
6. Do you have difficulty beginning a stream of urine or maintaining a stream?
7. Have you noticed a change in the force or shape of your urination stream?

8. Do you ever feel the need to urinate immediately?
9. Do you have difficulty controlling urination?
10. What color is your urine?
11. Is there an unusual odor associated with your urine?
12. Do you ever notice particles floating in your urine?
13. Have you experienced a large number of UTIs?
14. Have you ever been hospitalized or had surgery for a urinary tract problem?
15. Have you experienced any nausea, vomiting, or diarrhea?
16. Which prescription and nonprescription medications are you presently taking?

E. **Physical examination—appropriate sequence**
1. ABCs—vital signs
2. Inspection of the abdominal and flank areas for masses and other abnormalities
3. Palpation of the kidneys and bladder
4. Percussion of the kidneys over the posterior trunk, and bladder over the suprapubic area
5. Inspection of the perineum and urinary meatus
6. Palpation of the penis and perineum for masses or tenderness; palpation of the female perineal area for tenderness

IV. Pathophysiologic disorders

A. **Incontinence**
1. Definition—uncontrolled loss of urine from the bladder; two major classifications
   a. Acute—temporary incontinence associated with an acute illness or infective process
   b. Persistent (established)—continued incontinence after an acute illness has subsided. There are five subdivisions.
      (1) Stress—loss of urine during activities that increase abdominal pressure, such as coughing
      (2) Urge—incontinence after an immediate urge to void
      (3) Reflex—abnormal spinal cord reflex that causes a leakage of urine from the bladder
      (4) Total—continuous leakage of urine without knowledge of the need to void
      (5) Functional—incontinence related to a client who is unable to use accepted elimination methods owing to decreased cognition or mobility
2. Etiology
   a. Damage or weakness of the sphincter—may be due to injury during childbirth, damage during prostatectomy, or congenital weakness
   b. Deformity of the urethra—frequent UTIs, gynecologic surgery, or trauma

    c. Change in the angle between the bladder and urethra—the urethra normally lies at a 90-degree angle to the bladder. Pregnancy, surgery, or aging may decrease that angle to less than 90 degrees and allow the sphincter to open and become inefficient.

    d. Unstable detrusor muscle—bladder tumors and spinal cord lesions

    e. Weakened abdominal and perineal muscles—obesity, childbirth, and prostatectomy

3. Assessment
   a. Questions to ask
      (1) Do you ever have difficulty controlling your urine?
      (2) Do you wear any special pads or garments to keep you dry?
      (3) How frequently do you void?
      (4) How much do you void each time?
      (5) Do you ever feel burning when you void?
      (6) Do you drink a large amount of beverages that contain caffeine?
      (7) Are you being treated by a physician for any medical problems?
      (8) What color is your urine?
      (9) Does your urine have an unusual odor?
      (10) Are there any particles in your urine?
      (11) Is it difficult for you to get to the bathroom?
   b. Clinical manifestations
      (1) Stress incontinence—loss of urine during coughing, sneezing, and laughing
      (2) Urge incontinence—loss of urine associated with a feeling of **urgency**
      (3) Reflex incontinence—a regular loss of urine without awareness it is occurring
      (4) Total incontinence—continuous leakage of urine
      (5) Functional incontinence—loss of urine before the client can reach the appropriate facility because of decreased mobility or cognition
   c. Abnormal laboratory findings
      (1) Urinalysis—positive for bacteria, pyuria, and hematuria if incontinence is caused by UTI
      (2) Urine culture and sensitivity (C&S)—high colony count, positive for a specific bacteria; indicate which antibiotic is sensitive
   d. Abnormal diagnostic test results
      (1) Urodynamics—abnormalities in the voiding patterns indicative of incontinence
      (2) Intravenous pyelography (IVP)—identifies obstructions in the urinary tract
4. Expected medical interventions
   a. Surgical—bladder suspension
   b. Artificial urinary sphincter

    c. Pharmacologic therapies— Flavoxate (Urispas), Oxybutynin (Ditropan)

    d. Therapies such as bladder training and exercises such as pelvic floor exercises (also termed muscle exercises or Kegel or pubococcygeus exercises) to minimize incontinence

5. Nursing diagnoses

    a. Altered patterns of urinary elimination—incontinence related to muscle weakness and decreased ability to control bladder

    b. Body-image disturbance related to inability to control urinary elimination

    c. Social isolation related to fear of inability to control urinary elimination in public

    d. Impaired skin integrity related to skin in frequent contact with urine

6. Client goals

    a. Client will demonstrate decreased incidences of incontinence over a 24-hour period

    b. Client will state feeling more comfortable with body image as a result of being able to control incontinence

    c. Client will state having no hesitation leaving the home as a result of having more control of incontinence

    d. Client will indicate perineal skin is intact and free of breakdown

7. Nursing interventions

    a. Pelvic floor exercises; instruct client to

       (1) Tighten muscles in perineum—as if trying to stop the flow of urine

       (2) Hold tight muscles for 6 to 10 seconds

       (3) Repeat tightening 4 to 6 times

       (4) Repeat total exercise 3 to 4 times daily

    b. Bladder training; instruct client to

       (1) Void hourly throughout the day

       (2) Increase interval to 2 hours between voiding

       (3) Increase interval to 3 hours between voiding

    c. Incontinence garments

    d. External urinary drainage devices are available for men and women

    e. Skin care

       (1) Skin cleansed as necessary

       (2) Protective skin creams or ointments

       (3) Change damp underwear garments as soon as possible

    f. Client education related to specific medical regimen

8. Evaluation protocol

    a. How do I know that my interventions were effective?

       (1) Has client noticed decrease in incontinent episodes?

       (2) Has client felt comfortable in leaving the home and spending more time becoming involved outside of the home?

       (3) Is client having any difficulty in skin breakdown or redness?

  b. Which criteria will I use to change my interventions?
    (1) Increased episodes of incontinence
    (2) Client refusing to leave the home for any reason
    (3) Skin breakdown in the perineal area
  c. How will I know that my client teaching has been effective?
    (1) Client demonstrates effective technique for care of devices to be utilized
    (2) Client states correct regimen for medication administration
    (3) Client states correct individually developed bladder training or pelvic exercise sequence
  9. Older adult alert
    a. As a normal course of aging there is a decrease in the amount of urine clients can hold in the bladder and a decrease in the muscle strength of the detrusor muscle and muscles of the pelvis. This predisposes older adults to urinary incontinence.
    b. Nurses need to be careful not to assume, however, that incontinence is a normal part of the aging process. Instead, evaluation as to the cause of incontinence as it occurs is needed, and then an appropriate course of action should be implemented.
    c. An important reminder is that many of the medications older adults take can also predispose them to incontinence

B. Urinary Tract Infection (UTI)
  1. Definition—UTI is an infection at any point along the urinary tract; cystitis is an inflammation of the wall of the bladder
  2. Pathophysiology—as pathogens invade the urinary tract the bladder mucosa is affected and the wall loses its efficiency for contraction. Clients may complain of frequent voiding but still have the feeling the bladder is not empty. As the inflammation spreads across the bladder wall, clients complain of painful urination or **dysuria** and hematuria, or blood in the urine may be seen.
  3. Etiology—most common cause is bacterial, although other organisms can induce this disorder. Most UTIs occur because of contamination from the GI tract. Close proximity of the urethra to the rectum in women is the most commonly identified cause of UTI. Infections can descend or ascend from the origin of the infection, and thus, infect other internal structures if not treated properly.
  4. Assessment
    a. Questions to ask
      (1) Do you have pain when you urinate?
      (2) Do you have burning when you urinate?
      (3) Do you feel as if you must urinate frequently?
      (4) Do you feel as if you must run to the bathroom to urinate quickly?
      (5) Does your urine have an unusual smell?
      (6) Is there blood or other particles in your urine?
      (7) Have you been running a fever?

b. Clinical manifestations
   (1) **Frequency**
   (2) Urgency
   (3) **Dysuria** and burning
   (4) Suprapubic pain
   (5) Foul-smelling urine
   (6) Hematuria and pyuria
   (7) Fever
c. Abnormal laboratory findings
   (1) Urinalysis—positive for pathogen, blood, and possibly pus; RBCs and WBCs present
   (2) Urine culture and sensitivity—colony count over 100,000; pathogen identified, and sensitivity test identifies appropriate antibiotic therapy
d. Abnormal diagnostic test results
   (1) Cystoscopy—identifies inflamed bladder wall
   (2) Urodynamics—identifies voiding abnormalities with associated etiology; usually done if the client has frequent UTIs

5. Expected medical interventions
   a. Urinary analgesic for pain—phenazopyridine hydrochloride (Pyridium)
   b. Anti-infective therapy dictated by C&S test results
   c. Education for prevention
6. Nursing diagnoses
   a. Pain related to urinary tract inflammation
   b. Altered patterns of urinary elimination—urgency and frequency related to urinary tract inflammation
   c. Knowledge deficit—care of and prevention of UTI related to client teaching not yet completed
7. Client goals
   a. Client will state pain is relieved or reduced in level on a scale of 0 to 10
   b. Client will state frequency and urgency have subsided
   c. Client will state care procedure related to diagnosis and how to prevent the disorder in the future
8. Nursing interventions
   a. Acute care
      (1) Increase fluid intake up to 3000 ml/day to flush out the urinary tract
      (2) Void at least every 2 hours
      (3) Drink fluids free of caffeine and citrus because of the aggravating effect on the bladder
      (4) Use Sitz baths for perineal pain
   b. Home care regarding client education
      (1) Continue all interventions listed under acute care

(2) Instruct client on the importance of completing the antibiotic therapy

(3) Discourage use of bubble bath and any bathing products with perfume, such as soap, powder, or bath gels

(4) Instruct client on wiping the perineum from front to back only

(5) Instruct client on wearing only cotton underwear, which allows absorption of vaginal and urinary excretions, as opposed to nylon, which holds excretions close to urinary meatus. Wet nylon is a good medium for bacterial growth.

(6) Instruct client to void as soon as feasible after sexual intercourse—allows flushing of the urethra after mechanical friction, which may introduce bacteria

9. Evaluation protocol
   a. How do I know that my interventions were effective?
      (1) Does client still have pain when urinating?
      (2) Does client still have the urge to void immediately or void frequently?
      (3) Has client's urine returned to a normal color with normal odor?
      (4) How much fluid and which types of fluid is client drinking each day?
   b. Which criteria will I use to change my interventions?
      (1) Pain, frequency, and urgency continue
      (2) Hematuria and pyuria continue
      (3) Client begins to experience bladder spasms
      (4) Client's temperature is elevated or gets higher
   c. How will I know that my client teaching has been effective?
      (1) Client is voiding every 2 hours or at the first urge to void
      (2) Client urinates within 1 hour or sooner after sexual intercourse
      (3) Client is wearing only cotton underwear or cotton underwear under pantyhose
      (4) Client is careful to wipe only from front to back
      (5) Client has changed the brands of soaps and powders to those without perfume

10. Older adult alert
    a. UTIs in older adults may be asymptomatic
    b. In older adult clients the only manifestations of UTI may be anorexia, malaise, and low-grade fever
    c. Incontinence in older adults, especially those who are confused, may also be an indication of a UTI

C. **Bladder cancer**
   1. Definition—malignancy of the bladder
   2. Pathophysiology—most bladder tumors begin as papillomatous growths and at some point begin to invade the wall of the bladder.

Staging of the cancer is determined by the depth of infiltration into the bladder wall. Metastasis is generally to local lymph nodes, and to then to liver, lungs, and bones

3. Etiology—cigarette smoking has a high correlation with bladder cancer. Use of the drug phenacetin has been implicated. Exposure to aniline dyes (made synthetically or from poisonous liquid extracted from the indigo plant), rubber, and textiles also have been implicated.
4. Incidence—more common in the male population; accounts for approximately 2% of all deaths from cancer in the United States
5. Assessment
   a. Questions to ask
      (1) Do you experience pain when you urinate?
      (2) Do you ever see blood in your urine?
      (3) Do you feel as if you must void frequently?
      (4) Do you have an urge to void immediately at times?
   b. Clinical manifestations
      (1) *Painless hematuria*
      (2) Dysuria and burning
      (3) Frequency
      (4) Urgency
      (5) Pyuria
   c. Abnormal laboratory findings
      (1) Urinalysis—microscopic or gross hematuria
      (2) Urine cytology—malignant cells identified in voided specimen
   d. Abnormal diagnostic test results
      (1) Cystoscopy with biopsy—definitive diagnostic measure; positive for malignant cells
      (2) CT scan may be helpful with staging
6. Expected medical interventions
   a. Noninvasive tumors
      (1) Transurethral resection of tumors
      (2) Laser fulguration (burning away) of tumors
      (3) Intravesical chemotherapy
   b. Invasive tumors
      (1) Partial or radical cystectomy
      (2) Urinary diversion (Figures 8-1 and 8-2)
         (a) Ileal conduit—piece of ileum is dissected away and closed at one end. Ureters are implanted on top, and the other end of ileum is pulled out to the abdomen. A stoma is devised, and an appliance is required.
         (b) A Kock pouch—a continent ileal reservoir. Ureters are implanted on a 2-foot piece of the terminal ileum. The left ureter is attached to its blood supply. The ileum is formed into a reservoir with a nipple that is pulled out

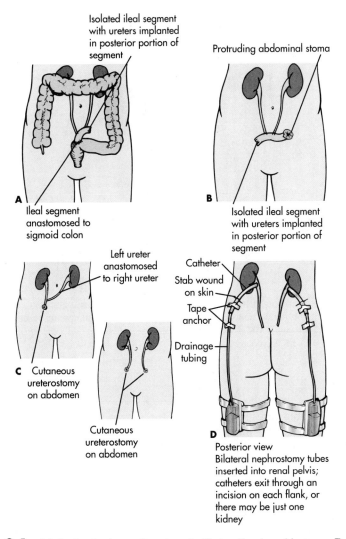

Isolated ileal segment with ureters implanted in posterior portion of segment

Protruding abdominal stoma

A

Ileal segment anastomosed to sigmoid colon

B

Isolated ileal segment with ureters implanted in posterior portion of segment

Left ureter anastomosed to right ureter

Catheter

Stab wound on skin

Tape anchor

Drainage tubing

C Cutaneous ureterostomy on abdomen

Cutaneous ureterostomy on abdomen

D

Posterior view
Bilateral nephrostomy tubes inserted into renal pelvis; catheters exit through an incision on each flank, or there may be just one kidney

Figure 8-1 Methods of urinary diversion. **A,** Ureteroileosigmoidostomy. **B,** Ileal loop (or ileal conduit). **C,** Ureterostomy (transcutaneous ureterostomy and bilateral cutaneous ureterostomies). **D,** Nephrostomy. (From Lewis SM, Heitkemper MM, Dirksen SR: *Medical-surgical nursing: assessment and management of clinical problems,* ed 5, St. Louis, 2000, Mosby.)

to the abdominal wall. The reservoir is catheterized every 3 to 4 hours, and no appliance is required.
   (3) Adjunct chemotherapy or radiation therapy
7. Nursing diagnoses
   a. Anxiety and fear related to the diagnosis and unknown outcome
   b. Pain related to the effects of surgery
   c. Body-image disturbance related to a change in the manner of urinary elimination

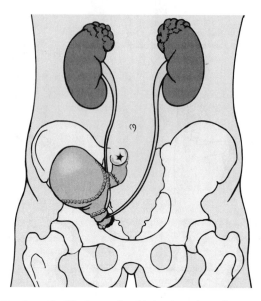

Figure 8-2.   Creation of a Kock pouch with implantation of ureters into one intussus-cepted portion of the pouch and creation of a stoma with the other intussuscepted portion. (From Lewis SM, Heitkemper MM, Dirksen SR: *Medical-surgical nursing: assessment and management of clinical problems,* ed 5, St. Louis, 2000, Mosby.)

      d. Sexual dysfunction related to nerve impairment secondary to bladder surgery
      e. Risk for impaired skin integrity related to urine contact with skin from stoma
   8. Client goals
      a. Client will state anxiety and fear has decreased in intensity
      b. Client will state pain has decreased on a scale of 0 to 10 or has been relieved
      c. Client will indicate by behavior and verbalization an acceptance of the change in body image and structure
      d. Client will indicate by verbalization an acceptance for alternative methods of sexual expression
      e. Client will have no skin breakdown around the stoma
   9. Nursing interventions
      a. Acute care
         (1) Preoperative education
            (a) Routine operative instructions
               (i) Instruct client to turn, cough, and breathe deeply every 2 hours; use incentive spirometer every 1 to 2 hours
               (ii) Instruct client to exercise leg muscles every hour while in bed; dorsi and plantar flexion of ankles

      (b) Teach client the procedures for the type of stoma and device

      (c) Introduce client to general care of the stoma and device if utilized

      (d) Advise client on the possibility of a NG tube

      (e) Arrange for stomal therapist to visit client before surgery

      (f) Instruct client on changes in sexual functioning and the possibility of impotence postoperatively

      (g) Provide bowel preparation before surgery

  (2) Postoperative care

      (a) Monitor vital signs

      (b) Carefully monitor I&O with strict attention to urinary output

      (c) Increase fluid intake as tolerated by the cardiovascular system

      (d) Carefully monitor for bleeding, and evaluate dressing and drainage from drains—drainage devices such as Jackson Pratt should be drained when half full or every 8 hours, whichever occurs first; document amount and color of drainage

      (e) Assess client's pain

      (f) Monitor stoma for bleeding and drainage

      (g) Monitor NG tube output

      (h) Ensure that client follows specific instructions from stomal therapist as to care of stoma and devices

         (i) Provide sexual counseling, and arrange for a visit from a member of an ostomy support group as the client progresses postoperatively

 b. Home care regarding client education

  (1) Incontinent urinary diversion care—the stoma and device or continent urinary diversion care

  (2) Need to be aware of findings associated with UTI and, on recurrence, to call physician

  (3) Use of straight drainage and gravity devices at night to prevent reflux into ureters with an incontinent urinary diversion

  (4) Need for follow-up care with physician and for chemotherapy or radiation therapy

10. Evaluation protocol

 a. How do I know that my interventions were effective?

  (1) Can client demonstrate exercises such as incentive spirometer use every 2 hours after surgery?

  (2) Client knows which type of stoma or device will be utilized?

  (3) Client's pain has decreased or been relieved?

    b. Which criteria will I use to change my interventions?
        (1) Vital signs are not within plus or minus 10% of baseline
        (2) Client has bleeding from operative site
        (3) Pain is not relieved or decreased
        (4) Client is not aware of postoperative regimen
        (5) Client is unclear as to why there is a stoma postoperatively
    c. How will I know that my client teaching has been effective?
        (1) Client states using a gravity drainage bag at night to prevent a kidney infection
        (2) Client demonstrates correct procedure for emptying a continent diversion and for applying a device on an incontinent diversion
        (3) Client states having an appointment to see physician in 2 weeks
        (4) Client states effective visits with a therapist for sexual counseling or attending a support group
11. Older adult alert
    a. The older adult population is the age group most likely to suffer from this disorder, and thus, careful attention must be paid to symptoms suggestive of cancer of the bladder
    b. Older adult clients' dexterity must be evaluated to determine capability of performing appropriate stomal care. Arthritis may cause some difficulty in preparing and applying the pouches. Because of impaired vision, older adults may need home visits from a nurse to perform ostomy care.

WEB Resources

http://www.wocn.org/
    Wound, Ostomy and Continence Nurses Society (WOCN)

REVIEW QUESTIONS

1. The nurse is caring for an older adult client who has become confused over the past 3 hours and is now incontinent for the first time. The nurse suspects
   1. Stress incontinence
   2. A CVA or a transient ischemic attack
   3. Urinary tract infection (UTI)
   4. Overflow from a distended bladder

2. A client requests guidelines for the irrigation of an ileal conduit. The nurse's most appropriate response would be
   1. Irrigation is done on a daily basis with 100 ml of water when the drainage is cloudy
   2. Technique is much like giving an enema with the use of a smaller tube
   3. Irrigation is done with sterile water on a weekly basis
   4. Irrigation is usually not done on an ileal conduit unless mucous plugs are suspected

3. When teaching an elderly female client how to prevent her frequent UTIs, it would be a priority to include instruction to
   1. Void immediately after intercourse
   2. Void every 4 hours
   3. Wipe, after toileting, from vagina to urinary meatus
   4. Wear only nylon underwear, especially under pantyhose

4. The definitive diagnostic test for a kidney infection is
   1. Urinalysis
   2. Intravenous pyelogram
   3. Kidneys, ureters, and bladder x-ray films
   4. Urine culture from a clean catch

5. When planning care for a client, who is taking sulfamethoxazole (Bactrim) for a UTI, the nurse is careful to instruct the client to include the need for
   1. Apple juice with all meals
   2. Meals with medications
   3. An increased fluid intake of at least 3000 ml/day
   4. Careful monitoring of intake only

6. The most definitive finding for bladder cancer is which of these complaints from a client?
   1. Urgency with frequency
   2. Cloudy urine
   3. Voiding blood in the urine without any pain
   4. Difficulty starting and stopping the urine stream

7. A client has had a Kock pouch formed. Which of these actions, specific to this situation, is required by the client for the remainder of life?
1. Application of an appliance around the opening
2. Catherization of the reservoir every 4 hours
3. Intake of at least 2500 ml of liquids daily
4. Ingestion of Vitamin C in quantities of 1000 mg/day

8. The major reason that the over-the-counter drug phenazopyridine (Pyridium), is recommended with UTIs is for its
1. Anesthetic effects on the urinary tract mucosa
2. Anti-inflammatory effects on the urinary tract mucosa
3. Antiseptic effects on the bladder mucosa
4. Antibiotic effects on the sites of infection

9. For which of these problems is the medication oxybutynin (Ditropan) typically prescribed?
1. Burning on urination
2. Bladder infections
3. Lazy bladder
4. Bladder spasms

10. A client is catheterized to check for retention of urine after spontaneously voiding. The residual amount of urine is 25 ml. Which of these nurses' notes appropriately describes this situation?
1. Client had adequate micturition with 25-ml residual
2. Client had 25 ml of urine output after urinary emptying
3. Absence of dysuria with voiding with minimal residual urine
4. Client voided well with a little amount of urine left in the bladder

ANSWERS, RATIONALES, AND TEST-TAKING TIPS

Rationales	Test-Taking Tips

1. Correct answer: 3

In an older adult client who has been continent and is now incontinent with confusion over a few hours, you must consider a UTI. Recall that with UTI and pneumonia, the temperature usually spikes. A temperature elevation would contribute to the confusion in this client. No information is given to support options 1, 2, and 3. If the information had only stated that the client was confused the best option would be option 2 that deals with neuropathology.

The question is asking about the urinary tract. Therefore, options 1 and 3 are the best choices. Of these two options, option 3 is the best. The clue given is that there is an acute change of client status, and infection typically can cause such an acute change, especially in elderly clients.

2. Correct answer: 4

Guidelines are centered on the fact that the output from an ileal conduit is liquid, the urine, and will not require routine irrigation. Irrigation would be done in situations of an increase of mucus production and mucous plugs with an evident decreased or cloudy urine output. Mucus comes from the mucosa of the piece of ileum that is used as a reservoir. The other options are incorrect information.

Note that a clue in the stem is that the client is asking for "guidelines", not steps in a procedure. If you have no clue as to a correct answer, cluster out options 1, 2, and 3 because they are quite specific, or cluster them under the theme of "irrigation is done." The odd option is 4. Select it as the correct answer.

3. Correct answer: 1

Both men and women clients should be urged to void immediately or within an hour of sexual intercourse to flush the urethra of any bacteria that may have been introduced through the friction of intercourse. Voiding should be

Do not let the word "immediately" distract you from the correct answer. The other options are obviously incorrect. Caution. Be aware of your bias from personal behaviors or thoughts associated with intercourse and the elderly that might lead you not to select 1 as

Rationales	Test-Taking Tips

every 2 hours to prevent UTIs. Wiping should be from front to back or from urethra to rectum. Cotton underwear should be worn because of its absorbency.

the correct answer. A clue in the stem is "prevent . . . frequent UTIs."

4. Correct answer: 4

A urine culture will tell which organism is the cause of infection in the urine. A urinalysis with the diagnosis of kidney infection would show the urine to be cloudy with WBCs or casts present but would not specify the type of organism. An IVP is helpful to diagnose kidney stones or tumors. A KUB, an X-ray, is a rough picture used to identify gross abnormalities of the urinary tract.

The clue "definitive" means with great certainty. Options 2 and 3 are test results that show which anatomic deviations are present or if stones are found in the kidney, ureters or bladder. A urinalysis is considered a screening test.

5. Correct answer: 3

Fluids should be increased to at least 3000 ml/day. The urine should be made alkaline. Sulfonamides such as Bactrim are most effective in alkaline urine. Thus, apple juice is inappropriate. Bactrim should be taken on an empty stomach. Sulfonamides, tetracycline, and Carafate are included in that group of medications that need to be taken on an empty stomach. Both intake *and output* require monitoring rather than just intake.

Eliminate option 4 with the absolute term "only" that makes this an incorrect answer. At this point, all of the other three options seem correct about a medicine given for a UTI. Reread the options to look for clues. In option 1 is the absolute term "all." This is probably an unlikely recommendation. Do not get this option confused with the thought to drink more juice with a UTI. Eliminate option 1. To decide between options 2 and 3 go with what you know and with what sounds reasonable. In situations of UTIs fluid intake is increased to keep the urinary system flushed. Whether or not the prescribed medication needs to be taken with meals is unknown because you do not probably specifically recall the given drug. Select option 3—what you are sure of.

6. Correct answer: 3

Painless hematuria is a classic finding associated with bladder cancer. Options 1 and 2 occur with bladder or kidney infections. Men with benign prostatic hypertrophy and women with decreased levels of estrogen or after numerous pregnancies commonly have difficulty starting and stopping the urine stream.

If you have no idea of a correct answer, associate that bladder cancer is a bad situation. Then select the worst finding given, which is option 3, blood in the urine. Go with what you know—that cloudy fluid or secretions from the body usually mean infection, and thus, eliminate option 2. The other findings are of no serious concern.

7. Correct answer: 2

A Kock pouch, also called a continent ileal reservoir, requires irrigation every 3 to 4 hours, and no appliance is required. A Kock pouch is a piece of ileum that is made into a reservoir internally within the lower abdominal cavity. An appliance is a collection bag for urine or stool that is attached to the skin and over a stoma site. Options 3 and 4 are considered general recommendations for persons with urinary problems. The question asks for an action specific to the given problem.

If you are stumped by this situation, ask yourself: "*How* can I figure it out?" and "What do I *know* about the words or options?" A clue in the stem is the word "pouch," which indicates that it will collect something rather than have it flow out. Then as you read the options, they have the clues that the problem presented is related to the urinary system. Ingestion of fluids, vitamin C, and catherization lead you to this conclusion. Connect your thoughts from the word "pouch" to the clues in the options about a urinary problem. Make an educated guess, and select option 2. Eliminate options 3 and 4 because they are general actions for a general renal situation, and the question asks about an action in a specific situation.

8. Correct answer: 1

Pyridium, a urinary analgesic, exerts an analgesic, anesthetic action on the mucosa of the

This is a frequently missed question because Pyridium is a commonly given drug for burning and

| Rationales | Test-Taking Tips |

urinary tract. A urinary anti-infective is given with it to fight the actual infection. The other options are incorrect answers.

frequency of urination. If you missed it, be thankful. Now you know the correct category for this drug and you will not miss it again!

9. Correct answer: 4

Ditropan, an antispasmodic or spasmolytic, relaxes smooth muscles in the urinary tract. It may have side effects similar to anticholinergics such as dry mouth and throat, restlessness, sinus tachycardia, blurred vision, and constipation. It is contraindicated in glaucoma because it increases intraocular pressure. Clients with neurogenic bladders commonly have this drug prescribed. Previous drugs given for bladder spasms were Banthine or Pro-Banthine. Banthine is more commonly given to children with neurogenic bladders. Pyridium is given for burning on urination. Anti-infective agents, such as urinary antiseptics and sulfonamides, are given for bladder infections. Cholinergic agents such as Urecholine may be given for lazy bladders to increase the bladder's detrusor muscle contraction.

If you had no idea of this drug's action, use your energy to determine *what you know about the options.* Most likely you have some degree of familiarity with drugs for situations in options 1 and 2 to eliminate these as choices for this unknown drug in the stem. Then think this—of the remaining options, bladder spasms are a more common problem than a lazy bladder. Take an educated guess that the test is more likely to test about common things. Select option 4.

10. Correct answer: 1

Option 1 is the best answer because it is the most objective, measurable, graphic, or specific description of what happened. From its wording, option 2 is confusing. What exactly does "urine output after

Documentation requires the characteristics of being measurable and objective. Use this guideline to select correct options for those documentation questions.

urinary emptying" mean? Option 3 addresses that there was no discomfort with voiding. It does not objectively state the residual amount when the word "minimal" is used. The words used in option 4 are neither objective nor measurable, that is, "voided well" and "little amount."

9

The Reproductive System

FAST FACTS

1. Many men and women avoid seeking medical care for reproductive disorders from embarrassment associated with the examination and a fear of the unknown.
2. Many women who have major misconceptions about gynecologic surgery must have these beliefs resolved to ensure trust and compliance of therapy.
3. Because many drugs can affect the male reproductive system, a thorough history of prescription and nonprescription drugs is imperative on the initial interview.
4. Clients' cultural, religious, socioeconomic, and educational backgrounds influence how they view reproductive health, illness, and the need to seek medical care for reproductive system problems.
5. Pelvic floor exercises, called Kegel or pubococcygeus exercises, are suggested for any client with dribbling or incontinence after surgery of reproductive areas.

CONTENT REVIEW

I. Definition
    A. The female reproductive system is responsible for
        1. Production of ova
        2. Provision for the means to fertilization, growth, and maturation of the embryo that will grow from a fertilized ovum
        3. Provision of milk for nutrition of the newborn
    B. The male reproductive system is responsible for
        1. Production of sperm
        2. Instillation of sperm into the female vagina so that fertilization can take place

II. Structure and function

A. Female

1. Ovaries—primary sex organs; two oval glands located on either side of the fallopian tubes that are responsible for production of the hormones estrogen and progesterone
2. Uterus—pear-shaped organ located in the pelvis that supports and nourishes a growing fetus
3. Fallopian tubes—hollow tubes situated between the ovaries and uterus that propel ova from ovaries to uterus
4. Vagina—an internal canal that accepts penile penetration during sexual intercourse and serves as the birth canal during childbirth
5. Breasts—mammary glands, which are responsible for milk production to nourish infants; found on each side of the chest between the second and sixth ribs

B. Male

1. Testes—two oval glands located in the scrotum, behind the penis in the perineal area, that are responsible for secretion of testosterone
2. Prostate gland—found just below the bladder, surrounding the urethra, this gland secretes fluid emitted with sperm during ejaculation that will ensure sperm motility
3. Penis—external reproductive and urinary organ responsible for urinary elimination and reproduction; ejaculates sperm into the female vagina during sexual intercourse for the purpose of fertilization of an ovum and subsequent reproduction

III. Targeted concerns

A. Pharmacology—priority drug classifications

1. Estrogens—hormones given through oral or dermal route
   a. Expected effects
      (1) Prostate cancer—causes tumor cells to atrophy
      (2) Menopause
         (a) Used as hormone replacement therapy
         (b) Reduces symptoms of dryness and resulting vaginitis
         (c) Prevents osteoporosis in menopausal women
   b. Commonly given drugs
      (1) Estradiol valerate (Delestrogen)
      (2) Ethinyl estradiol (Estinyl)
      (3) Diethylstilbestrol (DES)
   c. Nursing considerations
      (1) Warn clients about the possibility of dizziness
      (2) Teach clients to use a soft toothbrush and to floss regularly because gingival irritation can occur
      (3) Advise clients not to smoke cigarettes because of their vasoconstrictive effects and the thromboembolic effects of estrogen

2. Antiandrogenic agents—block the action of androgens, or the production of androgens
   a. Expected effects—used for palliative treatment of prostate cancer and to treat benign prostatic hyperplasia; prevent stimulation and growth of tissue
   b. Commonly given drugs
      (1) Flutamide (Eulexin)
      (2) Goserelin acetate (Zoladex)
      (3) Leuprolide acetate (Lupron)
      (4) Megestrol acetate (Megace)
      (5) Finasteride (Proscar)
   c. Nursing considerations
      (1) Instruct client about feeling hot flashes
      (2) Inform physician immediately if client has difficulty urinating
      (3) Instruct client that bone pain may increase initially but will subside; use analgesics to assist with pain relief
3. Alpha-adrenergic blockers—produce alpha$_1$ and alpha$_2$ blockade
   a. Expected effect—relaxation of bladder outlet to decrease symptoms of benign prostatic hyperplasia bladder outlet obstruction
   b. Commonly given drugs
      (1) Terazosin hydrochloride (Hytrin)
      (2) Prazosin hydrochloride (Minipress)
   c. Nursing considerations
      (1) Caution about orthostatic hypotension
      (2) Remind client about feeling fatigue for a period of time
4. Androgens—hormones administered to replace a lack of testosterone
   a. Expected effects—increase testosterone levels and promote male characteristics; used in breast cancer in postmenopausal women
   b. Commonly given drugs
      (1) Fluoxymesterone (Halotestin)
      (2) Testosterone (Histerone)
   c. Nursing considerations
      (1) Evaluate carefully for hypercalcemia
      (2) Monitor for edema

B. Procedures
1. Papanicolaou stain test (Pap test)—microscopic examination of cervical cells
2. Biopsies—removal of tissue for examination of cells for malignancy or other abnormalities
   a. Endometrial biopsy—removal of tissue from walls of the uterus by the aspiration method

    b. Cervical biopsy—removal of tissue from the cervix by the punch biopsy method or, if no specific lesion is identified, by cervical conization in which a cone of tissue is removed

    c. Breast biopsy—removal of tissue from a breast lesion by the open method or needle biopsy method

    d. Prostate biopsy—removal of tissue from the prostate gland by a needle biopsy using a transrectal or perineal approach

3. Fiberoptic examinations

    a. Colposcopy—direct visualization of vagina and cervix

    b. Culdoscopy—direct visualization of peritoneal cavity by way of an incision into the cul de sac of the vagina

    c. Laparoscopy—direct visualization of pelvic contents by way of an abdominal incision

    d. Hysteroscopy—direct visualization of the cervical canal and internal uterus; a scope is inserted through the cervix and into the uterus

4. Hysterosalpingography—contrast medium is injected into the uterus and fallopian tubes by way of a tube placed in the cervix to determine patency of the fallopian tubes and uterine abnormalities

5. Mammography—radiologic examination of breasts for abnormalities and lesions

6. Ultrasonography—sound waves used to emit images of the examined areas: abdominal cavity, pelvic cavity, breasts, prostate (transrectal), and the scrotum. This is the preferred method for evaluation of scrotal abnormalities.

7. Prostate-specific antigen (PSA)—elevated serum levels can be indicative of prostate cancer or inflammation

8. Testicular scintigraphy—nuclear medicine scan of the testicles that requires injection of radioactive contrast medium; helpful in identifying testicular torsion

C. Psychosocial concerns

1. Reproductive disorders can be associated with changes in self-concept, body image, personal identity, and role at home. Extreme sensitivity must be used when working with clients with reproductive disorders.

2. Sexuality and sexual functioning can be altered by a reproductive disorder

3. Fear and anxiety—the uncomfortable feeling associated with a real or unknown threat; commonly seen in clients with a reproductive disorder as a result of the changing effect the illness has on their lives

4. Embarrassment—related to the gynecologic and perineal examinations

5. Denial—commonly seen as a defense mechanism to protect one from the need to seek medical assistance, from intrusive perineal examinations, and from the fear of change in body image and self-concept

TABLE 9-1	**Physical Examination Assessments for Reproductive System**

Male	Female
Inspect breasts, palpate breasts for lumps	Same
Inspect abdomen, palpate abdomen for masses, tenderness	Same
Auscultate abdomen for bowel sounds	Same
Inspect pubic hair, skin, penis, and scrotum for abnormalities	Inspect pubic hair, skin, labia majora and minora, urethra meatus
Palpate penis and scrotum for lumps and tenderness	Palpate perineal area for lumps and tenderness

    D. Health history—question sequence
        1. What has been bothering you? Which problem are you seeking help for from the physician?
        2. Are you or have you ever been treated in the past for any illnesses?
        3. Do you have a history of disorders of the reproductive system?
        4. Is there a family history of disorders of the reproductive system?
        5. Have you ever had surgery involving the reproductive system?
        6. Which prescription or nonprescription medications are you currently taking?
        7. Do you suffer from allergies to any medications, foods, or substances?
        8. Have you experienced any breast tenderness, lumps, or nipple discharge? (Ask both females and males this question.)
        9. Are any of these findings associated with your menstrual cycle?
     10. Which type of contraception are you using? (Ask both male and female patients.)
     11. Tell me about your menstrual cycles
     12. Tell me about your pregnancies
    E. Physical examination—appropriate sequence
        1. ABCs—vital signs
        2. Selected assessments (Table 9-1)

IV. Pathophysiologic disorders
    A. Benign prostatic hyperplasia (BPH)
        1. Definition—enlargement of the prostate gland to the point of urethral obstruction with resultant urinary dysfunction
        2. Pathophysiology—circulating androgens decrease in the elderly male and may contribute to the incidence of BPH. As the prostate enlarges the urethra is compromised, and the male feels the need to exert more pressure to void. Total occlusion of the urethra may occur eventually, resulting in urinary retention.

3. Etiology—unknown or unclear
4. Incidence—one in every four men will require medical intervention for BPH; the incidence increases after the age of 50
5. Assessment
    a. Questions to ask
        (1) Have you noticed a decrease in the stream of your urine?
        (2) Have you felt as if your bladder was not empty when you were finished voiding?
        (3) Have you felt as if you must void frequently?
        (4) Do you waken at night with a need to void?
        (5) Have you had a normal appetite?
        (6) Have you noticed a weight loss or gain?
    b. Clinical manifestations
        (1) Change in urinary elimination pattern; decrease in force of the urinary stream; normal stream assessed for the following:
            (a) Force—enough to clear feet and reach toilet within several inches of penis
            (b) Caliber—stream diameter approximately equal to a pencil lead
            (c) Constancy—relatively constant stream
            (d) Trimness—stream constant and not spraying to the sides
        (2) Urgency frequent, yet difficulty starting and stopping stream
        (3) **Nocturia**
        (4) Urge incontinence
        (5) Inability to empty bladder (retention)
        (6) Frequent UTIs
        (7) Urinary calculi
        (8) Signs of renal insufficiency from an obstruction—nausea, vomiting, weight loss, edema with weight gain, oliguria, or polyuria
    c. Abnormal laboratory findings
        (1) Urinalysis—RBCs and WBCs indicative of infection
        (2) Urine culture—positive for specific pathogen; indicative of UTI
        (3) Creatinine and BUN—elevated if renal insufficiency is apparent
    d. Abnormal diagnostic test results
        (1) Urodynamics—voiding abnormalities
        (2) Prostatic ultrasonography—enlargement of gland; can differentiate between benign and malignant glands
        (3) Cystoscopy—visualization of urethra and bladder for decreased urethra size and bladder changes consistent with an obstructive disorder

6. Expected medical interventions
    a. Indwelling catheterization—allows for urinary drainage in the event of retention; may need to be long-term or repeated
    b. Pharmacologic interventions—antiandrogen agents, alpha-adrenergic blocking drugs to decrease size of gland
    c. Surgical interventions—approach depends on gland size and client's condition (Figure 9-1)
        (1) Transurethral prostatectomy
        (2) Suprapubic prostatectomy
        (3) Retropubic prostatectomy
        (4) Transurethral prostatic resection (TURP)
        (5) Microwave or hyperthermia of the prostate
        (6) Transurethral laser incision of the prostate
        (7) Transurethral balloon dilation
7. Nursing diagnoses
    a. Altered patterns of urinary elimination related to obstruction of flow through the urethra
    b. Urinary retention related to obstruction of the urethra
    c. Urge incontinence related to obstruction of the urethra
    d. Risk for infection related to retention of urine in bladder after voiding

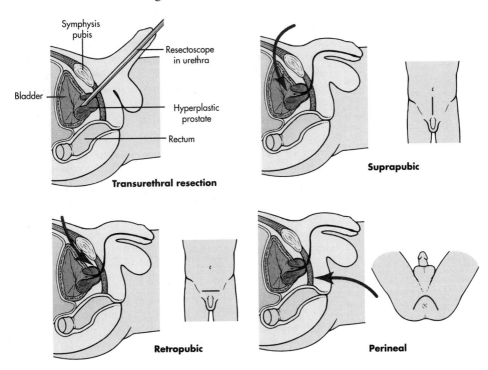

Figure 9-1   Four types of prostatectomy. (From Lewis SM, Heitkemper MM, Dirksen SR: *Medical-surgical nursing: assessment and management of clinical problems,* ed 5, St. Louis, 2000, Mosby.)

8. Client goals
   a. Client will return to previous urinary elimination pattern
   b. Client will state bladder is emptying completely
   c. Client will report incidence of urge incontinence gone
   d. Client will no longer exhibit factors associated with UTI (fever, burning, urgency, frequency)
9. Nursing interventions
   a. Acute care
      (1) Encourage fluid intake of 2000 to 3000 ml/day to prevent UTI
      (2) Discourage fluid intake 3 to 4 hours before bed to decrease nocturia
      (3) Note that intermittent catheterization or an indwelling catheter may be required. It is not uncommon to have a slight resistance from enlarged prostate to catheter insertion. Do not force the catheter. The physician may have to use special catheter.
      (4) Carefully assess the client for shock after inserting an indwelling catheter and draining the bladder. Shock can occur as a result of rapid blood flow into previously stretched, poorly perfused blood vessels of the bladder. Drain no more than 1000 ml at a time.
      (5) Postoperative care for a client having TURP
         (a) Maintain patency of three-way indwelling urinary catheter. Continuous bladder irrigation with normal saline should be done to maintain pink urine without clots; urine should return to a clear-yellow color within 24 to 48 hours (Figure 9-2).
         (b) Maintain traction on the catheter for 24 hours to decrease postoperative bleeding (Figure 9-3). During surgery the catheter will be firmly taped to the patient's leg, with traction applied by physician before taping.
         (c) Increase the rate of continuous bladder irrigation on any sign of increased bleeding or clots. If the increased rate does not diminish bleeding or clots, then monitor vital signs, validate patency of the urinary system, and notify physician.
         (d) Assess client carefully for transurethral resection (TUR) syndrome. TUR is caused by absorption of normal saline irrigation solution and results in electrolyte imbalance, which leads to bradycardia, hypertension, confusion, vomiting, headache, and tremors.
         (e) Assess I&O carefully to ensure that irrigation is draining from the bladder and urine output is adequate

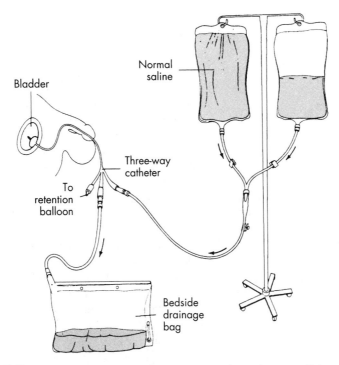

Figure 9-2   Continuous irrigation of the bladder requires a three-way Foley catheter that allows simultaneous infusion and drainage of an irrigating solution (normal saline) through the bladder. The solution is infused rapidly into the bladder, and the bedside drainage bag is assessed for evidence of excessive bleeding and then drained every 1 to 2 hours. (From Beare PG, Myers JL: *Adult health nursing,* ed 3, St. Louis, 1998, Mosby.)

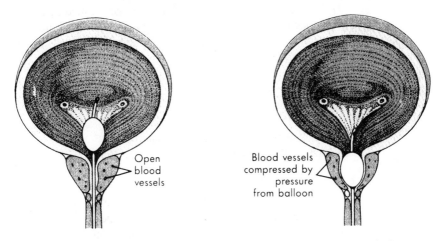

Figure 9-3   Gentle retraction is maintained against the prostatic vascular bed to prevent excessive bleeding after transurethral resection. (From Beare PG, Myers JL: *Adult health nursing,* ed 3, St. Louis, 1998, Mosby.)

(f) Stop continuous bladder irrigation after 24 hours, and remove the catheter within 72 hours

(g) Watch for dysuria, which is common after catheter removal. Urine will slowly return to normal yellow color in 7 to 10 days after surgery. Monitor color of urine carefully for onset of new bleeding and report bleeding to physician.

(h) Watch for bladder spasms, which are common and may be caused by obstruction of urinary flow by a clot. Belladonna and opium (B&O) suppositories are helpful to treat bladder spasms.

(i) Start pelvic floor exercises, called Kegel or pubococcygeus exercises, 48 hours after surgery to decrease postoperative dribbling. Instruct the client to

　(i) Tighten perineal muscles as if trying to stop urine flow

　(ii) Hold tightened muscles for 6 to 10 seconds

　(iii) Repeat exercise four to six times

　(iv) Complete total exercise three to four times daily

b. Home care regarding client education

(1) Encourage increase of fluid intake at home to 2000 to 3000 ml/day to decrease risk of UTI

(2) Instruct that after a prostatectomy the client will have retrograde ejaculation that will decrease his fertility yet not affect erection

(3) Resume sexual activity in 6 to 8 weeks

(4) Instruct client about pelvic floor exercises, called Kegel or pubococcygeus exercises, for dribbling or incontinence

(5) Advise client that small flecks of burgundy-colored "scabs" or clots may be shed 7 to 10 days after catheter removal and should clear within 24 to 48 hours of onset

10. Evaluation protocol

a. How do I know that my interventions were effective?

(1) Is client experiencing any pain?

(2) Does client know where he is, and the date?

(3) Assess the following:

　(a) Vital signs within 10% of baseline

　(b) Pink urine without clots

　(c) Fluid in drainage bag exceeds amount of irrigation—the difference is true urine output

b. Which criteria will I use to change my interventions?

(1) Vital signs not within 10% of baseline

(2) Bloody urine with clots

(3) Increased bladder spasms

(4) Drainage bag output less than irrigation intake

    c. How will I know that my client teaching has been effective?
      (1) Client states fluid intake is approximately 2000 ml/day
      (2) Client reports pelvic floor exercises are improving continence
      (3) Client states he will not have sexual intercourse for 6 to 8 weeks after surgery

11. Older adult alert
    a. It may be difficult to identify TUR syndrome in older adults, because the symptoms may be confused with anesthesia changes or confusion changes that could be considered normal in older adults
    b. Continue to reassure clients that incontinence can be controlled with continued exercise and does not have to be a part of their lives forever

B. Prostate cancer
1. Definition—malignancy of the prostate gland
2. Etiology—exact cause is unknown; prevailing theories include genetic tendency, multiple sexual partners, high fat consumption, chemical exposure, and a history of gonorrhea
3. Incidence—most common type of cancer in the male population. The black male population has the highest incidence.
4. Assessment
    a. Questions to ask
      (1) Do you have any rectal pressure?
      (2) Do you have any pain? Where?
      (3) Have you experienced painful ejaculation?
    b. Clinical manifestations
      (1) May be asymptomatic unless BPH is also present
      (2) May have no symptoms until symptoms of metastasis occur—hip or back pain
      (3) Rectal pressure may occur
      (4) Painful ejaculation may occur
    c. Abnormal laboratory findings
      (1) Acid phosphatase elevated
      (2) Alkaline phosphatase elevated
      (3) PSA elevated
    d. Abnormal diagnostic test results
      (1) Digital rectal examination—hard nodule
      (2) Transrectal ultrasonography—best test for early detection and identifies tumors twice as often as rectal examinations
      (3) Radionuclide imaging—bone metastasis
5. Expected medical interventions
    a. Radiation therapy with external beam or irradiated seeds, or both
    b. Radical prostatectomy by way of retropubic or perineal approach (see Figure 9-1, p. 301)

    c. Exogenous hormones

    d. Bilateral orchiectomy to remove androgens required by tumor to grow

    e. TURP is palliative

6. Nursing diagnoses

    a. Altered patterns of urinary elimination related to urethral obstruction

    b. Sexual dysfunction related to hormone administration or surgical disruption of the nerves necessary for erection

    c. Stress incontinence related to the effects of prostate surgery

    d. Chronic pain related to bone metastasis

    e. Anxiety and fear related to beliefs about the diagnosis of cancer

7. Client goals

    a. Client will report normal urinary elimination pattern

    b. Client will state use of alternative methods of sexual expression

    c. Client will reduce incontinence to two episodes daily

    d. Client will state pain is at a tolerable level

    e. Client will state a decrease in anxiety and fear

8. Nursing interventions

    a. Acute care

       (1) Preoperative—radical prostatectomy

          (a) Teaching regarding turning, coughing, deep breathing, and using the incentive spirometer every 2 hours

          (b) Leg exercises every 1 to 2 hours while in bed

          (c) Urethral catheter in place for 10 to 24 days

          (d) Bowel preparation—usually enemas until clear. Polyethylene glycol (Go-Lytely) induces rapid cleansing of bowel. Follow with neomycin (Mycifradin) for sterilization of bowel.

          (e) Reinforce teaching regarding the possibility of postoperative impotence and infertility

       (2) Postoperative—radical prostatectomy

          (a) Monitor vital signs

          (b) Monitor indwelling urinary catheter for bloody drainage and patency

          (c) Check dressing for bleeding and drainage

          (d) Administer pain medication as needed

          (e) Note: No foreign objects are to be inserted in the rectum for at least 5 days or until the anastomosis between the bladder and urethra heals

       (3) Radiotherapy therapy

          (a) Client must increase fluid intake to prevent dehydration because diarrhea may occur

          (b) Client should avoid fatty foods

  (4) Hormonal therapy
   (a) Discuss strategies for client and significant other to cope with impotence and infertility if that is of concern
   (b) Instruct client to take hormones with food to prevent nausea
   (c) Alert client that thromboembolism is a risk and instruct client on symptoms that should be reported to physicians
 b. Home care regarding client education
  (1) Available information on alternatives for sexual expression if dysfunction has not resolved after 12 months
  (2) Urinary dysfunction that has not resolved after 12 months should be brought to the attention of the urologist; medications may help in the interim
  (3) Chronic pain (Table 9-2)
   (a) Eliminate activities that exacerbate pain; prevention of pain in the first place is an effective way to treat chronic pain
   (b) Work with physician to find acceptable pain medication that is effective
   (c) Identify realistic goals for the client and have significant other assist with reorganizing activities so goals can be met
   (d) Refer client to a support group or a community agency
9. Evaluation protocol
 a. How do I know that my interventions were effective?
  (1) The client's pain has been decreased or relieved
  (2) Client recalls how long the catheter will stay in place
  (3) Client has increased fluid intake
  (4) Objective assessment
   (a) Vital signs stable within 10% of baseline
   (b) Urinary drainage pink without clots
   (c) Dressing dry and intact

TABLE 9-2 Characteristics of Acute and Chronic Pain

Acute	Chronic*
Short duration	Lasts more than several (usually 5 to 6) months
Usually well-defined cause	May or may not be well defined
Decreases with healing	Begins gradually and persists
Reversible	Exhausting and useless
Mild to severe	Mild to severe
May be accompanied by anxiety	May be accompanied by depression and fatigue

*Chronic malignant, chronic nonmalignant, and chronic intermittent pain.

  b. Which criteria will I use to change my interventions?
   (1) Unrelieved pain
   (2) Client is unaware of the amount of time the catheter will be indwelling
   (3) Vital signs are unstable or not within 10% of baseline
   (4) Urine is bloody with clots
  c. How will I know that my client teaching has been effective?
   (1) Client states adjustment of physical activities as needed to reduce chronic pain
   (2) Client states the finding of alternative methods of sexual expression with significant other
   (3) Client indicates regular performing of pelvic floor exercises as ordered, and incontinence is decreasing in incidence

10. Older adult alert
  a. Older male adults are the population most likely affected by this illness. Careful screening must be encouraged in this age group.
  b. Bone metastasis is very likely with prostate carcinoma. Older men should be evaluated for ambulatory stability as a result of the risk of falling and fractures.
  c. Homes of older adult men must be evaluated for potential causes of falls, such as the use of throw rugs in the home, poor lighting, and uneven steps

C. Testicular cancer
1. Definition—malignancy of the testes
2. Pathophysiology—testicular cancer arises from two components of the testes: germ cells that line the seminiferous tubules and cancers that originate from nongerm cells
3. Etiology—unknown; factors that may contribute are testicular atrophy, failure of testes to descend, and scrotal trauma
4. Incidence—second most common cancer in the male population; manifests between 20 and 35 years of age
5. Assessment
  a. Questions to ask
   (1) Have you noticed an increase in the size of your scrotum?
   (2) Have you noticed a full or heavy sensation in your scrotum?
   (3) Have you noticed an increase in the size of your breasts?
  b. Clinical manifestations
   (1) Testicular enlargement, unilateral or bilateral
   (2) A feeling of scrotal fullness, heaviness
   (3) Gynecomastia—enlarged, painful breasts
   (4) Hardness of testes or lumps on palpation; normally testes feel spongy on palpation
  c. Abnormal laboratory findings
   (1) Serum alpha-fetoprotein (AFP) elevated
   (2) Serum beta human chorionic gonadotropin elevated
   (3) Serum LDH elevated

      d. Abnormal diagnostic tests

        (1) Testicular ultrasonography—positive for tumor

        (2) Abdominal CT scan—nodal metastasis

6. Expected medical interventions

    a. Orchiectomy and lymph node dissection if lymph nodes are involved; prosthetic testes may be implanted

    b. Radiotherapy and chemotherapy if a tumor of the retroperitoneum is identified

7. Nursing diagnoses

    a. Pain related to stretching of scrotal sac and nerve pressure secondary to testicular tumor, or pain related to effects of surgery

    b. Body-image disturbance related to changes in sexuality secondary to surgery

    c. Sexual dysfunction related to the effects of surgery

    d. Anxiety related to beliefs about a diagnosis of cancer

8. Client goals

    a. Client will state pain is relieved or decreased

    b. Client will state feeling comfortable with bodily changes

    c. Client will state finding other ways of sexual expression

    d. Client will state anxiety is under control

9. Nursing interventions

    a. Acute care

      (1) Postoperative

        (a) Evaluate vital signs every 1 to 4 hours as client progresses postoperatively

        (b) Check dressing over scrotal wound or over abdomen if there is lymph node dissection with every set of vital signs

        (c) Evaluate urine output. Call physician if output is under 30 ml/hr

        (d) Maintain scrotal support to decrease edema

        (e) Administer pain medication as needed

    b. Home care regarding client education

      (1) Remind client of correct technique for monthly self-testicular examination for the remaining testicle

      (2) Provide information about what would be seen in the event of wound infection

      (3) Inform client that if chemotherapy or radiation therapy is used, decreased sperm counts may result. After treatment, sperm count may return to normal. Alternative fertilization techniques can be considered.

      (4) Refer client to support group or community agency

10. Evaluation protocol

    a. How do I know that my interventions were effective?

      (1) Client states pain is decreased or relieved

      (2) Vital signs are stable within plus or minus 10% of baseline

      (3) Urine output is at an acceptable level

      b. Which criteria will I use to change my interventions?
        (1) Pain is unrelieved or increased
        (2) Unstable vital signs are not within plus or minus 10% of baseline
        (3) Urine output is inadequate
      c. How will I know that my client teaching has been effective?
        (1) Client demonstrates correct technique for self-testicular examination
        (2) Client describes what a wound infection would look like
        (3) Client describes alternate techniques for fertilization to be used if needed
  11. Older adult alert
      a. Testicular cancer is rare in the older male adult. If suspicious symptoms occur, evaluation should be completed. Unfortunately, when testicular tumors do occur in older men they are almost always malignant.
      b. Scrotal enlargement in the older man is more often due to hydrocele, spermatocele, varicocele, or hernia

D. Cancer of the cervix
  1. Definition—a malignancy of the cervix
  2. Pathophysiology—usually squamous cell type. Spreads by direct extension or through the lymphatic system. Cervical cancer metastasizes to the liver, bones, and mediastinal nodes.
  3. Etiology—a major risk factor is intercourse at an early age. Other risk factors are multiple sexual partners, sexually transmitted diseases, pregnancies at an early age, and cigarette smoking.
  4. Incidence—seen more commonly in women of low socioeconomic status
  5. Assessment
      a. Questions to ask
        (1) Have you noticed any unusual bleeding from the vaginal canal?
        (2) Have you ever noticed bleeding after intercourse?
        (3) Have you noticed pain in your back, legs, or groin?
        (4) Have you had difficulty voiding?
      b. Clinical manifestations
        (1) Abnormal vaginal bleeding
        (2) Bleeding after intercourse
        (3) Unusual vaginal odor or brownish discharge between periods
        (4) Pain in the back, legs, or groin
        (5) Difficulty voiding
      c. Abnormal laboratory findings
        (1) CBC—anemia
        (2) Pap smear—abnormal cervical cells

    d. Abnormal diagnostic test results

      (1) Colposcopy—visualization of tumor or cells

      (2) CT scan of the abdomen—identification of tumor and its size

      (3) MRI scan of the abdomen—identification of tumor size and location

6. Expected medical interventions

    a. Treatment will depend on the stage of the cancer

    b. In the early stage, cryosurgery, electrocautery, laser surgery, and conization can be utilized

    c. Loop electrosurgery excision procedure (LEEP)—removes micro-invasive tissue

    d. Hysterectomy, removal of the uterus, is used for those clients not wishing to have more children

    e. For more extensive cancers, radical hysterectomy with pelvic lymphadenectomy

    f. Ovaries will be removed if determined to be necessary at the time of surgery (oopharectomy)

    g. External radiation and intracavitary radiation can be used at some stages

    h. Pelvic exenteration used if radiation therapy has failed, which includes removal of the perineum, pelvic floor, levator muscles, all reproductive organs, lymph nodes, rectum, distal sigmoid colon, and distal ureters. Colostomy and urinary conduit are created.

7. Nursing diagnoses

    a. Anxiety and fear related to beliefs about diagnosis of cancer

    b. Pain related to the effects of surgery or to the effects of the cervical tumor

    c. Fatigue related to anemia and anorexia

    d. Impaired skin integrity related to abnormal vaginal discharge

8. Client goals

    a. Client will state fear and anxiety are decreased to a manageable level

    b. Client will state pain has deceased or is relieved

    c. Client will state fatigue is diminishing

    d. Client will exhibit a perineal area that is clear and free of breakdown

9. Nursing interventions

    a. Acute care

      (1) Postoperative care (interventions for every client having surgery)

        (a) Monitor vital signs (normal routine: every 15 min $\times$ 4, every 30 min $\times$ 4, every hour $\times$ 4, every 2 hours $\times$ 4, and then every 4 hours)

        (b) Check dressing with every check of vital signs

        (c) Maintain IV rate as per physician's order

        (d) Monitor urine output for a minimum of 30 ml/hr

(e) Monitor NG drainage if present for amount and color. Irrigate NG tube PRN every 2 to 4 hours with 30 ml normal saline

(f) Monitor pain, and medicate as needed

    (i) If using a client-controlled analgesia (PCA) pump, evaluate the effectiveness of medication as well as the RR for depression

    (ii) If using a continuous epidural infusion pump, evaluate RR every hour with vital signs and urine output; also evaluate lower extremities for sensation, strength, and movement

(g) Instruct client to turn, cough, breathe deeply, and use the incentive spirometer every 2 hours

(h) Instruct client to perform leg exercises every 1 to 2 hours

    (i) Have client ambulate as soon as ordered by physician

  b. Home care regarding client education

    (1) Encouragement to keep follow-up appointments with physician

    (2) Information on how to balance rest and activity until strength has returned

    (3) Instruction on need for increased fluid intake at home to prevent urinary stasis—at least 2000 to 3000 ml/day

    (4) Referral to support groups and sexual counseling to improve self-image

10. Evaluation protocol

  a. How do I know that my interventions have been effective?

    (1) Client's vital signs are within 10% of baseline

    (2) The dressing is dry and intact

    (3) Client's urine output is at optimal level with input equal to output within plus or minus 300 ml

    (4) Client states that pain is decreased or relieved

    (5) Client is turning, coughing, deep breathing, using incentive spirometer, and ambulating without difficulty

  b. Which criteria will I use to change my interventions?

    (1) Vital signs are not within 10% of baseline

    (2) Bleeding is noted on dressings

    (3) Urine output has decreased; intake differs from output by plus or minus 300 ml

    (4) Pain is increased or not relieved

    (5) Client is reluctant to turn, cough, deep breathe, or ambulate, and lung sounds are decreased in the bases

  c. How will I know that my client teaching has been effective?

    (1) Client attends appointment with physician for follow-up examination

(2) Client reports drinking 2000 ml/day of fluid

(3) Client reports taking a 30-minute nap in the morning and afternoon, which results in the feeling of being stronger

(4) Client has contacted the American Cancer Society to locate a support group

11. Older adult alert

    a. The fatigue associated with the anemia in cervical cancer will be poorly tolerated by the older woman because of decreased stamina. Nursing interventions may require alterations at home, for example, changing the woman's ADL to include rest periods between activities, and moving the woman to an area of the house where there are no steps.

    b. If extensive surgery is required for an older woman, a careful medical workup must be completed to determine the woman's ability to withstand the surgery

E. Endometrial cancer

1. Definition—malignancy of the endometrium of the uterus

2. Pathophysiology—most are adenocarcinomas; metastases are usually to the pelvic and periaortic nodes

3. Etiology—many risk factors are acknowledged: obesity, nulliparity, late menopause, and use of estrogen therapy

4. Incidence—found most frequently in postmenopausal women; early diagnosis has significantly decreased the mortality rate

5. Assessment

    a. Questions to ask

        (1) Because menopause has started and you have stopped having periods, have you had any vaginal bleeding?

        (2) Have you noticed any unusual pain?

    b. Clinical manifestations

        (1) Postmenopausal bleeding

        (2) Pain in the lumbar area, hypogastric area, or pelvic area

    c. Abnormal laboratory finding—Pap test results may show malignant cells

    d. Abnormal diagnostic test results—endometrial biopsy shows malignancy

6. Expected medical interventions

    a. Total abdominal hysterectomy with bilateral salpingo-oophorectomy; pelvic and periaortic lymph node biopsies

    b. Preoperative intracavitary radiation (Figure 9-4)

    c. Postoperative external radiation

    d. Chemotherapy

7. Nursing diagnoses

    a. Pain related to pressure from tumor or to effects of surgery

    b. Fear and anxiety related to beliefs about diagnosis of cancer

    c. Body-image disturbance related to need for gynecologic surgery or need for surgery on a sexual organ

8. Client goals
   a. Client will state pain is decreased or relieved
   b. Client will state fear and anxiety are decreased and manageable
   c. Client will identify two ways to cope with changes in sexuality
9. Nursing interventions
   a. Acute care
      (1) See postoperative care guidelines under Nursing Interventions of the Client with Cervical Cancer on pp. 311-312
      (2) Care of client with intracavitary radiation—(see Figure 9-4)
         (a) Client must be in a private room
         (b) Nurse stands near the head of bed during care to reduce nurse's exposure to radiation
         (c) Visitors are limited to a 30-minute visit per day
         (d) Children and pregnant women are not allowed in the room
         (e) Client is on absolute bed rest
         (f) Client may be moved using "bedroll," and head of bed may be elevated but to no more than 45 degrees
         (g) Client should be encouraged to cough, breathe deeply, use the incentive spirometer, and perform leg exercises at least every 2 hours
         (h) Urinary catheter is in place and is patent to prevent a distended bladder from coming into contact with the radioactive source

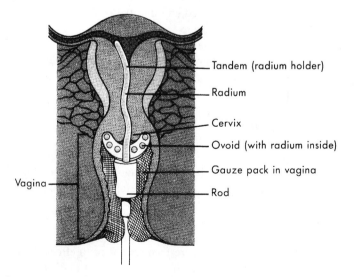

Figure 9-4 Intracavity irradiation of the cervix for treatment of cervical cancer. (From Beare PG, Myers JL: *Adult health nursing,* ed 3, St. Louis, 1998, Mosby.)

        (i) Client is assessed for temperature elevation, nausea, and vomiting, which may be indicative of uterine perforation or infection

        (j) Profuse vaginal drainage should be reported to physician immediately

        (k) Sexual activity can resume 1 week after therapy

        (l) Vaginal lubricant may be needed owing to dryness of vagina from effects of therapy

        (m) Vaginal dilator may be required owing to scarring from therapy

  b. Home care regarding client education

    (1) Postoperative teaching concerning diet, fluid, activity, and physician follow-up

    (2) Instruction on what occurs after intracavitary radiation

      (a) Fatigue is common; take frequent rest periods of 30 minutes every 2 hours

      (b) Diarrhea is a common occurrence; follow a low-fiber diet to decrease symptoms

      (c) Excessive nausea, vomiting, diarrhea, difficulty urinating, prolonged back, or abdominal pain should be reported to physician

      (d) Showers are preferred to baths because of the expected increase in vaginal discharge

10. Evaluation protocol

  a. How do I know that my interventions have been effective?

    (1) Client has not developed complications of bed rest while undergoing intracavitary radiation (DVT, atelectasis)

    (2) Postoperatively client demonstrates vital signs that are within 10% of baseline, with no bleeding

    (3) Client's postoperative pain has been controlled

  b. Which criteria will I use to change my interventions?

    (1) Client develops DVT or atelectasis

    (2) Postoperatively client has unstable vital signs or bleeding

    (3) Client's postoperative pain is increased or is not relieved

  c. How will I know that my client teaching has been effective?

    (1) Client is resting in the morning and afternoon, and has increased stamina and overall activity

    (2) Client has kept follow-up appointments

    (3) Client uses a water-soluble lubricant for intercourse

11. Older adult alert

  a. Endometrial cancer is a disorder most commonly seen in the older female client. Careful assessment for findings associated with this illness is imperative.

  b. An older adult woman who must have intracavitary radiation is at very high risk for complications, such as DVT, atelectasis, and pneumonia associated with bed rest. This client must be monitored carefully.

c. An older adult woman undergoing intracavitary radiation must also be monitored carefully for the development of fistulas

F. Ovarian cancer

1. Definition—malignancy of the ovary
2. Pathophysiology—risk factors are ovarian dysfunction and infertility. Most ovarian cancers are epithelial tumors. Ovarian cancer metastasizes through seeding and implantation commonly in the peritoneum, omentum, and bowel.
3. Etiology—unknown; however, there does seem to be a familial tendency
4. Incidence—seen in all age groups; most common in the white population
5. Assessment
   a. Questions to ask
      (1) Have you experienced abdominal or pelvic pain?
      (2) Have you been experiencing unusual vaginal bleeding?
      (3) Have you had any GI complaints?
      (4) Have you noticed any changes in urinary function or any unusual symptoms with urination?
   b. Clinical manifestations
      (1) Manifestations are most often seen in advanced cases
      (2) Ascites
      (3) Pelvic or abdominal pain
      (4) Abnormal uterine bleeding
      (5) Persistent GI complaints
      (6) Urinary complaints
   c. Abnormal laboratory findings—elevated cancer antigen 125 (CA-125)
   d. Abnormal diagnostic tests
      (1) Bimanual examination—results of palpation of the ovaries in postmenopausal women are abnormal; any ovarian mass should be considered suspicious
      (2) Ultrasonography—identification of a mass or enlarged ovaries
6. Expected medical interventions
   a. Total abdominal hysterectomy with bilateral salpingo-oophorectomy and omentectomy as soon as diagnostic workup is completed
   b. Radiation and chemotherapy may follow surgery; intraperitoneal and systemic chemotherapy may be done
7. Care of this client will be very much the same as for the client with endometrial and cervical cancers; refer to those nursing interventions and evaluations

G. **Breast cancer**
 1. Definition—malignancy of the female or male breast
 2. Etiology—familial tendency, history of fibrocystic disease, and hormonal influence
 3. Incidence—breast cancer is now the second leading cause of cancer deaths in women; it is rare in men
 4. Assessment
    a. Questions to ask
       (1) Has your mother or a sister ever been diagnosed with breast cancer?
       (2) Do you routinely perform self-examination of your breasts? When in relation to your periods?
       (3) Do you have mammographies? How often?
       (4) Did you find this lump during self-examination?
    b. Clinical manifestations
       (1) Single lump or thickening on one breast—earliest finding
       (2) Painless lump
       (3) Lump is irregular and nonmobile
       (4) Nipple discharge
       (5) Skin dimpling on the breast
       (6) Change in breast shape
       (7) Skin ulcerations (late finding)
    c. Abnormal diagnostic test results
       (1) Mammography—defined mass with size and shape
       (2) Biopsy—identification of malignant or benign cells
       (3) Sentinel lymph node biopsy—identifies nodes that drain first from the tumor site
       (4) Estrogen-progesterone receptor assays—show well-differentiated tumors
 5. Expected medical interventions
    a. Lumpectomy—removal of tumor with surrounding healthy tissue followed by radiation therapy
    b. Mastectomy
       (1) Modified radical—breast and axillary lymph nodes are removed
       (2) Radical—breast, pectoral muscles, and axillary nodes are removed
       (3) Simple—breast is removed
       (4) Quadrantectomy—quadrant of breast that houses the lesion is removed
       (5) Breast reconstruction is done at the initial surgery in many cases
    c. Radiation therapy—internal implants or external radiation
    d. Chemotherapy
    e. Hormonal therapy—given to women who have tumors that are estrogen or progesterone receptor positive. Tamoxifen

citrate—blocks estrogen receptor sites on the tumor and prevents tumor growth.

    f. Autologous bone marrow or stem cell transplantation—high-dose radiation therapy preceded by harvesting the client's bone marrow, freezing it, and returning it to the client after chemotherapy is completed. This procedure replenishes bone marrow destroyed by the chemotherapy. Client can also donate a blood specimen from which stem cells are harvested and returned to the client after chemotherapy.

6. Nursing diagnosis
    a. Body-image disturbance related to surgical changes in the breast
    b. Impaired skin integrity related to the effects of radiation therapy
    c. Impaired physical mobility related to acute pain after surgery extending into the axilla
    d. Pain related to pressure from the tumor or to the effects of surgery
    e. Fear and anxiety related to beliefs about the diagnosis of cancer
    f. Altered nutrition (less than body requirements) related to anorexia, nausea, and vomiting caused by chemotherapy

7. Client goals
    a. Client will state feeling comfortable with the new body image that is going to occur
    b. Client will maintain clean, dry, intact skin in association with radiation therapy
    c. Client will be able to have full, active, range of motion of the affected arm
    d. Client will indicate pain is decreased or relieved
    e. Client will state that fear and anxiety have decreased to a manageable level
    f. Client will maintain present body weight or will not lose over half a pound per week

8. Nursing interventions
    a. Acute care
        (1) Postoperative care
            (a) Maintain usual postoperative care
            (b) Empty drains and continuous portable suction devices when half full or every 8 hours, whichever occurs first
            (c) Elevate and abduct the affected arm above the level of heart when the client is sitting or lying
            (d) Begin arm exercises as soon as the client is awake enough to cooperate
                (i) Encourage client to perform wall-walking with fingertips—up the wall so that the arm extends above the head
                (ii) Encourage client to squeeze a ball

        (e) Have client begin full range-of-motion exercises with the affected arm after drains are removed

        (f) Give client pain medication as needed to ensure exercise regimen is carried out

    (2) Have a volunteer who has experienced breast cancer visit the client while still hospitalized. Volunteers (e.g., from Reach for Recovery or another organization affiliated with the American Cancer Society) can assist in postoperative adjustment and even offer a temporary prosthesis to wear home.

  b. Home care regarding client education

    (1) Carry out required care for the arm on the surgical side

        (a) Avoid burns, insect bites, cuts, scrapes, and scratches if there is a loss of lymph nodes in the axilla. The greater the number of nodes removed, the greater the risk for infection.

        (b) Avoid procedures on the arm such as BPs, injections, and blood drawing

        (c) Carry heavy objects in the unaffected arm. Usually 3 weeks after surgery, items weighing less than 5 pounds can be carried in the affected arm and driving is permitted.

        (d) Wear a medical-alert bracelet to inform caregivers of the disorder

9. Evaluation protocol

  a. How will I know that my interventions were effective?

    (1) Client indicates pain is decreased or tolerable

    (2) Affected arm does not become edematous

    (3) Client is able to perform assisted active range-of-motion exercises effectively

  b. Which criteria will I use to change my interventions?

    (1) Client's pain is increased or unrelieved

    (2) Affected arm becomes edematous

    (3) Client is unable to perform assisted active range-of-motion exercises

  c. How will I know that my client teaching has been effective?

    (1) Client protects the affected arm from trauma and exposure to infection

    (2) Client carries packages with the unaffected side

    (3) Client wears medical-alert bracelet

10. Older adult alert—treatment plan for the older adult client may be modified to hormonal manipulation or radiation therapy, or both, if the client cannot tolerate surgery

WEB Resources

http://www3.cancer.org/cancerinfo/res_home.asp?ct=5 Breast Cancer: Resource Center
http://www3.cancer.org/cancerinfo/res_home.asp?ct=36 Prostate Cancer: Resource Center
http://www.cancerlinksusa.com/testicular Testicular Cancer, CancerLinksUSA.com

REVIEW QUESTIONS

1. While caring for a client who had a TURP, the nurse understands that the urinary catheter is pulled tight and taped to the leg to
    1. Minimize bladder spasms
    2. Encourage compression of the prostatic area and further dilate the urethra
    3. Decrease the incidence of postoperative excessive blood loss
    4. Prevent edema in the area from which the prostate was removed

2. A client asks why his bladder must be continuously irrigated. The best reply by the nurse is
    1. "The irrigation keeps your urine clear."
    2. "The irrigation clears any clots and blood out of your bladder."
    3. "The room temperature continuous saline drip decreases swelling and inflammation in the area of the surgery."
    4. "The normal saline promotes an increase your urine output."

3. An important teaching need of the postoperative TURP client is
    1. Pelvic tilt exercises
    2. Bladder training after the urethral catheter is removed
    3. Pubococcygeus exercises
    4. Fluid restriction for items such as coffee, water, and tea

4. When assessing a client with prostate cancer who has suffered with metastasis to the bones for over 4 months, the nurse would expect to see what kind of assessment findings indicative of pain?
    1. Facial grimacing
    2. No physiologic findings
    3. Clenched fists
    4. Fetal position with a tight muscle tone

5. A clinical manifestation associated with the diagnosis of testicular cancer is
    1. Anemia
    2. Impotence
    3. Scrotal pain
    4. Gynecomastia

6. The most common problem reported by clients after intracavitary radiation therapy is
    1. Difficulty voiding
    2. Diarrhea
    3. Abdominal pain
    4. Low back pain

7. A friend asks a nurse about her risk of having ovarian cancer, since she just lost her mother to ovarian cancer. The nurse's best response would be
1. The cause of ovarian cancer is unknown, so that risk is also unclear
2. Ovarian cancer is so difficult to identify in the early stages that physicians are unsure of what risks might be associated with the illness
3. There is a familial tendency for ovarian cancer; so having routine complete gynecologic examinations would be wise
4. There is no known link to family heredity in ovarian cancer

8. The nurse knows that a client has grasped the concept of arm exercises after a modified radical mastectomy when the client says she will
1. Wear her sling when up and about until her incision is healed
2. Perform wall-walking exercises with her fingertips above her head every 2 to 4 hours after pain medication
3. Exercise only her wrist until she is at home
4. Do her exercising by using the movements when showering and caring for her hair as her exercises exclusively

9. The nurse explains to a client that the major reason the client must not have injections, BPs, or venipunctures in the affected arm after a modified radical mastectomy is
1. The lymph drainage from the arm is seriously impeded and may make the arm extremely edematous with nonabsorption of any medication if any of those procedures would occur
2. There is an incision in the axilla that must heal before any of those procedures can be performed owing to possible impaired healing of the incision
3. Pressure from the tourniquet for venipuncture and increased fluid load from injections can impede healing of the mastectomy scar and increase the risk of infection
4. Lymphatic fluid pooling from the surgery makes veins impossible to find on the affected arm and injections impossible to be absorbed

10. When positioning a client immediately postoperatively after a lumpectomy, the nurse would use which position?
1. Supine with the affected arm elevated on a pillow in a position of comfort for the client
2. Side-lying, nonsurgical side only with the affected arm elevated
3. Low Fowler's position with the affected arm elevated on two pillows, above the level of the heart
4. Whichever position is comfortable for the client

ANSWERS, RATIONALES, AND TEST-TAKING TIPS

Rationales	Test-Taking Tips

1. Correct answer: 3

The urinary catheter is pulled tight to decrease bleeding by the traction to put direct pressure on the surgical site of the prostate removal. Remember that the prostate is one of the more vascular areas of the body. A TURP removal is by pieces, and thus a small piece could be retained and result in hemorrhage postoperatively. Option 1 is incorrect. The large 30-ml balloon causes bladder spasms. Options 2 and 4 are incorrect statements.

The key words in the stem are "pulled tight." This clue helps you associate this action with the prevention of bleeding. Recall actions in first aid—apply pressure.

2. Correct answer: 2

Continuous bladder irrigation is initiated after a TURP to flush blood and clots out of the bladder. This irrigation process ensures free draining of the urine. Option 1 might be a correct answer but is not the best answer. It is a general statement and not as specific as option 2. The statements in options 3 and 4 are not correct information.

The question asks about irrigation. Therefore, the options can be narrowed to option 1 or 2. The concept of irrigation means, "to remove."

3. Correct answer: 3

After TURP the client must be taught how to perform pubococcygeus exercises so that urinary control can be achieved as quickly as possible after catheter removal. Option 1 is taught to clients with low back pain. Option 2 is usually needed when urinary catheters

If you read quickly, you may have narrowed the options to 3 and 4. Fast reading may have resulted in a focus on the coffee and tea in option 4. If you missed the word "water," it makes the question much harder than it is. When you feel this way, let it be a signal to you to go back and reread the options in a

are in for over 1 or 2 weeks. With most TURPs the urinary catheter is in for 2 to 3 days. This time period typically does not result in a change of the bladder tone to flaccid. Option 4 would have been a correct answer if it did not include "water." Water is not to be restricted in these clients. However, even if the water were not included, option 3 would still be the best answer. Exercises have better long-term effect for urinary control than does specific fluid restriction, which provides control on only a daily basis.

reverse manner. You will be sure to identify your error and then select the correct option with confidence.

4. Correct answer: 2

A client who has suffered pain for that length of time typically will not show physical evidence of pain. The client will control any physical evidence either consciously or unconsciously. All of the other options may be findings of acute pain.

The time element is important here—chronic pain is commonly defined as that which lasts for longer than 3 to 4 months. Chronic pain is best assessed by use of client complaints and not physical findings. Chronic pain may be less intense than acute pain.

5. Correct answer: 4

Gynecomastia quite frequently accompanies the diagnosis of testicular cancer. This finding is from tumors that produce either estrogen or progesterone hormones or cause a decrease in the normal levels of testosterone hormone production. Anemia is often a result of cancer therapy. Impotence would more likely be an effect of surgery or a change in mental thoughts of clients. Pain generally is not present in testicular cancer. The most common complaint is a feeling of heaviness or fullness in the scrotal sac.

Associate that tumors typically produce or inhibit hormonal production. The only option with an indication of a hormonal influence is option 4. Some lung tumors produce insulin and others produce ADH, antidiuretic hormone.

Rationales	Test-Taking Tips

6. Correct answer: 2

Diarrhea is a problem after intracavitary radiation therapy that must be treated to prevent dehydration. Difficulty voiding may occur after removal of urinary catheters that have been in for one or more weeks. Abdominal pain is more likely a finding in clients with adhesions after radical surgeries in the abdominal cavity. Low back pain has many causes, from abnormal bone and muscle structure to normal events in life such as scoliosis, poor posture, being overweight, or being pregnant.

The clue is the key word in the stem, "common." Think anatomy—this radiation is for the uterus and the only option that is anatomically close is diarrhea—the bowel. Another thought is that radiation, internal or external, like chemotherapy will affect the most rapidly producing cells, both normal and tumor, with the result of irritation or inflammation. The only option suggestive of irritation is diarrhea.

7. Correct answer: 3

Ovarian cancer has a familial tendency. The other options are incorrect statements.

If you have no idea of an answer, make an educated guess by looking for clues in each option. Cluster the common themes in the options 1, 2, and 4—key words: "unknown," "difficult to identify . . . unsure" and "no known link." Select option 3. It gives specific information.

8. Correct answer: 2

Wall-walking exercises using fingertips and walking fingers above the head are appropriate exercises for this client. Every 2 to 4 hours would be appropriate after PRN pain medication, which would allow for less discomfort during the exercises. Slings are usually not encouraged. Rather, clients are taught to prop their affected arm in an elevated and abducted position when sitting or lying. Option 3 is an

Careful reading alerts you to immediately eliminate options 3 and 4 with absolute words "only" and "exclusively." Options with absolutes are usually incorrect answers. With options 1 and 2 left, go with what you know, that is, to exercise the surgical area after any type of surgery is more likely than to keep the area immobile. You may have also remembered that one common problem after a radical mastectomy is the decreased range of motion of the affected shoulder

incorrect action. In option 4 the exercises are appropriate but to use only these exercises is incorrect information.

from clients wanting to roll the shoulder inward and adduct the arm to minimize their postsurgical pain. Use imagery. Close your eyes and picture option 1 and then option 2. That option 2 is correct becomes evident.

9. Correct answer: 1

Removal of the lymph glands from the axilla will prevent lymph drainage from the affected arm. BP readings, venipunctures, or injections will further hinder lymph drainage from the arm. The contents in options 2, 3, and 4 are incorrect, except for the second part of option 3. These actions do increase the risk of infection in the affected arm. Remember that a modified radical mastectomy is the removal of lymph nodes and breast tissue. A radical mastectomy is the additional removal of the pectoral muscle.

Avoid the temptation to select option 1 and not to read the other options. If you had this action, force yourself to recognize this bad habit. Then proceed to read option 4; then read option 3; then read option 2. Reread option 1. Only at this point, after reading all of the options, make your selection. The error of not reading all of the options puts you at high risk to fail tests. Be aware that you are likely to revert to this error when options have a lot of verbiage, as in this instance. You get tired of reading. This is why you need to change the way you read—go from options 4 to 1 for better concentration.

10. Correct answer: 4

A lumpectomy is the removal of the tumor—lump—with a margin of the surrounding healthy tissue. It does not involve the removal of lymph nodes from the axilla. Remember "lumpectomy = lymph still intact." Thus, arm positioning is not crucial. A position of comfort is best in the given situation. Options 1 and 2 are not used for any specific surgeries. Option 3 is a correct position immediately after a modified radical mastectomy. After a radical mastectomy, clients usually

If you have no idea of a correct answer, use the theme approach. Cluster the options 1, 2, and 3 under the theme of very specific information. Option 4 is the odd man out with general information. Select option 4.

have their arm positioned
across their chest in the
immediate postoperative
period. With removal of the
pectoral muscle the client
would have poor control of the
affected arm at this time. Note
that in this question the time is
not as important as is the type
of surgery.

10

The Endocrine System

FAST FACTS

1. Identification of endocrine disorders is difficult because assessments cover many body systems.
2. Vital signs and body weight are essential in the *initial* assessment and *later* during therapy evaluation for the client with an endocrine disorder.
3. The glands or tissues affected by hormones may be distant from the parent organ.
4. *Hypofunction* of an organ results in a diminished level of a hormone (think hypodermic or under the skin).
5. *Hyperfunction* of an organ results in an excess level of a hormone (think hyperactivity equals excess activity).
6. Most hormones have a diurnal production pattern or an increase or a decrease in serum hormonal levels within a 24-hour period. Blood samples usually are drawn in the morning and afternoon.
7. Endocrine glands secrete hormones directly into the blood or lymph systems.
8. Exocrine glands secrete hormones through a duct into the GI tract.
9. The pancreas functions as both an endocrine and exocrine gland. As an endocrine gland it secretes insulin and glucagon into the blood. As an exocrine gland it secretes bicarbonate, lipase, amylase, and trypsin into the duodenum.

CONTENT REVIEW

I. The endocrine system in association with the nervous system is responsible for controlling homeostasis

II. Structure and function (Table 10-1, Figures 10-1 and 10-2)

TABLE 10-1 Major Endocrine Glands, Hormones, Target Tissues, and Functions

Hormones	Target Tissue	Functions
Anterior Pituitary (adenohypophysis)		
Growth hormone (GH) or somatotropin	All body cells	Promotes protein anabolism (growth, tissue repair) and lipid mobilization and catabolism
Thyroid-stimulating hormone (TSH) or thyrotropin	Thyroid gland	Stimulates synthesis and release of thyroid hormones, growth and function of thyroid
Adrenocorticotropic hormone (ACTH) or corticotropin	Adrenal cortex	Fosters growth of adrenal cortex; stimulates secretion of glucocorticoids
Gonadotropic hormones	Reproductive organs	Stimulates sex hormone secretion, reproductive organ growth, reproductive processes
• Follicle-stimulating hormone (FSH)		
• Luteinizing hormone (LH)		
Melanocyte-stimulating hormone (MSH)	Melanocytes in skin	Increases melanin production in melanocytes to make skin darker in color
Prolactin	Ovary and mammary glands in females	Stimulates milk production in lactating women; increases response of follicles to LH and FSH; has unclear function in men
Posterior Pituitary (neurohypophysis)		
Oxytocin	Uterus; mammary glands	Stimulates milk secretion, uterine motility
Antidiuretic hormone (ADH) or vasopressin	Renal tubules, vascular smooth muscle	Promotes reabsorption of water
Thyroid		
Thyroxine (T_4)	All body tissues	Precursor to T_3
Triiodothyronine (T_3)	All body tissues	Regulates metabolic rate of all cells and processes of cell growth and tissue differentiation
Calcitonin (CT)	Bone tissue	Regulates calcium and phosphorus blood levels, lowering of blood Ca^{2+} levels

Parathyroids

Hormone	Target Tissue	Functions
Parathyroid hormone (PTH) or parathormone	Bone, intestine, kidneys	Regulates calcium and phosphorus blood levels (bone demineralization and increased intestinal absorption)

Adrenal Medulla

Hormone	Target Tissue	Functions
Epinephrine (adrenalin)	Sympathetic effectors	Enhances and prolongs effects of sympathetic nervous system
Norepinephrine	Sympathetic effectors	Response to stress; enhances and prolongs effects of sympathetic nervous system

Adrenal Cortex

Hormone	Target Tissue	Functions
Corticosteroids (e.g., cortisol, hydrocortisone)	All body tissues	Promotes metabolism, response to stress
Androgens (e.g., testosterone and androsterone and estrogen)	Sex organs	Promotes masculinization in men, growth and sexual activity in women
Mineralocorticoids (e.g., aldosterone)	Kidney	Regulates sodium and potassium balance and thus water balance

Pancreas

Hormone	Target Tissue	Functions
Islets of Langerhans		
Insulin (from beta cells)	General	Promotes movement of glucose out of blood and into cells
Glucagon (from alpha cells)	General	Promotes movement of glucose from storage and into blood
Somatostatin	Pancreas	Inhibits insulin and glucagon secretion

Gonads

Hormone	Target Tissue	Functions
Women: Ovaries Estrogen	Reproductive system, breasts	Stimulates development of secondary sex characteristics, preparation of uterus for fertilization and fetal development; stimulates bone growth
Progesterone	Reproductive system	Maintains lining of uterus necessary for successful pregnancy
Men: Testes Testosterone	Reproductive system	Stimulates development of secondary sex characteristics, spermatogenesis

From Lewis SM, Heitkemper MM, Dirksen SR: *Medical-surgical nursing: assessment and management of clinical problems*, ed 5, St. Louis, 2000, Mosby.

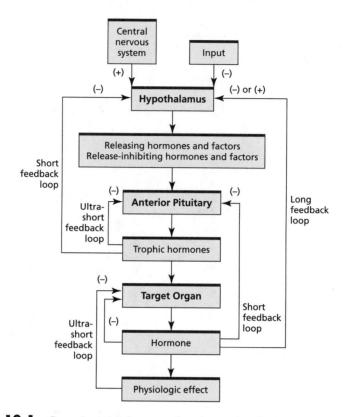

Figure 10-1 General model for control and negative feedback to hypothalamus-pituitary target organ systems. Negative feedback regulation is possible at three levels: target organ (ultra short feedback), anterior pituitary (short feedback), and hypothalamus (long feedback). (From Lewis SM, Heitkemper MM, Dirksen SR: *Medical-surgical nursing: assessment and management of clinical problems,* ed 5, St. Louis, 2000, Mosby.)

III. Targeted concerns

A. Pharmacology—priority drug classifications

1. **Hormones**—synthetic or naturally occurring substances used to treat hypoactive states of the various endocrine organs

   a. Expected effect—replacement of insufficient hormones

   b. Commonly given drugs

      (1) Insulin (see Table 10-2)

      (2) Glucagon

      (3) Adrenocorticotropin hormone (ACTH)

         (a) Corticotropin

         (b) Cosyntropin (Cortrosyn)

      (4) Androgens

         (a) Testosterone (Histerone)

         (b) Danazol (Danocrine)

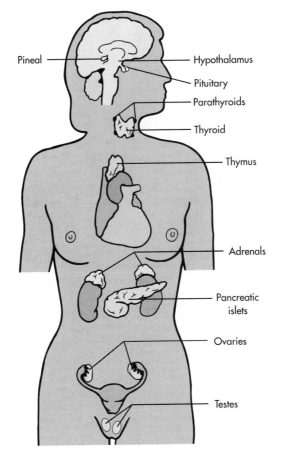

Figure 10-2   Location of the major endocrine glands. The parathyroid glands actually lie on the posterior surface of the thyroid. (From Lewis SM, Heitkemper MM, Dirksen SR: *Medical-surgical nursing: assessment and management of clinical problems,* ed 5, St. Louis, 2000, Mosby.)

(5) Antidiuretic hormone (ADH)
    (a) Desmopressin (DDAVP)
    (b) Vasopressin (Pitressin)
(6) Estrogens
    (a) Diethylstilbestrol (DES)
    (b) Conjugated estrogens (Premarin)
(7) Oxytocin (Pitocin)
(8) Progestin
    (a) Medroxyprogesterone acetate (Provera)
    (b) Progesterone (Gestrol)
(9) Thyroid
    (a) Levothyroxine sodium (Synthroid)
    (b) Thyroid (Thyrar)

TABLE 10-2	Hypoglycemic Medications		

Medication	Onset Hours	Peak Hours	Duration Hours
Insulin Analog			
Humalog, insulin lispro	15 min	45 min-1	1-1.5
Rapid Acting Insulins:			
Regular	0.5-1	2-4	6-8
Iletin, zinc suspension	0.5-1	2-8	8-16
Humulin R	30 min	1-3	3-5
Semilente	1-3	2-8	12-16
Intermediate Acting Insulins:			
Isophane insulin suspension (NPH)	1-2	6-12	18-26
Insulin zinc suspension (Lente)	1-3	6-12	18-26
Humulin N	1-2	8-12	26-30
Long-Acting Insulins:			
Protamine zinc (PZI)	4-6	18-24	28-36
Insulin zinc suspension extended (Ultra-lente)	4-6	16-24	36
Humulin U	4-6	16-24	24-30
Insulin Mixture			
70% NPH 30% Regular	30 min	2-12	18-24
Oral Hypoglycemic Agents: First Generation			
Tolbutamide (Orinase)	1	4-6	6-12
Tolazamide (Tolinase)	1	1-6	12-24
Acetohexamide (Dymelor)	1	3-6	12-24
Chlorpropamide (Diabinese)	1	3-6	24

c. Nursing considerations
   (1) Client must understand dosage schedule
   (2) Follow-up examinations must be emphasized to determine the effectiveness of the therapy
   (3) Client must be aware of adverse reactions to report to physician
   (4) Dosage cannot be abruptly stopped but must be tapered
   (5) Client should avoid alternating between brand name and generic medication
2. Glucocorticoids—used as replacement therapy when client is lacking in glucocorticoids. They also are used in connection with

TABLE 10-2   Hypoglycemic Medications—cont'd

Medication	Onset Hours	Peak Hours	Duration Hours
Oral Hypoglycemic Agents: **Second Generation**			
Glyburide (Micronase, Diabeta)	45 min-1	1.5-3	24
Glipizide (Glucotrol)	15-30 min	1-2	24
Glimepriride (Amaryl)	15 min	1-2	24
New Classifications:			
Meglitinides			
Repaglinide (Prandin)	30 min	1-1.5	2-3
Biguanides			
Metformin (Glucophage)	Several days	2-4 wk	12-24
Thiazolidinediones			
Troglitazone (Rezulin)	Unknown	2-3	>24
Alpha Glucosidase Inhibitors			
Acarbose (Precose)	Unknown	1	Affects
Miglitol (Glyset)	Unknown	1	postprandial
Pioglitazone Hydrocholoride			absorption of
(Actos)	Unknown	1	carbohydrates

Nursing Considerations

Assess client carefully for hypoglycemic reactions, especially when starting a new medication or changing dosages

Check for sulfa allergies before administering oral hypoglycemic agents

Regular insulin is the only insulin that can be administered intravenously

Tablets may be crushed if client has difficulty swallowing pills

Make sure client has insulin on board at all times. Know the peak and duration times for insulins given to client.

Regular insulin should be given 30 min before a meal

Blood glucose monitoring should be done 30 min to 60 min before giving ordered insulin

Humalog must be given 15 min before or with the meal to coincide with peak sugar levels

many other disorders for their immunosuppressive and anti-inflammatory properties.

   a. Expected effects—replacement of hormones; immunosuppressive and anti-inflammatory properties

   b. Commonly given drugs

      (1) Cortisone acetate (Cortone)

      (2) Hydrocortisone sodium succinate (Solu-Cortef)

      (3) Methylprednisolone (Medrol)

      (4) Prednisolone (Predalone)

      (5) Prednisone (Deltasone)

      (6) Dexamethasone (Decadron)

      (7) Beclomethasone dipropionate (Vanceril)

    c. Nursing considerations
- (1) Client must take medication with meals to prevent gastric ulcers
- (2) Warn client never to skip a dose or stop taking medication—adrenal crisis may be the result: severe hypotension, sinus tachycardia, and tachypnea
- (3) Instruct client to report sudden weight gain, black-tarry stools, edema, infection, or increased thirst to physician
- (4) Advise client to wear a medical-alert bracelet indicating that the medication is taken

    d. Common side effects
- (1) Hyperglycemia
- (2) Weight gain, moon face from sodium and fluid retention, and edema
- (3) Mood swings
- (4) Increased frequency of infections or colds
- (5) Higher risk for hypokalemia

3. Hypoglycemic agents (see Table 10-2, p. 333)
- a. Expected effect—to modulate serum glucose levels
- b. Commonly given drugs
- c. Nursing considerations (see also pp. 355, 357)
- d. Common side effect—hypoglycemia

4. Antithyroid agents—used to treat hyperthyroidism; inhibit formation of thyroid hormone
- a. Expected effect—decreased symptoms of hyperthyroidism
- b. Commonly given drugs
  - (1) Potassium iodide (Pima Syrup)
  - (2) Lugol's solution
  - (3) Saturated solution of potassium iodide (SSKI)
  - (4) Methimazole (Tapazole)
  - (5) Propylthiouracil (PTU)—takes about 3 months to be effective
- c. Nursing considerations
  - (1) Warn client not to miss doses—may trigger hyperthyroidism
  - (2) Ask client to confer with physician about eliminating foods high in iodine. Iodine is needed to manufacture thyroid hormone; however, these clients have too much hormone. Therefore, decreasing iodine intake may cause a decrease in the amount of thyroid hormone created.
  - (3) Teach findings of hypothyroidism because medication may destroy too much of the gland

B. Procedures
1. Serum and urinary measurement of hormone levels—vital in diagnosing a disorder
2. Radioactive iodine uptake (RAIU)—radioactive iodine administered, then thyroid scanned for uptake of radioactive iodine

3. Thyroid ultrasonography—evaluation of thyroid using ultrasonic sound waves for detection of fluid or tissue-filled tumors
4. Thyroid biopsy—tissue sample evaluated for benign or malignant tissue type
5. Serum calcium and phosphorus—evaluated in suspected parathyroid disorders
6. Skeletal X-ray films—identify loss of calcium in bones of the client with a parathyroid disorder
7. CT scan of adrenal glands—helpful in identifying tumors and gland enlargement
8. Adrenal arteriography—identification of tumors
9. Dexamethasone suppression test—confirms Cushing's syndrome. Client is given high or low doses of dexamethasone, and a 24-hour urine specimen is evaluated for response to the medication.
10. Urine and plasma catecholamines—helpful in identifying pheochromocytoma
11. Fasting blood sugar (FBS)—helpful in screening for diabetes mellitus
12. Two-hour postprandial glucose test—determines level of glucose in the body 2 hours after a meal; screens for diabetes mellitus
13. Glucose tolerance test (GTT)—the definitive test for diabetes mellitus
14. Glycosylated hemoglobin (Ghb/Hb A_{1C})—measurement of time-averaged values of blood glucose over the preceding 2 to 4 months; assay of Hb A_{1C}. Blood can be drawn without regard to meals or insulin therapy.

C. Psychosocial concerns
1. Anxiety—uncomfortable feeling associated with an unknown direct cause. It may be difficult for clients to verbalize their anxiety but they can tell you they are uneasy about the outcome of their disorder.
2. Fear—uncomfortable feeling associated with a direct cause, such as change in lifestyle, body changes, or death
3. Social isolation—may occur if clients have a significant change in their body or disease symptoms make it more comfortable for them to stay home
4. Dietary restrictions—many restrictions are associated with disorders of the endocrine system, and thus eating outside the own home is difficult and may be provoke anxiety
5. Lifestyle changes—many changes are needed, especially for clients with diabetes mellitus. Health maintenance must be very intense and clients must learn how to maintain correct medication administration and correct dietary intake.

D. Health history—question sequence
1. Would you please describe the problem you have been experiencing?
2. Do you tire easily?
3. Do you find that you must sleep or take rest periods more than you used to?

4. Do you wake up frequently at night? Do you sleep restlessly?
5. Does cold or heat bother you?
6. Have you noticed weight gain or loss? Over what period of time?
7. Have you noticed a loss of hair? Where? How long has this been occurring?
8. Have you noticed puffiness in your face, eyes or hands? Do you notice this when you wake up or all the time?
9. Do you ever have heart palpitations?
10. Which medications do you take for constipation or diarrhea? How often?
11. Do you ever feel very thirsty or void large amounts of urine?
12. Do you ever feel nervous or jittery for days rather than hours?
13. Do your muscles ever feel weak or painful?

E. **Physical examination—appropriate sequence**
1. ABCs—vital signs
2. Height and weight
3. Inspect skin for integrity, turgor, and lesions
4. Inspect hair and nails for distribution, quantity, and quality; inspect nails for thickness and clubbing
5. Inspect head and face for edema and *exophthalmos*—eyes bulging out of the sockets
6. Inspect neck for any asymmetry, especially in the thyroid area
7. Palpate the thyroid for abnormalities
8. Inspect the chest for any heaves or thrusts in the area of the heart, and inspect for gynecomastia in males
9. Palpate the anterior chest for thrills and for position of the apical impulse
10. Auscultate heart sounds
11. Inspect extremities—note any tremors, asymmetry, or disproportion to the trunk
12. Inspect the abdomen for striae or scars
13. Auscultate for bowel sounds
14. Palpate the abdomen for painful areas
15. Inspect the genital area for abnormal pubic hair distribution and abnormal genitalia

IV. **Pathophysiologic disorders**
A. **Hyperthyroidism (thyrotoxicosis or Plummers Disease)**
1. Definition—a metabolic imbalance resulting from an excess of thyroid hormone. Grave's disease is a form of hyperthyroidism with four components: enlarged thyroid (goiter), increased thyroid production, exophthalmos, and skin changes.
2. Etiology—autoimmune process from an as yet unidentified cause. Possible viral cause. There is a familial tendency toward hyperthyroidism.
3. Incidence—more common in females and usually occurs between 20 and 40 years of age

4. Pathophysiology—thyroid gland is stimulated to oversecrete thyroid hormone by circulating immunoglobulins
5. Assessment
   a. Questions to ask
      (1) Have you noticed an enlargement of your neck or difficulty swallowing?
      (2) Have you been losing weight lately?
      (3) Have you experienced diarrhea?
      (4) Do you find you are unable to tolerate heat?
      (5) Do you tire easily?
      (6) Do you ever have difficulty sleeping?
      (7) Have you noticed a dryness of your eyes or difficulty focusing your eyes?
      (8) Have you experienced heart palpitations?
   b. Clinical manifestations
      (1) Easily tired
      (2) Fine tremors
      (3) Tachycardia with palpitations
      (4) Hypertension
      (5) Heat intolerance
      (6) Thin, brittle hair
      (7) Thick skin and subcutaneous tissue, especially over the tibia
      (8) Exophthalmos—bilateral bulging of the eyes from the sockets
   c. Abnormal laboratory findings
      (1) T_4 (thyroxine) total—elevated
      (2) T_3,T_3 radioimmunoassay (triiodothyronine; RIA)—elevated T_3
      (3) Thyroid-stimulating hormone (TSH) assay—decreased
   d. Abnormal diagnostic test results
      (1) Thyroid scan—abnormal uptake of radioactive iodine
      (2) Thyroid ultrasonography—differentiates a cyst (fluid filled) from a tumor (tissue growth)
      (3) Thyroid biopsy—identifies thyroid tissue as malignant or benign
6. Expected medical intervention
   a. Antithyroid drugs to bring the client to a euthyroid state before additional therapy
   b. A beta-blocker, propranolol (Inderal), to decrease sympathetic symptoms associated with hyperthyroidism
   c. Radioactive iodine (^{131}I)—quickly picked up by the thyroid and destroys thyroid tissue. Within 6 to 12 weeks the thyroid becomes euthyroid. The major complication is hypothyroidism because the radiation dosage is difficult to prescribe accurately.
   d. Thyroidectomy or partial thyroidectomy with preservation of parathyroid glands

7. Nursing diagnoses
   a. Altered body nutrition (less than bodily requirements) related to increased metabolic rate
   b. Diarrhea related to increased peristalsis
   c. Potential for fluid volume deficit related to diarrhea
   d. Risk for injury—corneal ulceration related to inability of client to close eyelids
8. Client goals
   a. Client will not lose any additional weight; begins to gain a quarter pound per week
   b. Client will have only four liquid stools per day, with frequency decreasing by one episode of diarrhea per day then stools of normal consistency after the fifth day
   c. Client will show a balanced I&O and will have acceptable skin turgor and moist mucous membranes
   d. Client will maintain moist-appearing cornea, with no evidence of corneal ulceration
9. Nursing interventions
   a. Acute care
      (1) Quiet, restful environment
      (2) Carefully balanced rest and activity
      (3) Diet high in calories, protein, and carbohydrates
      (4) Daily weights, with strict I&O
      (5) Care after thyroidectomy
         (a) Use semi-Fowler's position with no high Fowler's position to prevent strain on incision and neck
         (b) Evaluate dressing for tightness or bleeding
         (c) Check back of neck for bleeding; blood may trickle down neck folds and pool behind the neck
         (d) Ensure that a tracheostomy set is at the bedside at all times
         (e) Evaluate client for hoarseness that is worsening, which is indicative of laryngeal nerve damage. The ability to talk in a whisper may be normal for 3 to 5 days after surgery.
         (f) Assess for tetany owing to accidental removal of parathyroid glands
            (i) Tingling around mouth and in fingers is the first indication
            (ii) Muscle spasms and twitching
            (iii) Positive Chvostek's sign and Trousseau's sign (Figure 10-3)
            (iv) Palpitations
         (g) Encourage client to support head and neck when moving

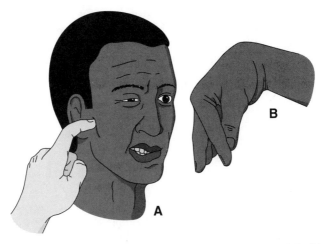

Figure 10-3 **A,** Chvostek's sign: a contraction of facial muscles elicited in response to a light tap over facial nerve in front of the ear. **B,** Trousseau's sign: a carpopedal spasm induced by inflating a blood pressure cuff above systolic pressure for one minute with a slow cuff deflation. (From Beare PG, Myers JL: *Adult health nursing,* ed 3, St. Louis, 1998, Mosby.)

       (h) Have calcium gluconate available because of the possibility of tetany from accidental removal of parathyroid glands

    (6) Assess and intervene in client with thyrotoxic crisis—fever, tachycardia, flushing, sweating, dysrhythmias, shock, delirium, or coma

       (a) Slow IV infusion of propranolol (Inderal) to control sympathetic response

       (b) IV propylthiouracil to prevent further release of hormones

       (c) Possible steroid administration to support stress response

  b. Home care regarding client education

    (1) Therapy with ^{131}I

       (a) Isotope is administered by way of a tasteless, colorless liquid in a single dose

       (b) NPO after midnight

       (c) For the first 24 hours after medication ingestion the client should not be in contact with infants, children, or pregnant women

       (d) Fluids should be increased to 2000 to 3000 ml/day for several days

       (e) Toilet should be flushed several times after each use for 2 to 3 days to decrease exposure to family members

    (2) Care of client with exophthalmus

       (a) Restrict sodium

       (b) Elevate head of bed

         (c) Have client use eye drops for moistness

         (d) Have client wear sunglasses for photophobia

      (3) Evaluation of client in 6 months after therapy for the need for replacement thyroid therapy, such as T_3, T_4

      (4) Instruction of client regarding findings associated with hypofunction of the thyroid gland

         (a) Constant fatigue

         (b) Sustained constipation

10. Evaluation protocol

  a. How do I know that my interventions have been effective?

    (1) Is client having any difficulty in breathing or swallowing?

    (2) Has the client complained of a hoarse voice?

    (3) Does client feel any tingling around the lips or fingers?

    (4) Is client able to rest? Is room temperature conducive to sleep?

  b. Which criteria will I use to change my interventions?

    (1) Difficulty breathing or swallowing

    (2) Bleeding on the dressing or pooling of blood behind neck

    (3) Evidence of thyrotoxic crisis

    (4) Tingling around mouth or fingers

    (5) Uncomfortable environment as stated by the client

  c. How will I know that my client teaching has been effective?

    (1) Client demonstrates appropriate eye care for exophthalmos

    (2) Client states appropriate precautions to be taken in the home after initiation of radioisotope therapy

11. Older adult alert

  a. Many older adult clients are misdiagnosed because they may not present with classic findings. Their complaints many times fit nicely into a cardiac picture and will not stimulate the physician to perform thyroid testing.

  b. Treatment of choice for the older adult client with hyperthyroidism is radioactive iodine

B. Hypothyroidism

1. Definition—decreased metabolism related to decreased thyroid hormone

  a. *Myxedema,* a complication of hypothyroidism, is a generalized hypometabolic state

  b. Myxedema coma is a life-threatening hypometabolic state

2. Pathophysiology—iodine is required for the thyroid gland to synthesize and secrete its hormone. Insufficient dietary iodine causes the thyroid gland to enlarge in an attempt to compensate for the deficiency. When the pituitary gland identifies insufficient thyroid hormone, it increases secretion of TSH. Increased TSH is responsible for the enlarging thyroid gland, also known as a *goiter.*

3. Etiology—most common cause is *Hashimoto's thyroiditis,* an autoimmune disorder that leads to deterioration of the thyroid gland. Other etiologies are iodine deficiency, congenital defects, or ineffective hormone synthesis.
4. Incidence—more common in the female population and between 30 and 60 years of age
5. Assessment
   a. Questions to ask
      (1) Do you find that the cold really bothers you?
      (2) Have you been gaining weight without a change of diet or exercise?
      (3) Is your hair and skin very dry or oily?
      (4) Do you have trouble remembering things?
      (5) Do you tire easily?
   b. Clinical manifestations
      (1) Lethargy
      (2) Sinus bradycardia
      (3) Cold sensitivity
      (4) Weight gain
      (5) Constipation
      (6) Dry skin
      (7) Brittle hair
      (8) Forgetfulness
      (9) Depression
   c. Abnormal laboratory findings
      (1) TSH increased, pituitary is attempting to stimulate thyroid to produce more hormone
      (2) T_3 and T_4 decreased because thyroid gland is not producing them
      (3) H&H decreased owing to the decreased metabolic rate, which affects RBC production
      (4) Cholesterol and triglycerides elevated owing to decreased metabolic rate, resulting in disorders of lipid metabolism
      (5) Blood glucose decreased
   d. Abnormal diagnostic test result—radioactive iodine uptake (RAIU) decreased
6. Expected medical interventions
   a. For myxedema coma—resuscitative measures include synthroid IV, glucose, and corticosteroids
   b. Lifetime replacement drug therapy—the most commonly used drug is levothyroxine sodium (Synthroid)
   c. Diet high in iodine, which is easily accomplished with iodized salt
7. Nursing diagnoses
   a. Altered nutrition—more than bodily requirements related to decreased body metabolism

     b. Activity intolerance related to decreased metabolic rate

     c. Constipation related to decreased peristalsis secondary to decreased metabolic rate

     d. Hypothermia related to decreased metabolic rate

8. Client goals

     a. Client will have balanced nutrition in relation to metabolic demands as evidenced by weight within 2 to 4 lb of baseline

     b. Client will increase activity by 10 minutes each day

     c. Client will have a daily bowel movement of soft consistency

     d. Client will maintain a temperature between 36.8° C and 37° C

9. Nursing interventions

     a. Acute care

        (1) Assess vital signs every 2 to 4 hours

        (2) Assess lung and heart sounds every 2 to 4 hours. Be alert for heart failure: crackles, and S_3 and S_4 sounds

        (3) Maintain warm environment to meet client's needs

        (4) Balance rest and activity as required by client's needs

        (5) Meticulous skin care, paying attention to moisturizing the skin and preventing skin tears

        (6) Request an order for a stool softener to alleviate constipation. Increasing fluids or activity may not be effective in hypothyroidism.

        (7) Take client's daily weight to identify fluid retention, and report a loss or gain of more than 2 lb/wk to physician

     b. Home care regarding client education

        (1) Inform client of lifetime medication regimen and follow-up care

        (2) Instruct client on the need to take medications at same time each day and on an empty stomach

        (3) Teach client to take pulse biweekly and report a resting pulse rate of over 100 to physician

        (4) Inform client of symptoms associated with too much medication to report to physician: chest pain, SOB, palpitations or "heart racing," insomnia, or feeling jittery

        (5) Teach client that diet should be high in fiber and bulk, and low in calories, fat, and cholesterol

        (6) Inform client of the need to increase fluid intake to at least 2000 ml/day

        (7) Teach client to take weights biweekly on the same days and times of the day

        (8) Inform client to use moisturizers to counteract dry skin

10. Evaluation protocol

     a. How do I know that my interventions have been effective?

        (1) Does client feel short of breath?

        (2) Has client noticed any palpitations?

        (3) Is client warm enough?

        (4) Is client feeling overly tired with usual activities?

b. Which criteria will I use to change my interventions?
   (1) Chest pain and SOB
   (2) S_3 and S_4 heart sounds, pulmonary crackles
   (3) Client expresses feeling cold
   (4) Client expresses feeling exhausted even after minimal activity
   (5) New skin tears or breakdown areas noted

c. How will I know that my client teaching has been effective?
   (1) Client demonstrates correct technique for taking pulse and weight
   (2) Client gives correct time span for taking pulse and weight
   (3) Client repeats correct adverse reactions to be reported to physician
   (4) Client shows a food diary that indicates correct food and fluid choices
   (5) Client reports using a moisturizer especially after bathing, and no skin breakdown is evident

11. Older adult alert
   a. Hypothyroidism should be considered by health care providers when ruling out a wide variety of illnesses
   b. The older adult client who is placed on drug therapy for hypothyroidism is at risk for developing ischemic heart disease because of the sudden increase in the metabolic rate. The client must be monitored carefully for cardiac complaints.
   c. Subclinical hypothyroidism is not uncommon in postmenopausal women and should be evaluated appropriately if complaints are suggestive of hypoactive thyroid

C. Hyperparathyroidism

1. Definition—oversecretion of parathyroid hormone
2. Pathophysiology—parathyroid hormone in its overstimulated state will function at an accelerated rate. Increased loss of calcium from the bone, which leads to bone resorption; increased renal retention of calcium; and increased GI absorption of calcium occurs. The excess calcium is responsible for the clinical manifestations of the disease.
3. Etiology—benign adenoma in most cases
4. Incidence—more common in the female population especially after age 50. It is one of the most frequently identified endocrine disorders.
5. Assessment
   a. Questions to ask
     (1) Have you experienced weakness or fatigue?
     (2) Have you noticed that you feel drowsy or sleepy a great deal of the time?
     (3) Is your appetite normal?
     (4) Have you been experiencing constipation?

(5) Have you been excreting a great deal of urine?

(6) Have you experienced pain in your bones?

b. Clinical manifestations (Table 10-3)

c. Abnormal laboratory finding—serum calcium elevated

d. Abnormal diagnostic test—parathyroid hormone RIA elevated (most specific)

6. Expected medical interventions (see Table 10-3)

7. Nursing diagnoses

a. Constipation related to decline in peristalsis

b. Risk for injury—pathologic fractures related to resorption (loss) of calcium from bones

c. Activity intolerance related to fatigue

8. Client goals

a. Client will have a soft, formed stool at least every other day

b. Client will not demonstrate any findings of pathologic fractures or renal calculi

c. Client will increase activity level by 10 minutes each day

9. Nursing interventions

a. Acute care—client will be hospitalized for surgical removal of the parathyroid glands. See Care of the Client after a Thyroidectomy, p. 338.

b. Home care regarding client education

(1) Balanced activity and rest. Be aware that too much bed rest is not helpful in moving calcium back into the bones. Weight bearing or resistance exercises promote calcium return to the bone.

(2) Maintain a low calcium diet—limit dairy products

(3) Increase fluid intake to 2000 to 3000 ml/day to prevent renal calculi

(4) Increase fiber and bulk in diet

10. Evaluation protocol—How will I know that my client teaching has been effective?

a. Client indicates naps are taken in the morning and afternoon

b. Client shows a food diary indicating a low-calcium, high-fiber, high-fluid diet

c. Client reports normal pattern of bowel elimination without use of evacuation aids

11. Older adult alert—this disorder is commonly dismissed as the effects of aging in the older adult client. Be alert to significant findings that could lead you to be suspicious of hyperparathyroidism.

D. Hypoparathyroidism

1. Definition—undersecretion of the parathyroid hormone

2. Pathophysiology—parathyroid hormone normally acts to increase bone resorption and maintain an appropriate balance between calcium and phosphate. A decrease in this hormone leads to a decrease in serum calcium and decreased renal excretion of phosphate. Hypocalcemia, hyperphosphatemia, and the resulting

TABLE 10-3	Parathyroid Gland Disorders, Symptoms, Client Management		
Disorder	**Description**	**Symptoms**	**Client Management**
Hyperparathyroidism	Disorder of calcium, phosphate, and bone metabolism characterized by hypersecretion of PTH from increased gland mass. May be caused by benign adenomas or secondary responses to hypocalcemic states. Incidence increases sharply after age 50.	Usually detected on routine chemistry profiles because most clients are asymptomatic. If present, symptoms are related to excess calcium and include hypertension, renal stones, muscle weakness, GI distress, constipation, and bone pain.	Surgical removal of affected gland; low-calcium diet, fluids, and calcium-blocking agents
Hypoparathyroidism	May be produced by a variety of disease states associated with impaired section of PTH. Rare disorders and autoimmune involvement are likely.	Symptoms are variable and primarily relate to the severity and rapidity of the deficiency. Calcium deficiency is a primary aspect with muscle tetany and abdominal cramping. Cardiac depression and seizures may occur.	Medications to replace calcium and vitamin D and control phosphate levels.

From *AJN Mosby Nursing boards review*, ed 9, St. Louis, 1994, Mosby.

alkalosis lead to an extreme in neuromuscular excitement and eventually tetany if not treated. Make the connection between low calcium and tetany.

3. Etiology—most common cause is accidental removal of the parathyroid glands during thyroidectomy or damage to the glands during the thyroidectomy
4. Incidence—more common in the female population
5. Assessment
   a. Questions to ask
      (1) Have you noticed any numbness or tingling around your mouth or in your fingertips?
      (2) Have you experienced any abdominal cramping?
   b. Clinical manifestations (see Table 10-3)
      (1) Numbness or tingling around mouth or fingertips
      (2) Cardiac dysrhythmias
      (3) Positive Chvostek's sign and Trousseau's sign (see Figure 10-3, p. 339)
   c. Abnormal laboratory findings
      (1) Serum calcium decreased
      (2) Serum phosphate elevated
      (3) Urinary calcium low or absent
6. Expected medical interventions (see Table 10-3, p. 345)—tetany is considered a medical emergency. Laryngeal spasms and subsequent respiratory obstruction may occur, which require immediate intervention to maintain a patent airway. Tetany must be treated with intravenous calcium immediately to return calcium to normal levels; calcium gluconate is the drug of choice.
7. Nursing diagnosis—risk for injury related to seizures or tetany caused by hypocalcemia
8. Client goal—Client will have no injury from the seizure activity or from the effects of hypocalcemia
9. Nursing interventions
   a. Acute care—monitor for the emergence of tetany
      (1) Evaluate airway and breathing frequently
      (2) Monitor client for numbness or tingling around the mouth and fingertips—first sign
      (3) Evaluate for Chvostek's sign and Trousseau's sign
      (4) Have IV calcium gluconate readily available
      (5) Place client on cardiac monitor if calcium gluconate administration is required

⚠ Warning!

When calcium gluconate is given by IV push method, rapid administration may cause vasodilation, decreased BP, cardiac arrhythmias, syncope, and cardiac arrest. Push very slowly. Do not exceed 200 mg/min.

  b. Home care regarding client education
   (1) Oral calcium and concurrent vitamin D administration to enhance absorption through the intestines
   (2) Diet high in calcium and low in phosphorus
   (3) Phosphate binder [aluminum hydroxide gel (Amphojel)] before meals
   (4) Physician follow-up to monitor calcium levels
 10. Evaluation protocol
  a. How do I know that my interventions have been effective?
   (1) Vital signs are within 10% of baseline
   (2) Client is free of assessment findings indicating tetany, such as numbness or tingling around lips
   (3) Imminent tetany is treated promptly to prevent respiratory difficulty
  b. Which criteria will I use to change my interventions?
   (1) Vital signs are not within expected parameters
   (2) Assessment findings indicate tetany, such as numbness and tingling around mouth and in fingertips
   (3) Client experiences respiratory distress
  c. How will I know that my client teaching has been effective?
   (1) Client shows a food diary indicating appropriate food and beverage choices
   (2) Client indicates making a follow-up appointment with physician and identifying the importance of continuing the follow-up visits
   (3) Client states that aluminum hydroxide gel (Amphojel) is taken before each meal
 11. Older adult alert—the nurse must emphasize to the older adult client that this disorder requires lifelong care and follow-up with a health care practitioner
E. **Adrenal insufficiency (Addison's disease)**
  1. Definition—insufficient release of hormones from the adrenal cortex (associate cortex with corticosteroids)
  2. Pathophysiology—results in a decrease in mineralocorticoids (aldosterone), glucocorticoids (cortisol), and androgens. See Figure 10-4 for more information regarding the effects of adrenal insufficiency.
  3. Etiology—autoimmune adrenalitis is a common cause. Also can be caused by a dysfunction of the adrenal gland or by a deficiency in ACTH. Seen in the client removed from exogenous steroid use after long-term therapy.
  4. Incidence—rare illness that affects men and women equally
  5. Assessment
   a. Questions to ask
    (1) Have you been feeling increasingly fatigued lately?
    (2) Have you noticed weight loss recently?

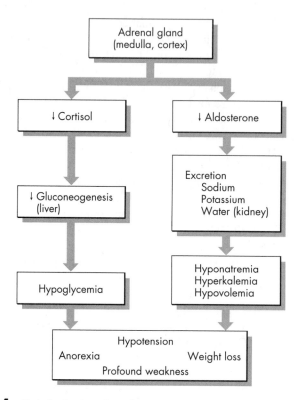

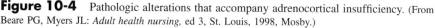

Figure 10-4 Pathologic alterations that accompany adrenocortical insufficiency. (From Beare PG, Myers JL: *Adult health nursing,* ed 3, St. Louis, 1998, Mosby.)

    (3) Has your abdomen bothered you lately?

    (4) Have you experienced any nausea, vomiting, diarrhea, or constipation?

    (5) Have you experienced any dizzy spells?

  b. Clinical manifestations

    (1) Progressive weakness

    (2) Abdominal complaints—pain, anorexia

    (3) Nausea, vomiting, diarrhea, and constipation

    (4) Amber coloration of the skin—called *bronzing*

    (5) Postural hypotension

    (6) Decreased pubic and axillary hair in the female population

  c. Abnormal laboratory findings

    (1) Electrolytes—sodium is low, potassium and calcium are increased

    (2) ACTH stimulation test—most reliable. A baseline cortisol level is taken, ACTH is administered intravenously, and 45 minutes later another cortisol level is taken. The resulting level of ACTH is abnormally low.

    (3) Fasting Blood Sugar (FBS)—low

(4) Melanocyte-stimulating hormone (MSH)—elevated; results in bronzed skin and hyperpigmentation
6. Expected medical intervention
   a. Lifelong glucocorticoid and mineralocorticoid administration
   b. Acute Addisonian crisis, which causes vascular collapse, is treated with
      (1) Rapid infusion of saline and 5% dextrose
      (2) IV dexamethasone
      (3) Hemodynamic monitoring
7. Nursing diagnoses
   a. Activity intolerance related to decreased glucose available for metabolism, secondary to decreased cortisol levels
   b. Risk for injury—falls related to decreased CO
   c. Risk for fluid volume deficit related to decrease in aldosterone production
8. Client goals
   a. Client will increase activity by 10 minutes each day without expression of excessive fatigue
   b. Client will not suffer falls or injuries
   c. Client will maintain a balanced I&O: input equals output within 300 ml/day
9. Nursing interventions
   a. Acute care—Addisonian crisis
      (1) Evaluate ABCs every 10 to 15 minutes until stable
      (2) Institute IV access
      (3) Institute cardiac monitoring to observe for cardiac dysrhythmias
      (4) Monitor serum electrolytes
   b. Home care regarding client education
      (1) Teach client that replacement of glucocorticoids and mineralocorticoids is lifelong
      (2) Inform client that glucocorticoid dosage should be increased, as directed by physician, during minor illnesses or stressful life situations
      (3) Instruct client that medication supply is always a priority; therefore, client needs to ensure a sufficient supply, especially for extended travel
      (4) Instruct client to obtain a medical-alert bracelet or necklace
      (5) Show client how to use injectable cortisone for emergencies
10. Evaluation protocol
    a. How do I know that my interventions have been effective?
       (1) Vital signs are within 10% of baseline
       (2) Input equals output within 300 ml/day
       (3) Electrolytes are within acceptable limits

    b. Which criteria will I use to change my interventions?
       (1) Vital signs are over 10% of baseline
       (2) Output is not equal to intake within 300 ml/day
       (3) Electrolytes are not within acceptable levels
    c. How will I know that my client teaching has been effective?
       (1) Client states that these medications must be taken for life
       (2) Client states that illness or extreme stress will increase the need for medication, and that any increase in dose must be on the advice of a physician
       (3) Client demonstrates correct use of a self-injector for an acute crisis

11. Older adult alert
    a. Generally adrenal insufficiency is not a disease seen in the older adult population
    b. When it is seen in older adults, remember that older adults' symptoms may be more pronounced because they may already have decreased adrenal function as a normal course of aging
    c. The older adult client may also be more sensitive to the side effects of corticosteroids because some of the symptoms may already be apparent as a normal course of aging, such as hypertension

F. Adrenal hyperfunction (Cushing's syndrome)
    1. Definition—increased secretion of glucocorticoids from the adrenal cortex or as a result of exogenous steroid administration
    2. Pathophysiology—increased glucocorticoid production has an effect on every system in the body (Table 10-4)
    3. Etiology
      a. ACTH-producing pituitary or hypothalamus lesion
      b. Extrapituitary malignancies producing ACTH
      c. Adrenal adenomas
      d. Adrenal carcinoma
      e. Exogenous steroid administration
      f. Alcohol intake
    4. Incidence—more common in the female population, 20 to 40 years of age
    5. Assessment
      a. Questions to ask
        (1) Have you noticed a change in the shape of your face?
        (2) Have you noticed stretch marks on your abdomen?
        (3) Has your hair begun to thin?
        (4) Have you noticed that it takes a long time for cuts to heal?
      b. Clinical manifestations (see Table 10-4 and Figure 10-5)
      c. Abnormal laboratory findings
        (1) Urinary 17-hydroxysteroids—elevated
        (2) Plasma cortisol levels—elevated throughout the day with a loss of normal **diurnal** rhythm. Normal rhythm is high

TABLE 10-4	Cushing's Syndrome: Pathophysiologic Changes and Clinical Manifestations

Pathophysiologic Changes	Clinical Manifestations
Increased cortisol levels	Depression, apathy, mood changes, psychosis, cataracts
Sodium and water retention, potassium excretion	High BP, hypokalemia, increased urinary potassium, metabolic alkalosis, edema
Increased androgen production	Acne, hirsutism, virilization, hyperpigmentation, amenorrhea, menstrual changes
Immunosuppression	Poor wound healing, leukocytosis, decreased lymphocyte and eosinophil production, increased erythropoiesis
Body fat redistribution	Moon face, truncal obesity, "buffalo hump"
Increased protein catabolism and collagen loss	Skin and hair thinning, abdominal striae, muscle weakness, atrophy
Capillary fragility	Easy bruising
Gastric hyperacidity	Peptic ulcer formation
Increased calcium loss	Increased urinary calcium, osteoporosis, backache, pathologic fractures
Increased gluconeogenesis	Hyperglycemia

From Beare PG, Myers JL: *Adult health nursing,* ed 3, St. Louis, 1998, Mosby.

       levels in the morning, decreasing in the evening, and becoming lowest near midnight.

      (3) Urinary-free cortisol—elevated

      (4) Low-dose dexamethasone suppression test—elevation of blood and urine cortisol

    d. Abnormal diagnostic test results

      (1) Adrenal CT scan—identifies adrenal tumor

      (2) X-ray films—used to identify tumors in other areas of the body that could be causing the disorder

6. Expected medical interventions

    a. Surgery to remove adrenal tumors

    b. Radiation therapy for pituitary tumors or tumors in other areas of the body

    c. Drug therapy to suppress the release of ACTH or the synthesis of corticosteroids

    d. Monitoring of use of exogenous steroids

7. Nursing diagnoses

    a. Activity intolerance related to weakness and fatigue

    b. Risk for fluid volume excess related to increased corticosteroid production

    c. Risk for infection related to increased production of corticosteroids causing a suppressed immune system

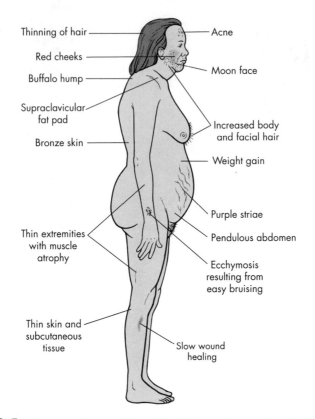

Thinning of hair

Red cheeks

Buffalo hump

Supraclavicular fat pad

Bronze skin

Thin extremities with muscle atrophy

Thin skin and subcutaneous tissue

Acne

Moon face

Increased body and facial hair

Weight gain

Purple striae

Pendulous abdomen

Ecchymosis resulting from easy bruising

Slow wound healing

Figure 10-5 Common characteristics of Cushing's syndrome. (From Lewis SM, Heitkemper MM, Dirksen SR: *Medical-surgical nursing: assessment and management of clinical problems,* ed 5, St. Louis, 2000, Mosby.)

    d. Body-image disturbance related to changes in fat deposits and hair distribution secondary to increased glucocorticoid production

8. Client goals

    a. Client will tolerate activity, 10 minutes more each day without stated excessive fatigue

    b. Client will have input equal to output within 300 ml/day

    c. Client will be free of infection as evidenced by normal WBC and differential within accepted parameters

    d. Client will state feeling comfortable with bodily changes

9. Nursing interventions

    a. Acute care—postoperative. See Postoperative Care, Chapter 9, pp. 311-312.

    b. Home care regarding client education

       (1) Instruction that steroid replacement therapy is lifelong if treatment has left client in a state of adrenal insufficiency

       (2) Warning of the risks associated with abruptly stopping steroid medication

(3) Instruction on the need for increasing steroid dose during times of stress or illness, if client requires lifelong steroid replacement

(4) Instruction on how client should protect self from infection; careful hand washing

(5) Instruction on daily weight monitoring and reporting of weight gain or loss of 2 lb/wk to physician

(6) Advice on maintaining a diet low in sodium and high in potassium

(7) Advice on the need to take steroids with food or milk

10. Evaluation protocol
   a. How do I know that my interventions have been effective? See Evaluation Protocol for Adrenal Insufficiency on p. 349.
   b. Which criteria will I use to change my interventions? See Evaluation Protocol for Adrenal Insufficiency on p. 349.
   c. How will I know that my client teaching has been effective?
      (1) Client indicates correct drug administration regimen and precautions about not stopping medication abruptly
      (2) Client states risks of infection from increased steroid production or administration
      (3) Client demonstrates correct method for daily weight
      (4) Client shows a food diary with appropriate food and beverage choices

11. Older adult alert—may present with an excessive number of assessment factors because many older adults already manifest these symptoms as a result of the normal changes associated with aging

G. Diabetes mellitus
   1. Definition—a metabolic disorder affecting a wide variety of systems; the most commonly affected is glucose metabolism
      a. Diabetic ketoacidosis—life-threatening disorder caused by an ineffective level of insulin and resulting hyperglycemia; average of 600 mg/dl or higher
      b. Hyperglycemic hyperosmoler nonketotic (HHNK) syndrome—life-threatening disorder associated with an extremely high blood glucose level; average of 1100 mg/dl or higher; dehydration and coma may occur
      c. Hypoglycemia—low blood glucose level; average less than 50 mg/dl
   2. Pathophysiology
      a. Type I—a deficiency of insulin noted as well as an increase in counterinsulin hormones: glucagon, epinephrine, cortisol, somastostatin, and growth hormone. (These hormones stimulate the release of glucagons and break down or antagonize the effects of insulin.)
         (1) Lack of insulin causes a decreased utilization of serum glucose by the cells, allowing the serum and urine glucose to increase

      (2) Lack of glucose for cellular nutrition forces the body to mobilize fat and protein stores for metabolism

      (3) This results in ketone buildup in the blood and urine

      (4) Glucose is hypertonic and pulls fluid out of the extracellular space, resulting in increased urine output, thirst, and sodium and potassium losses

   b. Type II—insulin levels may be low, normal, or elevated; several factors are believed to contribute to the pathophysiology: slower response of insulin release, decreased number of insulin receptors, and reduced responsiveness to glucose by the beta cells in the pancreas. A major factor in the advent of Type II diabetes is obesity.

3. Etiology—several theories are presently being evaluated, including autoimmune, viral, environmental, and genetic etiologies

4. Incidence—over 12 million Americans are affected, with over 500,000 new cases reported each year. Most are diagnosed with Type II diabetics.

5. Assessment

   a. Questions to ask

      (1) Have you noticed that you are urinating more than usual?

      (2) Have you been very thirsty lately?

      (3) Have you been losing weight, even when eating the same amount of food or more?

      (4) Do you ever feel very tired and weak?

   b. Clinical manifestations

      (1) Polyphagia—increased appetite

      (2) Polyuria—increased urination

      (3) Polydipsia—increased thirst

      (4) Weight loss

      (5) Fatigue

      (6) Weakness

      (7) Clients with Type II diabetes may not show the symptoms listed above but may be initially diagnosed with complications

      (8) DKA (Table 10-5), HHNK (Table 10-6)

   c. Abnormal laboratory findings

      (1) Blood glucose—elevated

      (2) Fasting blood glucose—elevated

      (3) Postprandial blood glucose—elevated

      (4) Glucose tolerance test—elevated with a longer time period for return to normal. This is the definitive test to diagnose diabetes.

      (5) Urine ketones elevated

6. Expected medical interventions

   a. Individualized treatment

   b. Insulin administration

   c. Oral hypoglycemic agents

TABLE 10-5	**Differentiating Hypoglycemia from Ketoacidosis (Hyperglycemia)**	
	Hypoglycemia (Insulin Reaction)	**Ketoacidosis (Diabetic Coma)**
Causes	Delayed or missed meals, excess insulin, excess exercise (glucose <50 mg/dl)	Inadequate insulin, too much food, infection, injury, physical or emotional stress (glucose >350 mg/dl)
Clinical findings	Anxiety, irritability, weakness, sweating, hunger, tremor, nausea, headache (severe confusion, unconsciousness); moist, cool skin; "feels shaky"	Thirst, increased urination, weakness, nausea, abdominal pain (classic: acetone breath odor, Kussmaul's respirations, decreased consciousness); hot, dry skin
Treatment	5-15 g carbohydrate as 4- to 8-oz soft drink (regular, not diet) 4-oz orange juice 6-8 Life Savers 1-1.5 Tbs honey 1-2 Tbs jam Administer glucagons IM or SQ (0.5-1.0 mg) if client is unable to swallow *Give some complex carbohydrates from meal plan within 1 hr after initial treatment*	Correct volume depletion with IV fluids, 0.9% NS initially Administer regular insulin by infusion Replace electrolytes as volume is restored Monitor vital signs I&O, blood glucose, and LOC

Modified from *AJN/Mosby nursing board review,* ed 9, St. Louis, 1994, Mosby.

    d. Diet therapy—American Diabetic Association diet; calorie intake is individualized

    e. Exercise—recommended six to seven times per week at approximately the same time each day

    f. Hypoglycemia (see Table 10-5)

    g. Ketoacidosis (see Table 10-5)

    h. HHNK (see Table 10-6)

7. Nursing diagnoses

    a. Risk for infection related to impaired leukocyte function and high glucose content in tissues

    b. Potential for injury or trauma related to inability to feel pain secondary to peripheral nerve degeneration

    c. Risk for impaired peripheral tissue integrity related to micro- and macrocirculatory changes

    d. Knowledge deficit—medication and dietary regimen related to need for additional teaching

TABLE 10-6	**Hyperglycemic Hyperosmolar Nonketotic Coma (HHNK)**

A life-threatening condition characterized by severe elevation of blood glucose, dehydration and stupor or coma. It occurs primarily in elderly Type II or previously undiagnosed diabetics. It has a 15% to 20% mortality rate.

Pathophysiology:
The crisis is frequently caused by an infection or stressor that causes an outpouring of steroids and increases the blood glucose. Enough insulin is produced to prevent ketosis but hyperglycemia and dehydration become life-threatening, especially if the client cannot take oral fluids.

Clinical Findings:
Severe dehydration
Hypothermia, hypotension
Severe weakness and lethargy
Depressed mental status to coma
Blood glucose greater than 600 mg/dl; usually around 1100 mg/dl
Elevated serum sodium
Serum osmolality above 350 mOsm/kg
Ketones—negative

Treatment:
IV fluid replacement, 0.9% NS initially
Low-dose IV insulin
Careful monitoring for complications (e.g., CHF, pulmonary edema, electrolyte imbalance, seizures)

Modified from *AJN/Mosby Nursing boards review,* ed 9, St Louis, 1994, Mosby.

8. Client goals
   a. Client will show no evidence of infection as evidenced by normal WBC with being afebrile
   b. Client will show no evidence of burns, abrasions, or cuts to extremities and will carefully assess extremities for injury several times per day
   c. Client will have appropriate tissue integrity as evidenced by intact skin without ulcerations
   d. Client will demonstrate knowledge and skills necessary to follow appropriate diet and take insulin or hypoglycemic agents as ordered
9. Nursing interventions
   a. Acute care
      (1) Ketoacidosis (serum glucose over 600 mg/dl and ketones present) and HHNK (serum glucose over 1100 mg/dl and ketones absent)
         (a) Maintain ABCs; monitor lung sounds frequently, especially the bases for the advent of CHF

       (b) Evaluate neurologic status frequently for changes

       (c) Maintain IV access and prepare to administer fluids in large quantities. It is not uncommon to administer 8 to 12 L in the first 24 hours of care. Fluid of choice is 0.9% saline followed by 0.45% saline.

       (d) Evaluate serum glucose levels as ordered or indicated. Administer insulin bolus IV initially followed by insulin drip or SC injections as blood glucose levels decrease to a more acceptable range.

       (e) Monitor urine output—anticipate large urine output until blood glucose has returned to baseline

       (f) Evaluate electrolyte levels as ordered—potassium and phosphorus abnormalities may not be seen immediately in the serum levels. Potassium and phosphorus will be replaced as indicated by results of serum levels as pH is corrected.

    (2) Hypoglycemia (insulin shock)—serum glucose less than 50 mg/dl

       (a) If client can tolerate PO fluids, administer approximately 15 g of carbohydrate such as soda, sugar, candy, or orange juice

       (b) If unconscious, administer IM or SQ glucagon

       (c) Note that physician may order an IV to be started and 50% dextrose administered

       (d) Evaluate blood sugar levels frequently to ensure a return to the client's baseline

  b. Home care regarding client education

    (1) Instruct client about medication administration

       (a) Instruct client to keep insulin vial currently used at room temperature and to refrigerate other vials

       (b) Instruct client that insulin must be at room temperature before administration

       (c) Teach client to roll the vial and not to shake it

       (d) Teach client the correct technique for drawing insulin from the vial

       (e) Instruct client that if two insulins are to be mixed, place the short-acting insulin in the syringe first, followed by the long-acting insulin—from clear to cloudy. (Tell client to associate this technique with bath water—first clear then cloudy.)

       (f) Inform client to rotate injection sites (Figure 10-6), so that all sites are used within a week

       (g) Show client how to inject the insulin at a 45- to 90-degree angle, depending on the amount of subcutaneous tissue

       (h) Tell client not to rub the site after administration but to press on it lightly as desired

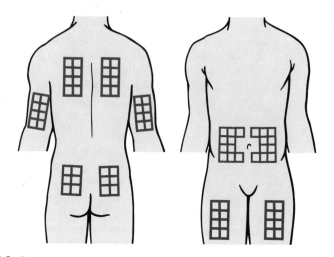

Figure 10-6 Injection sites for insulin. (From Lewis SM, Heitkemper MM, Dirksen SR: *Medical-surgical nursing: assessment and management of clinical problems,* ed 5, St. Louis, 2000, Mosby.)

       (i) Inform client not to smoke cigarettes for 30 minutes after administration because smoking causes vasoconstriction, which reduces insulin absorption

       (j) Teach another person living with or near client how to inject the medication in the event the client is unable to inject own medication

    (2) Glucose and ketone monitoring

       (a) Teach urine testing procedure for evaluating ketones—test before meals and at bedtime if required; document in percentages

       (b) Teach proper needle stick technique for blood glucose monitoring

          (i) Use correct timing as per manufacturer's requirements

          (ii) Use earlobes and sides of fingertips

       (c) Notify physician if levels are higher or lower than physician recommends

    (3) Diet therapy

       (a) Instruct client to follow the individualized meal plan

       (b) Inform client to carefully follow the exchange list of the diet

       (c) Teach client not to skip meals

       (d) Teach client how to modify diet for illness

          (i) Drink fluids hourly to replace lost fluid

          (ii) Make sure there is an intake of simple sugars that can be digested easily

(4) Exercise requirements
    (a) Carefully plan exercise; suggest 6 to 7 days a week at the same time each day to facilitate glucose control
    (b) Explain to client that exercise enhances the effects of insulin, and thus may cause hypoglycemia
    (c) Monitor blood glucose before and after exercise
    (d) Eat at least 1 hour before exercise, and make sure insulin has been taken
    (e) Carry a quick-acting carbohydrate in case of hypoglycemic reaction
    (f) Always wear a medical-alert bracelet or necklace case of hypoglycemic reaction
(5) Teach client the relationship between diet, exercise, and medication administration
(6) Instruct client how to identify when ketoacidosis and hypoglycemia occur and the interventions that should be taken (see Table 10-5, p. 355)
(7) Teach diabetic foot care
    (a) Inspect feet daily for dryness, cracks, and ingrown toenails
    (b) Thoroughly cleanse and dry feet and between toes daily
    (c) Place skin moisturizer on feet to prevent cracking
    (d) Never walk around barefooted
    (e) Always wear socks with shoes
    (f) Allow only a podiatrist to care for corns, callouses, and toenails
    (g) Be aggressive in treating even minor breakdown in the feet to prevent local infection and subsequent bone infection
(8) Changes that must occur in the event of illness or surgery
    (a) Continue to take medication
    (b) Increase the amount of insulin
    (c) Increase the frequency of blood glucose monitoring
    (d) If unable to eat, take in increased fluids and simple carbohydrates
(9) Health care maintenance
    (a) Careful daily hygiene is imperative
    (b) Frequent checkups with dentist are required
    (c) At least yearly evaluation by an ophthalmologist is required

10. Evaluation protocol
  a. How do I know that my interventions have been effective?
    (1) Client exhibits patent airway, acceptable breathing pattern, and circulation
    (2) Client maintains appropriate neurologic status—client is awake, oriented ×3

    (3) Client exhibits urine output of 30 ml/hr or more, and input equals output within 300 ml/day

    (4) Client exhibits decreasing or increasing blood glucose levels with a return to client's baseline level

    (5) Client exhibits normal electrolyte balance

  b. Which criteria will I use to change my interventions?

    (1) Unstable airway, breathing, or circulation

    (2) Decreased or decreasing neurologic status

    (3) Unbalanced I&O

    (4) Blood glucose levels that are resistant to therapy without a return to or near baseline levels

    (5) Abnormal electrolyte balance

  c. How will I know that my client teaching has been effective?

    (1) Client demonstrates the correct technique and timetable for medication administration

    (2) Client produces a food diary that exhibits correct dietary management

    (3) Client demonstrates the correct technique for blood glucose monitoring

    (4) Client produces a plan for exercise, indicating that exercise will occur after a meal and after insulin administration at the same time each day

    (5) Client correctly identifies factors to watch for that could indicate ketoacidosis or hypoglycemia is about to occur, and which interventions should be used

    (6) Client demonstrates proper foot care

    (7) Client states changes that must be made in the event of illness, surgery, or any other stressful life events

    (8) Client states the frequency of appointments with dentist and ophthalmologist for examinations

    (9) Client shows a medical-alert bracelet

    (10) Client states the conditions that need to be reported to physician

11. Older adult alert

  a. Type II diabetes mellitus is more common in the older adult client

  b. The older adult client is at great risk for complications associated with diabetes that would require hospitalization

  c. The symptoms commonly associated with diabetes mellitus may be masked by other illnesses in the older adult client. An example is polyuria, which may manifest itself as incontinence.

  d. Many older adult clients have unusual or erratic eating patterns that must be considered when planning a diet

e. Keep in mind there may be decreased visual acuity or manual dexterity in older adult clients that may decrease their ability to prepare and administer insulin

f. Proper foot care may not be possible with their decreased mobility and visual acuity

WEB Resources

http://www.diabetes.org/default.asp
   American Diabetes Association

http://www.niddk.nih.gov/
   National Institute of Diabetes and Digestive and Kidney Diseases

REVIEW QUESTIONS

1. A client is admitted to the hospital with a tentative diagnosis of Grave's disease. The nurse would expect to assess for which finding?
   1. Hypotension
   2. Bradycardia
   3. Client sleeps when undisturbed
   4. Client complains of the room being cold

2. When caring for a client who has received radioactive iodine therapy for hyperthyroidism, the teaching interventions must include all but which of these actions?
   1. The client should keep regular eating and sleeping habits
   2. The client should avoid close contact with children and pregnant women
   3. The client should use a bathroom separate from the rest of the family members
   4. The client should flush the toilet several times after each use

3. In a client with hypothyroidism the nurse would expect to see which group of laboratory values?
   1. Increased T_3, increased T_4, increased TSH
   2. Decreased T_3, decreased T_4, decreased TSH
   3. Decreased T_3, decreased T_4, increased TSH
   4. Increased T_3, increased T_4, decreased TSH

4. A major complication likely to occur in a client with hyperparathyroidism is
   1. Repeat occurrences of urinary calculi
   2. Muscle weakness over a period of a few weeks
   3. Intermittent fatigue
   4. Constipation alternated with diarrhea

5. An assessment appropriate for a client believed to be entering the beginning stages of tetany would be
   1. Allen's test
   2. Range of motion with resistance test
   3. Reflex evaluation
   4. Evaluation for Trousseau's sign

6. A client having surgery, who is taking corticosteroids for Addison's disease, will require
1. A smaller dose the day of surgery owing to the effects of anesthesia
2. A much larger dose from the increased need associated with the stress of surgery
3. More frequent doses given over several days before surgery
4. A larger dose the day of surgery followed by withholding the usual dose for 48 hours

7. Addisonian crisis requires which initial nursing assessment skill?
1. Evaluation of arterial monitoring results
2. Monitoring for dysrhythmias
3. Checks of BP for drastic changes
4. Complete an overall pulmonary function status

8. In the client with Cushing's syndrome, it is imperative that cortisol levels be evaluated twice a day. Expected normal plasma cortisol level is at its highest
1. At noon
2. At midafternoon
3. After eating
4. On wakening

9. The exercise regimen suggested for the client with diabetes mellitus is
1. At the same time each day and 3 times per week
2. Without concern as to the time of day and 4 times per week
3. At available free times of the client and 6 to 7 times per week
4. At the same time each day and 6 to 7 times per week

10. The purpose for administration of low-dose IV insulin in the event of hyperosmolar nonketotic coma is to
1. Have the availability of glucose to the cells for the prevention of severe hypotension
2. Encourage the passage of glucose into the cells slowly to prevent lysis of cells
3. Return blood glucose to an acceptable level for the client slowly to prevent profound shock
4. Return electrolyte imbalance to normal for the client and prevent a rapid change in this balance

ANSWERS, RATIONALES, AND TEST-TAKING TIPS

Rationales	Test-Taking Tips

1. Correct answer: 3

A client with Grave's disease may exhibit fatigue or exhaustion from a hypermetabolic state. Grave's disease is a form of hyperthyroidism with four attributes: enlarged thyroid or goiter, excess production of thyroid hormones, exophthalmos or bulging eyes, and skin changes. Other findings are hypertension, tachycardia, and heat intolerance. An inability to sleep occurs more during the onset of the disease process. If undiagnosed the disease progresses with the client becoming exhausted. Options 1, 2, and 3 are findings in hypothyroidism.

Beware of a tendency to select something you know is incorrect based on the fact you cannot find "your answer." Even if you could not recall what Grave's disease is, make an educated guess. Cluster options 1, 2, and 3 under the theme of a slow metabolism or slow body function. Option 3 would not be included in that theme because it indicates the client is alert when stimulated. If the metabolic functions were extremely slow the client would sleep all the time and be difficult to arouse. Select option 3.

2. Correct answer: 3

These clients do not have to use a separate bathroom from the rest of the family members. All of the other items need to be included in home care instructions. Avoidance of extended contact with children, pregnant women, or spouse is suggested for at least 1 week. The radioactive iodine is excreted in the urine, sweat, feces, breast milk, and saliva. Clients should avoid expectorating for the initial 24 hours because the saliva and any emesis are highly radioactive for 6 to 8 hours after the drug is ingested.

This question is in the harder category because it has an awkward structure "all but which." This is a format different from the usual "except" questions. Your best approach is to reword the question for clarity of thought. For example: which of these information statements should not be included?

Flushing the toilet several times after each use dilutes radiation that may be excreted in urine or feces.

3. Correct answer: 3

The T_3 and T_4 would be low from the inability of the thyroid to produce the hormones. The pituitary hormone TSH, thyroid-stimulating hormone, would be high in an attempt to stimulate the thyroid to produce more hormones.

The key word in the stem is "hypothyroidism." Therefore, read down vertically through the first item in these series. The options immediately can be narrowed to 2 and 3. Use common sense to think that T_3 and T_4 will be low but the TSH, thyroid-stimulating hormone, will be increased because it will try to get the thyroid to produce more hormones.

4. Correct answer: 1

Urinary calculi are common in clients with hyperparathyroidism. Bone demineralization occurs from increased levels of PTH. Recall that the balance of calcium and phosphorus can be thought of as a seesaw—when calcium is up phosphorus is down. And in parathyroid problems the calcium follows the direction of the imbalance: hyper equals increased calcium, decreased phosphorus; hypo equals the opposite. All of the other options are not complications of this problem. However, *acute* muscle weakness and fatigue or persistent constipation may be indications of high serum calcium levels and require immediate attention. High levels of calcium may have a paralysis type of effect.

Recall that the parathyroid deals with the balance of two minerals, calcium and phosphorus. Then associate that the only option given that might deal with mineral accumulation—since the question is asking about hyperfunction—would be the formation of kidney stones. Option 1 is correct.

Rationales	Test-Taking Tips

5. Correct answer: 4

Trousseau's sign is a carpal pedal spasm of the fingers when a blood pressure cuff is inflated for at least 1 minute on the arm. If positive with these spastic findings, it is indicative of impending tetany. Allen's test is used to evaluate collateral arterial blood flow through the ulnar artery. This is done prior to the needle stick of the radial artery for obtaining an ABG sample. ROM with resistance test is to determine clients' muscle strength and joint motion at the selected joint. Reflex evaluation would be to test the deep tendon reflexes or the knee reflex. It would not give you useful information in this type of client.

Options 2 and 3 are too general to be answers to a question about a specific assessment. Remember that the A in Allen's test is a clue that the test assesses Arterial collateral circulation to the hand. And last, the T in Trousseau's sign indicates Tetany if the sign is present or positive.

6. Correct answer: 2

The stress of surgery increases the client's need for corticosteroids and thus a higher dose is appropriate before or during surgery. Remember the S for Steroids: they need to be given Steadily, with more given in Stress, and cannot be Stopped abruptly. Option 1 and 3 are incorrect. In option 3 avoid an interpretion that more frequent doses mean an increased dosage. In option 4, the first part could be correct if it stood alone. However, the second part "withholding the usual dose for 48 hours" is incorrect.

Common sense about stress is to recall that more hormones are needed in the entire body when a person has stressful events; thus, the options can be narrowed to either 2 or 4. If you read option 4 too quickly, the key words "withholding the usual dose for 48 hours" were probably missed. If you got stuck on these two options, simply note that option 4 is a two-part option. Read the second part first, and then read the first part. With this action, it will become evident quickly that option 2 is the correct answer.

7. Correct answer: 3

A severe lack of corticosteroids, or Addisonian crisis, will cause cardiovascular collapse, a decrease in BP, and cardiac dysrhythmias. The other options are correct actions but are not the best answer to the question.

The key word is "initial." The nurse would assess options 1, 2, and 3. However, initially the BP would be the most important to be done first because arterial monitoring and dysrhythmia detection require more sophisticated equipment, which causes the loss of time before an action can occur.

8. Correct answer: 4

Cortisol is highest in the morning because there has been little use of it during sleep. Associate the levels of cortisol with most people's energy level throughout the day: highest energy in the morning and lower in the afternoon or early evening.

Avoid misreading the question as asking when the levels would be drawn. If you had no idea of a correct answer, think it through. Options 1 and 2 are fairly close together. Eliminate them. Option 3 is quite global—after eating. You think, Eat what? When? Eliminate it. Select option 4.

9. Correct answer: 4

Exercise in the client with diabetes must be consistent, the same time each day and at least 6 to 7 days per week. The cardiac client is advised to exercise three times a week. The diabetic needs to exercise every day to facilitate the best control of serum glucose levels with minimal fluctuations. The time of the exercise needs to fit the client's needs, with consideration given to when the daily oral hypoglycemic or insulin injection is taken.

Everything in life increases the need for insulin, except exercise, which decreases the need for insulin. Therefore, to have a better steady dosage of insulin the exercise needs to be consistent in terms of days and time of day.

10. Correct answer: 3

It is preferable to bring the glucose levels down slowly to prevent profound shock. Options 1 and 4 are incorrect statements. The beginning of option 2 is correct; however the second part is incorrect.

If you had no idea of what the diagnosis is, ask yourself What do I know from the given information. Note an important clue in the stem: low-dose insulin. After you read the options you get a sense that the problem is with a higher glucose

Rationales	Test-Taking Tips
	level. Eliminate option 4 because electrolytes have nothing to do with insulin. Think of what you know about the relationship between glucose and insulin—neither have an association with severe hypotension or cell lysis. Eliminate options 1 and 2. A final point is to remember that serum glucose and electrolyte levels require slow changes to avoid acute pathology in clients in most given situations. Note the important clues in the stem: insulin given in a high-glucose situation. Recall the basic information that insulin lowers glucose levels. Select response 3.

11

The Musculoskeletal System

FAST FACTS

1. Rest, an essential therapy in the care of clients with a musculoskeletal disorder, promotes the healing process.
2. Rest or immobility predisposes clients to complications of which pneumonia, also referred to as hypostatic pneumonia, is usually the first to occur.
3. Other complications of immobility are constipation, thrombophlebitis, pulmonary embolism, and renal calculi.
4. Elevation of the affected body part above the level of the heart decreases edema associated with trauma or an inflammatory process.
5. Body parts must be kept in proper body alignment or in the functional position of the body part.
6. High-top sneakers alternated on and off every 2 hours are the best intervention for prevention of drop foot.
7. Log-rolling or turning a client "all in one piece" is accomplished with two nurses and one or two pillows under the client's head and between the legs.

CONTENT REVIEW

I. Definition—the musculoskeletal system is responsible for support and movement of the body, protection of internal organs, storage of minerals, and the process of hematopoiesis

II. Structure and function
   A. **Bones**
      1. A total of 206 in various sizes and shapes

2. The outer layer of the bones is called the *periosteum*
3. Bones are held in alignment by ligaments

B. **Joints—formed where two bones come into contact with one another**
   1. Fibrous joints—no movement, such as in the suture lines of cranial bones
   2. Cartilaginous joints—small amount of movement, such as between vertebrae
   3. Synovial joints—move freely, such as the elbow
      a. The articulating surfaces of bones at the joint are covered with hyaline cartilage
      b. The joint capsule is lined with synovial membranes
      c. The joint cavity is filled with synovial fluid to decrease friction

C. **Muscles—muscle fibers are the actual working unit; skeletal muscle contraction and relaxation are accomplished by innervation by nerve impulses**
   1. Skeletal muscles are commonly attached to two bones and cross a joint
      a. some muscles form sphincters
      b. some muscles connect bone with skin such as in the cheek
   2. When a bone breaks, the muscle contracts and the extremity shortens

III. Targeted concerns

A. **Pharmacology—priority drug classifications**
   1. Salicylates—inhibit prostaglandin synthesis. Aspirin irreversibly inhibits platelet aggregation for the life of a platelet (7 to 10 days).
      a. Expected effects—antipyretic, analgesic, anti-inflammatory, and antiplatelet
      b. Commonly given drugs
         (1) Aspirin
         (2) Diflunisal (Dolobid)
         (3) Choline magnesium trisalicylate (Trilisate)
      c. Nursing considerations
         (1) Monitor for dizziness or ringing in ears, called *tinnitus,* which may indicate toxicity
         (2) Do not give to children or teenagers because of the risk of Reye syndrome
         (3) Do not give to clients with bleeding tendencies
         (4) Assess for bleeding
   2. NSAIDs—inhibit prostaglandin synthesis
      a. Expected effects—antipyretic, anti-inflammatory, and analgesic
      b. Commonly given drugs
         (1) Ibuprofen (Motrin)
         (2) Naproxen (Naprosyn)
         (3) Sulindac (Clinoril)
         (4) Piroxicam (Feldene)
         (5) Ketorolac tromethamine (Toradol)

    c. Nursing considerations

        (1) If client is unable to tolerate one type of NSAID, a different NSAID may be tolerated

        (2) Administer NSAIDs with food to decrease gastric distress

3. Corticosteroids—(see Chapter 10, pp. 332-334, and Chapter 13, pp. 425-426)

4. Central-acting muscle relaxants—mechanism of action unknown; possibly related to sedative effect

    a. Expected effect—relieves muscle spasm

    b. Commonly given drugs

        (1) Carisoprodol (Soma)

        (2) Cyclobenzaprine (Flexeril)

    c. Nursing considerations

        (1) Evaluate client carefully for lethargy because drug may impair mental functioning

        (2) Instruct client to avoid alcohol, CNS depressant medications, and hazardous tasks

5. Direct-acting muscle relaxants—act on a site within the muscle

    a. Expected effect—relaxation of tense skeletal muscles

    b. Commonly given drug—dantrolene sodium (Dantrium)

    c. Nursing considerations

        (1) Instruct client to avoid concurrent use of CNS depressant drugs

        (2) Monitor liver function studies when ordered

        (3) Evaluate for findings associated with hepatotoxicity—rash, pruritus, bruising, tarry stools, and jaundice

6. Acute anti-gout medication—specific action not understood

    a. Expected effect—decreases inflammatory response associated with acute gout

    b. Commonly given drug—colchicine

    c. Nursing considerations

        (1) Begin at first sign of gout attack; do not delay even an hour

        (2) For IV use, dilute only in normal saline; give over 2 to 5 minutes

        (3) Medication also may be given orally

        (4) Store medication in a tight dark container

7. Uricosuric drugs—increase renal excretion of uric acid

    a. Expected effect—prevents precipitation of uric acid in joints

    b. Commonly given drugs

        (1) Probenecid (Benemid)

        (2) Sulfinpyrazone (Aprazone)

        (3) Allopurinol (Zyloprim)

    c. Nursing considerations

        (1) Client must drink at least 2 to 3 L/day of water to prevent formation of uric acid kidney stones

        (2) Advise client that aspirin reduces the drug's effectiveness

(3) Instruct client to use caution when driving or using machinery because the drug may cause drowsiness for as long as 12 hours after it is taken

8. Gold compounds—mechanism unknown
   a. Expected effect—stops bone destruction and articular destruction in rheumatoid arthritis
   b. Commonly given drugs
      (1) Auranofin (Ridaura)
      (2) Aurothioglucose (Solganal), gold sodium thiomalate (Myochrysine) deep IM
   c. Nursing considerations
      (1) Assess if client is pregnant—contraindicated in pregnancy
      (2) Evaluate for normal or near normal baseline levels of urinalysis, CBC, platelet count, and liver function studies before beginning treatment
      (3) Avoid exposure to sunlight and ultraviolet light; use sunscreens
      (4) Report skin or mucous membrane lesions
      (5) Instruct client that the drug's effects may not be seen for 6 weeks to 6 months

9. Immunosuppressive agents (see Ch. 13, p. 425)

10. Cytotoxic drugs—interfere with folic acid metabolism; use only in clients with severe cases of rheumatoid arthritis
    a. Expected effect—immunosuppression
    b. Commonly given drugs
       (1) Methotrexate (Rheumatrex)
       (2) Cyclophosphamide (Cytoxan)
    c. Nursing considerations
       (1) Monitor client carefully for findings associated with GI tract lesions and bone marrow suppression
       (2) Instruct client that NSAIDs should not be taken during this therapy
       (3) Monitor client for symptoms of gout—severe pain in one joint. Increase fluid intake to at least 2000 ml/day to reduce risk of gout.

11. Gastric acid secretion inhibitor
    a. Expected effect—prevention of gastric ulceration secondary to administration of NSAID and aspirin
    b. Commonly given drug—misoprostol (Cytotec)
    c. Nursing considerations
       (1) Must not be taken if pregnant
       (2) May decrease the effects of aspirin

B. Procedures
1. Bone and joint X-ray films—identify irregularities in bones and joints

2. Magnetic resonance imaging (MRI)—produces body tissue images through the use of electromagnetic waves
3. Computed tomography (CT) scan—serial radiographic images of bone and tissue taken in cross sections
4. Bone scan—scanning of bones after an injection of a radioisotope to evaluate its distribution throughout the bone
5. Arthroscopy—direct examination of a joint using a lighted fiber-optic scope
6. Electromyography—evaluates nerve transmission and checks for muscle impulse response
7. Myelography—radiographic studies after injection of a radiopaque solution into the spinal canal to evaluate spinal conditions
8. Arthrography—radiographic studies of a joint after injection of a radiopaque solution to evaluate joint integrity
9. Biopsies of bone, muscle, and synovium—evaluate for malignancies or other disorders

C. Psychosocial concerns
1. Anxiety—uncomfortable feeling associated with an unknown direct cause. Common in these clients related to the unknown outcome of the illness and the threat to financial stability.
2. Anger—related to forced lifestyle changes, most often seen after trauma
3. Lifestyle changes—in response to changes in **mobility** or ability to continue working
4. Body-image change—usually related to structural changes as a result of trauma or malignancy
5. Isolation—may be related to decreased mobility or self-inflicted by client who is uncomfortable with the new body image

D. Health history
1. What exactly is the problem you are experiencing?
2. Are you having pain? Point to the pain with one finger.
3. Describe the pain. Is it achy, throbbing, stabbing, or sharp?
4. Does anything make the pain worse or better?
5. Is your pain worse during or damp or rainy weather?
6. Does the pain awaken you at night?
7. Have you recently had an injury to the area?
8. Point to which joints are stiff. Are your joints always stiff? How long do they feel stiff each day? In the morning only?
9. Has your joint ever locked and you could not move it?
10. Do you feel any weakness in your muscles? Which muscles?
11. How long have you had this swelling? Is there pain associated with the swelling?
12. Do you have any difficulty walking?
13. Do you have a loss of sensation, or burning and tingling in your extremities?
14. Which past medical problems have you experienced?

15. Have you had any injuries or surgeries in the past?
16. Which medical problems are you being treated for presently?
17. Which prescription and over-the-counter medications are you taking presently?
18. Is there a family history of any bone, joint, or muscle problems?
19. Are you having any difficulties taking care of your personal hygiene?
20. Are you able to do the work of your occupation?

E. Physical examination
1. ABCs—vital signs
2. Inspect and palpate each body part—examine when client is at rest and then while performing range-of-motion exercises
3. Observe general appearance
4. Observe posture
5. Observe gait
6. Observe for any deformities
7. Observe client in supine position for body alignment and deformity
8. Inspect and palpate each muscle group
9. Palpate each bone and joint
10. Evaluate for *crepitus* (grating sound or feeling in joint) in joints with movement

IV. Pathophysiologic disorders

A. **Fractures** (Figure 11-1)
1. Definition—a break in a bone. There are five categorizations of fractures.
   a. When the skin is open, it is called an open fracture; when the skin is intact, it is called a closed fracture
   b. Line of fracture—transverse, oblique, spiral, or linear
   c. Broken into pieces—comminuted
   d. Position of distal fragment—displaced or angulated
   e. Fracture involving the joint—intraarticular or extraarticular
2. Pathophysiology—stress placed on bone will result in fracture. Stress includes direct blows; twisting; severe muscle contractions; or as in a malignancy or severe osteoporosis, the bone may crumble.
3. Etiology—usually a result of trauma in the workplace or during sports activities. In older adult clients the cause may be osteoporosis or calcium loss from bones
4. Incidence—most commonly seen in young males and older adults
5. Assessment
   a. Questions to ask
      (1) Do you have pain at the site?
      (2) Do you feel as if the area is swollen?
      (3) Can you move the area?

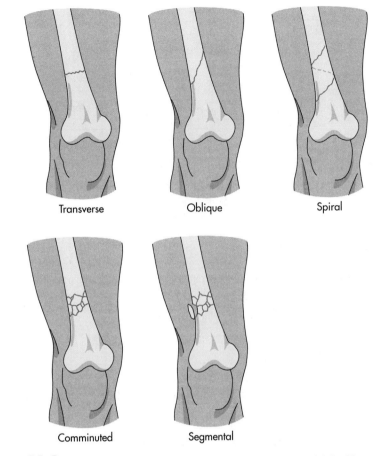

Transverse   Oblique   Spiral

Comminuted   Segmental

Figure 11-1   Five types of fractures. (From Beare PG, Myers JL: *Adult health nursing*, ed 3, St. Louis, 1998, Mosby.)

    b. Clinical manifestations—depend on cause, classification, type, and site
       (1) Pain with or without movement or bearing weight
       (2) Swelling
       (3) Inability to move
       (4) Discoloration at the area
       (5) Crepitus
       (6) Deformity
       (7) In hip fractures, the affected leg is
          (a) Shortened
          (b) Abducted
          (c) Externally rotated

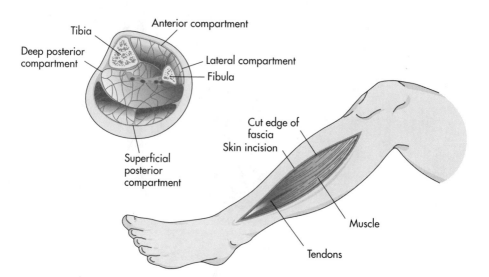

Figure 11-2 Compartment syndrome. Often more than one compartment is involved, and the anterior compartment is especially vulnerable. Causes include trauma, severe burns, or excessive exercise. A single incision may open more than one compartment. (From Beare PG, Myers JL: *Adult health nursing,* ed 3, St. Louis, 1998, Mosby.)

   c. Complications
     (1) Arterial damage—hemorrhage
     (2) Nerve damage—burning pain or loss of sensation or movement
     (3) Bleeding—hematoma
     (4) Avascular necrosis—loss of blood supply to the bone, resulting in death of bone; usually found at head of femur
     (5) Compartment syndrome—poor venous return in an area results in edema, which becomes so great in one of the compartments that arterial flow and nerve impulse transmission are impeded. Absence of or decreased pulses and paresthesia are common manifestations (Figure 11-2). Clients with crush injuries are at the greatest risk for this problem.
     (6) Fat emboli—usually with a femur fracture and less common after trauma to adipose tissue or a fatty liver. Fat globules enter the vascular space and become emboli, eventually entering the lung (see Chapter 5, Pulmonary Embolism, pp. 176-180). This event occurs 12 to 36 hours after the injury, with the classic signs of petechial hemorrhages on the neck, shoulders, axillae, and conjunctivae.
     (7) Osteomyelitis—infection of the osseous tissue of the bone
   d. Abnormal diagnostic test results
     (1) Bone X-ray films—show fracture

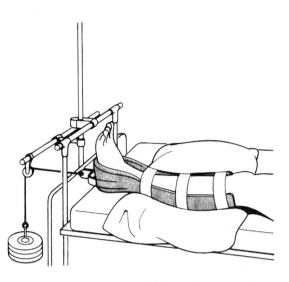

Figure 11-3   Buck's traction. (From Beare PG, Myers JL: *Adult health nursing,* ed 3, St. Louis, 1998, Mosby.)

       (2) Arthroscopy—determines extent of joint involvement, if applicable

       (3) Bone scans—determine extent of pathologic fracture, if applicable

  6. Expected medical interventions

    a. Closed reduction—bones manually manipulated back into alignment

    b. Open reduction—surgical incision; bone fragments held in place by plates, screws, pins, rods, wires, or a combination of these

    c. Casting once reduction is completed

    d. Traction

       (1) Skin traction—Buck's traction is used to decrease edema and muscle spasms before open reduction of a hip fracture (Figure 11-3)

       (2) Skeletal traction—pins are inserted through the distal end of the femur; traction is then applied to pins to pull the bones back into alignment (Figure 11-4)

    e. External fixation devices—metal frame with pins inserted through the bone to hold the fracture in position; commonly used for multiple fractures in a long bone or in the forearm

  7. Nursing diagnoses

    a. Pain related to injury of soft tissue and bone

    b. Impaired physical mobility related to restriction of cast, fixation device, or traction

    c. Risk for impaired skin integrity related to decreased mobility secondary to cast, traction, or fixation device application

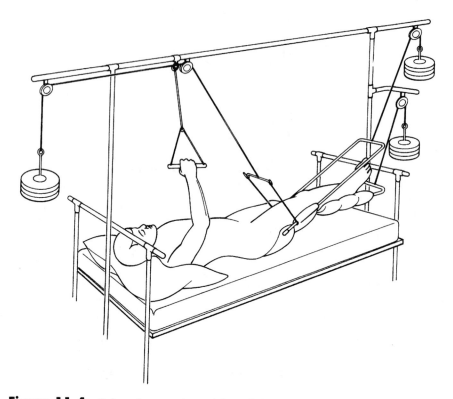

Figure 11-4 Balanced suspension traction (skeletal). (From Beare PG, Myers JL: *Adult health nursing,* ed 3, St. Louis, 1998, Mosby.)

8. Client goals
   a. Client will state pain is decreased or relieved
   b. Client will demonstrate appropriate mobility of extremities that can be moved and range of motion of joint that can be moved
   c. Client will not have skin breakdown at high-risk areas
9. Nursing interventions
   a. Care of the client after surgical hip fracture repair (pinning or prosthesis)
      (1) Routine postoperative care
      (2) Assess the five Ps of neurovascular status with routine postoperative checks
         (a) Pain
         (b) Pallor
         (c) Paralysis
         (d) Paresthesia
         (e) "Pulselessness"
      (3) Assess surgical drainage devices—empty hemovac or Jackson-Pratt drains when half full or once every shift, whichever occurs first, and then recharge the drainage device

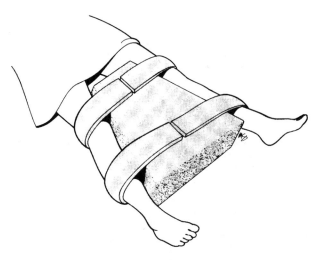

Figure 11-5   Abduction pillow used after total hip replacement. (From Beare PG, Myers JL: *Adult health nursing,* ed 3, St. Louis, 1998, Mosby.)

(4) Notify physician if drainage is over 150 ml/hr

(5) Monitor H&H for an additional decrease, and monitor electrolytes for any changes

(6) Administer antiembolism stockings or sequential compression device to the unaffected leg as per physician's order

(7) Institute exercises—have client perform
  (a) Ankle rotations
  (b) Dorsiflexion and plantar flexion of the ankle

(8) Maintain abductor pillow while the client is confined to bed (Figure 11-5)

(9) Turn client every 2 hours to unaffected side and back only

(10) Do not allow hip flexion greater than 40 degrees

b. Care of the client in a cast (plaster or synthetic—Box 11-1)

(1) Check neurovascular status every 30 minutes for 4 hours, then every 2 hours for 4 hours, then every 4 hours

(2) Evaluate increase in drainage through the cast by using a pen to draw a circle around the drainage perimeter and write down the time on the cast

(3) Elevate casted extremity on a pillow to promote venous return and prevent edema

(4) Apply ice to the cast over the affected area, and be sure to protect the cast from moisture

(5) Assess the cast for areas of increased heat, which may indicate an infection under the cast

(6) Assess the cast for foul odor

Box 11-1
Client Education Guide to Cast Care

Do Not

- Get cast wet*
- Remove any padding
- Insert any foreign object inside cast
- Bear weight on new cast for 48 hr (not all casts are made for weight bearing; check with health care provider when unsure)
- Cover cast with plastic for prolonged periods

Do

- Apply ice directly over fracture site for first 24 hr (avoid getting cast wet by keeping ice in plastic bag and protecting cast with cloth)
- Check with physician before getting cast wet†
- Dry cast thoroughly after exposure to water:
  Blot dry with towel
  Use hair dryer on low setting until cast is thoroughly dry
- Elevate extremity above level of heart for first 48 hr
- Move joints above and below cast regularly
- Report signs of possible problems to health care provider
  Increasing pain
  Swelling associated with pain and discoloration of toes or fingers
  Pain during movement
  Burning or tingling under cast
  Sores or foul odor under cast
- Keep appointment to have fracture and cast checked

*Plaster of Paris cast.
†Synthetic cast.
From Lewis SM, Heitkemper MM, Dirksen SR: *Medical-surgical nursing: assessment and management of clinical problems,* ed 5, St. Louis, 2000, Mosby.

    (7) Use the palms of your hands to handle a wet cast. Using your fingers may cause indentations that could impair the skin.

    (8) Do not cover the cast; let it air-dry for the first 24 hours

    (9) Petal the edges of the cast to prevent rough edges from breaking down the skin

  c. Care of the client in traction (skeletal and skin)

    (1) Use fracture bedpan for elimination

    (2) Assess neurovascular status of the extremity every 1 to 2 hours

    (3) Maintain body alignment

    (4) Keep weights off floor, and use the correct weight size ordered

    (5) For skeletal fractures, perform pin care every 8 hours with solution as ordered by physician

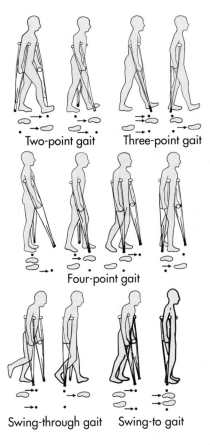

Two-point gait   Three-point gait

Four-point gait

Swing-through gait   Swing-to gait

Figure 11-6   Crutch gaits. (From *Mosby's Medical, nursing, and allied health dictionary,* ed 5, St. Louis, 1998, Mosby.)

   d. Home care regarding client education
     (1) Care of the cast (see Box 11-1)
       (a) Do not insert anything between the cast and the skin
       (b) Bear weight only when physician indicates it is safe
       (c) Call physician if there is a foul odor or if an area of the cast feels warm
       (d) Call physician if the cast becomes tight because it may require cutting the cast in half, or bivalving it, with windows cut out over pressure areas to assess circulation
     (2) Use of assistant devices
       (a) Crutch walking (Figure 11-6 for crutch walking gaits)
         (i) Non-weight-bearing using three-point gait
         (ii) Appropriate crutch fit. Bottom of crutches should have rubber tips and be 6 to 8 inches from

client's side or feet; top of crutches should be 2 inches below the axilla crease.
    (iii) Weight on hands not axilla
    (iv) Elbows slightly bent
  (b) Cane carried in hand opposite the affected leg for greater support and balance
  (c) Walker—with arms bent slightly, position the walker ahead of gait to a comfortable length of the arms and walk into walker; repeat
  (3) Physician follow-up—very important—first visit is usually within 1 week of the traumatic event

10. Evaluation protocol
  a. How do I know that my interventions have been effective?
    (1) Neurovascular status is maintained—palpable pulse, warm extremity with color equivalent to opposite extremity, appropriate sensation and movement, and brisk capillary refill of less than 3 seconds
    (2) Pain is relieved
    (3) Cast is drying and intact
    (4) Skeletal traction is appropriate with correct body alignment
    (5) Traction pin sites are not infected; drainage, if any, is serous
    (6) Hip prosthesis is in appropriate alignment
    (7) Assessment findings do not indicate a tight cast or compartment syndrome
  b. Which criteria will I use to change my interventions?
    (1) One aspect of neurovascular status has deteriorated
    (2) Pain has increased
    (3) Cast is tight, and skin is breaking down
    (4) Skeletal traction is out of alignment
    (5) Pin sites have purulent drainage
    (6) Hip prosthesis has left the acetabulum
    (7) Client assessment findings indicate possible complication—most often identified by a change in neurovascular status or increasing pain
  c. How will I know that my client teaching has been effective?
    (1) Cast has dried appropriately without neurovascular impairment
    (2) Client can state symptoms that should be reported to physician
    (3) Client demonstrates appropriate use of assistant device

11. Older adult alert
  a. The older adult client is more susceptible to fractures as a result of osteoporosis. Teaching should be aimed at preventing accidents.

b. The older adult client who is confined to bed will be at a much higher risk for complications than the younger adult

B. Ruptured lumbar intervertebral disc (herniated disc)
1. Definition—displacement of intervertebral disc material
2. Pathophysiology—most often occurs in the back of a disc where the outer ring of tissue holding the disc in place is the weakest; most often involves a tear in this outer tissue and the interior contents. The *nucleus pulposus* (pulpy center) bulges outward, putting pressure on the spinal nerve roots. Pain and paresthesia result from compression of nerve roots.
3. Etiology—most clients report a previous back injury that involved flexion or rotation of the back in such a way as to cause disc displacement
4. Incidence—more than 10% of clients who seek medical advice for back pain have a herniated disc
5. Assessment
   a. Questions to ask
      (1) Where is your pain? Point to it with one finger.
      (2) Does the pain travel anywhere else?
      (3) Have you noticed any feeling other than pain?
   b. Clinical manifestations
      (1) Lower back pain
      (2) Radiation of pain into the posterior thigh
      (3) Muscle spasms
      (4) Decreased deep tendon reflexes
      (5) Numbness along nerve roots
   c. Abnormal diagnostic test results
      (1) Spinal X-ray films—narrowed disc space
      (2) MRI—spinal stenosis and herniated material from disc
      (3) Myelography—narrowed disc space and herniation at a specific level
6. Expected medical interventions
   a. Anti-inflammatory agents
   b. Muscle relaxants
   c. Analgesics
   d. Decreased activity; bed rest if necessary
   e. Pelvic traction
   f. Back brace
   g. Percutaneous lateral diskectomy
   h. Microsurgical diskectomy
   i. Laminectomy and spinal fusion
7. Nursing diagnoses
   a. Pain related to pressure on nerve roots or to the effects of surgery
   b. Impaired mobility related to lumbar pain secondary to pressure on nerve roots

8. Client goals
   a. Client will state pain is relieved or decreased
   b. Client will increase mobility by 10% to 20% daily
9. Nursing interventions
   a. Acute care—postoperative
      (1) Perform routine postoperative care
      (2) Perform neurovascular assessment with each set of vital signs
      (3) Empty and evaluate drainage from the continuous portable suction device (hemovac or Jackson-Pratt drain) when half full or every shift, whichever occurs first
      (4) Logroll client every 2 hours
      (5) Evaluate lumbar and iliac incisions if a bone graft has been performed
      (6) Get client out of bed into a straight-back chair, with feet on the floor, usually the evening of surgery, for 30 to 60 minutes as tolerated
      (7) If a spinal fusion has been done, ensure that client stays in bed for 24 to 48 hours. Logroll client every 2 hours.
      (8) Evaluate client for urinary retention if indwelling urinary catheter is not in place
   b. Home care regarding client education
      (1) Instruct client about when and how to take all medications
      (2) Teach client to clean the incision with soap and water at least once a day and to report redness, swelling, or drainage from the incision to physician
      (3) Instruct client on the principles of correct body mechanics
         (a) Use leg muscles, not back muscles, when lifting
         (b) Always get help in lifting
         (c) Do not turn and lift at the same time
      (4) Do not twist the back, especially when getting out of bed
      (5) Sleep on a firm mattress
      (6) Avoid sitting for longer than 1 hour at a time
      (7) Maintain or achieve ideal body weight
      (8) Do not climb steps for at least 2 to 3 weeks
      (9) Do not attempt to lift any weight until the first visit to physician. At that time, the physician may tell the client to lift only 5 pounds at a time, slowly increasing by ½ pound at a time over the next 4 weeks.
      (10) Inform client that he or she may be able to return to work in 3 to 4 weeks, depending on the type of work
10. Evaluation protocol
    a. How do I know that my interventions have been effective?
       (1) Neurovascular status is intact
       (2) Drains are intact, with minimal drainage

    (3) Incisions are approximated, clean, and dry
    (4) Client is turned every 2 hours using logrolling technique
    (5) Client is out of bed as ordered
    (6) Client does not have urinary retention
  b. Which criteria will I use to change my interventions?
    (1) Neurovascular status is impaired
    (2) Drains are not intact or have increased bloody drainage
    (3) Client is trying to turn without using the logrolling technique
    (4) Urinary retention is identified
  c. How will I know that my client teaching has been effective?
    (1) Client correctly states medication regimen
    (2) Client demonstrates correct body mechanics
    (3) Client indicates sleeping on a firm mattress
    (4) Client indicates appropriate weight changes: has lost weight, is losing weight, or is maintaining ideal weight
    (5) Client follows regimen for postoperative activity
    (6) Client indicates that the incision is clean and dry, and that the edges are together
11. Older adult alert—older adult clients must be evaluated carefully for the complications associated with immobility during the recovery phase of this surgery

C. Arthritis
1. Definition
  a. Osteoarthritis—a nonsystemic, degenerative disorder of the weight-bearing joints
  b. Rheumatoid arthritis—a systemic inflammatory disorder of the connective tissue that is chronic; exacerbations and remissions are characteristic
  c. Gouty arthritis—inflammatory changes evident in one joint in response to high uric acid levels
2. Pathophysiology
  a. Osteoarthritis—wearing down and breakdown of the articular cartilage of the joints. Cracks occur in the surface of cartilage, spurs form, and pain is the result.
  b. Rheumatoid arthritis—synovial lining of the joint becomes inflamed, granulation tissue forms, cartilage is destroyed, and fibrous tissue is left in place of cartilage
  c. Gouty arthritis—increase in purine metabolism results in excess uric acid. Uric acid crystals form in a joint and connective tissue, resulting in inflammation and pain. Gout, a unilateral problem, most often affects the great toe or the ankle.
3. Etiology
  a. Osteoarthritis—unknown; aging is considered a risk factor
  b. Rheumatoid arthritis—unknown; theories suggest autoimmune disorder and infectious agents

TABLE 11-1	Comparison of Arthritis Types		
	Osteoarthritis	Rheumatoid Arthritis	Gouty Arthritis
No. of joints affected	1 or 2	Multiple	One
Joint deformity?	Yes	Yes	Possible
Pain with movement?	Yes	Decrease with movement	Pain all the time
Morning stiffness?	Yes	Yes	No
Fever, increased WBC?	No	Yes	Fever
Symptoms increase with humidity?	Yes	Yes	No
Exacerbations and remissions?	No	Yes	If medications and diet are not followed

    c. Gouty arthritis—increase in purine metabolism, for example, in clients on antineoplastic therapy, with a high purine diet, or those ingesting excess alcohol

4. Incidence

    a. Osteoarthritis—common after the age of 35; more common in females over the age of 55

    b. Rheumatoid arthritis—more common in female population

    c. Gouty arthritis—more common in male population

5. Assessment

    a. Questions to ask

        (1) When does your pain occur?

        (2) Do you have swelling of your joints?

        (3) Does the weather make your pain worse?

        (4) What makes your pain worse?

        (5) What makes your pain better?

    b. Clinical manifestations (Table 11-1)

    c. Abnormal laboratory findings

        (1) Osteoarthritis—none specific for this disorder

        (2) Rheumatoid arthritis

            (a) Rheumatoid factor—positive

            (b) ESR—elevated

        (3) Gouty arthritis

            (a) Serum uric acid—elevated

            (b) CBC—elevated WBC

            (c) Sedimentation rate—elevated

    d. Abnormal diagnostic test results

        (1) Osteoarthritis

            (a) Joint X-ray films—narrowed joint space, bone cysts, and sharpened articular surfaces

      (2) Rheumatoid arthritis

          (a) Joint aspiration—increased synovial fluid volume, and fluid is cloudy

          (b) Joint X-ray films—eroded joint surfaces, joint space narrowing, and unstable joint

      (3) Gouty arthritis

          (a) Joint aspiration—presence of uric acid crystals

          (b) Joint X-ray films—radiolucent *urate tophi* (nodules of urate)

6. Expected medical interventions

    a. Osteoarthritis

      (1) Rest for affected joints

      (2) Weight reduction if necessary

      (3) Moist heat

      (4) Intraarticular steroids

      (5) NSAIDs

      (6) Joint replacement surgery

      (7) Range-of-motion exercises, passive and active

    b. Rheumatoid arthritis

      (1) Rest, especially during exacerbations; splints may be used

      (2) Range-of-motion exercises, passive and active

      (3) Cold therapy during acute exacerbations and moist heat for stiffened joints

      (4) Aspirin

      (5) Gold salts (Myochrysine)

      (6) Corticosteroids

      (7) Methotrexate (Rheumatrex)

    c. Gouty arthritis

      (1) NSAIDs

      (2) Colchicine for acute episodes

      (3) Uricosuric agents—allopurinol (Zyloprim)

      (4) Low purine diet

      (5) Gouty tophi excision if eroding through skin

7. Nursing diagnoses

    a. Acute pain related to inflamed joint spaces

    b. Impaired physical mobility related to joint pain

    c. Fatigue related to prolonged immobility and increased metabolic demands

8. Client goals

    a. Client will state pain has decreased or has been relieved with the use of specified interventions

    b. Client will demonstrate active range of motion exercises for all joints daily

    c. Client will state fatigue has decreased

9. Nursing interventions
   a. Acute care
      (1) Postoperative joint replacement—care will be the same as for the client following hip surgery (pp. 378-379)
   b. Home care regarding client education
      (1) Adhere to medication regimen
      (2) Fulfill need for daily activity, and avoid overexertion
      (3) Apply heat for analgesia
      (4) Exercise joints to the point of pain but not past the point of pain
      (5) Use splints on affected joints during acute exacerbations
      (6) Prevent gout by a low purine diet
      (7) Increase fluid intake to prevent uric acid urinary calculi with gout
      (8) Control weight if indicated
10. Evaluation protocol
      (1) How will I know that my client teaching has been effective?
         (a) Client states performance of range-of-motion exercises three times a day
         (b) Client demonstrates correct medication regimen and verbalizes side effects to relate to physician
         (c) Client loses weight with maintenance of appropriate weight
         (d) Client demonstrates correct procedure for moist heat application
11. Older adult alert—this is a disorder of older adults and should be evaluated for when assessing older adult clients

D. Amputation
   1. Definition—removal of a limb
   2. Pathophysiology—would be the pathophysiology of the disorder that led to the need for amputation
   3. Etiology—traumatic injury; surgical removal as a result of a gangrenous process, cancerous tumor, osteomyelitis, and so forth
   4. Assessment
      a. Clinical manifestations
         (1) Traumatic
            (a) Discoloration of the limb
            (b) Muscle loss and vascular impairment
            (c) Neurovascular compromise
         (2) Surgical—(see Peripheral Arterial Occlusive Disorders, Chapter 3, p. 103)
      b. Abnormal diagnostic test results
         (1) Angiography—shows inadequate circulation
         (2) CT scan—evaluates for extensive neoplasm or osteomyelitis

(3) Doppler ultrasonography—indicates degree of inadequate circulation

5. Nursing diagnoses

   a. Pain related to the effects of trauma or the surgical procedure

   b. Impaired physical mobility related to the loss of the lower extremity and the need to learn how to use the prosthesis

   c. Pain related to phantom limb syndrome or *pseudesthesia*—sensation or discomfort experienced in the missing limb

   d. Body-image disturbance related to the loss of a body part

6. Client goals

   a. Client will state pain is relieved or decreased

   b. Client will demonstrate range-of-motion exercises for the remaining extremities

   c. Client will attempt to maintain independence

   d. Client will state phantom pain is relieved

   e. Client will state feeling comfortable with changes in body and is adapting to trauma

7. Nursing interventions

   a. Acute care

      (1) Routine postoperative care

      (2) Maintain immediate postoperative prosthesis (IPOP) as ordered by physician—cast applied over postoperative dressing and prosthesis applied to cast, which increases early ambulation and decreases edema. Use until permanent prosthesis is ready.

      (3) Air splints and ace bandage wraps may be used to decrease stump edema

      (4) Elevate the stump with physician's order for the initial 24 hours to hasten a decrease in edema

      (5) After the first 24 hours, assist client into a prone position, if tolerated, for 1 hour, three times a day, to prevent hip and knee contractures

      (6) Treat phantom pain as needed

         (a) Physician may prescribe beta-blockers to increase serotonin level and decrease pain

         (b) Use distraction therapy and massage therapy

         (c) Use transcutaneous electrical nerve stimulation (TENS) unit

         (d) Maintain epidural anesthesia postoperatively—very effective for reducing phantom pain

      (7) Encourage client to look at stump and touch it to begin acceptance

   b. Home care regarding client education

      (1) Stump care before and after prosthesis use

      (2) Indications of wound infection

  (3) Exercise regimen

  (4) Ambulation with assistant devices

 8. Evaluation protocol

  a. How will I know that my interventions have been effective?

   (1) Stump does not become edematous

   (2) Hip and knee contractures do not occur

   (3) Phantom pain is controlled

   (4) Client is accepting of stump; looks at it and begins to care for the incision

  b. Which criteria will I use to change my interventions?

   (1) Edematous stump

   (2) Hip or knee contractures

   (3) Uncontrolled phantom pain

   (4) Refusal by client to look at or touch stump

  c. How will I know that my client teaching has been effective?

   (1) Client demonstrates the correct technique for stump care

   (2) Client states findings associated with wound infection

   (3) Client demonstrates the correct exercise regimen

   (4) Client demonstrates the correct technique for use of assistant devices

 9. Older adult alert

  a. The older adult client will be more difficult to return to a preamputation mobility status because of joint changes that may be present in the other extremities

  b. It is more difficult for older clients to use a prosthesis. They often have impaired mobility in other extremities or difficulty placing and removing the prosthesis because of decreased dexterity or vision.

E. Osteoporosis

 1. Definition—metabolic bone disease that results in bone demineralization and subsequent fractures

 2. Pathophysiology and etiology—loss of bone density that begins in the third and fourth decades

  a. Because of aging, impaired osteoblasts are unable to form bone at the same rate as bone resorption occurs

  b. Because of decreased estrogen, less vitamin D is available, resulting in impaired calcium absorption

  c. Decreased intake of dietary calcium causes bone loss

  d. Decreased weight-bearing exercise causes bone loss

  e. Smoking more than 10 cigarettes per day decreases serum estrogen

  f. Alcohol and caffeine intake can increase daily calcium loss

 3. Incidence—approximately 50% to 60% of women over the age of 65 have osteoporosis; more common in women

 4. Assessment

  a. Questions to ask

   (1) Do you ever have pain in your back or hip?

      (2) Have you noticed that your height has decreased over the past 3 years?

      (3) Do you have difficulty walking?

  b. Clinical manifestations

      (1) Many clients are asymptomatic until a fracture occurs

      (2) Hump or *kyphosis* at the top of the spine

      (3) Shortened height

      (4) Pain, worsened by activity

  c. Abnormal laboratory findings

      (1) Serum calcium—high

      (2) Alkaline phosphatase—low

  d. Abnormal diagnostic test results

      (1) Bone X-ray films—show demineralization and fractures

      (2) CT scan—shows demineralization in the cancellous bone, which may allow early diagnosis

      (3) Single-photon absorptiometry—measures skeletal density in two dimensions, showing a loss of density

5. Expected medical interventions

  a. Balanced diet with at least 1500 mg/day of elemental calcium

  b. Moderate daily exercise, walking and swimming

  c. Back or neck support to prevent fractures

  d. Calcium carbonate supplementation

  e. Vitamin D supplementation, one to two times per week

  f. Estrogen-progestin combinations

6. Nursing diagnosis

  a. Risk for injury (fracture) related to falls and bumping into objects

  b. Impaired physical mobility related to changes in vertebral column and decreased muscle tone

  c. Pain related to fracture

7. Client goals

  a. Client will not injure self, as evidenced by absence of bruises or fractures

  b. Client will demonstrate mobility as evidenced by walking for 10 minutes each day or swimming for 10 minutes each day

  c. Client will state pain has decreased to a 2 on a pain scale of 0 to 10

8. Nursing interventions

  a. Acute care—would be the nursing care of the client with fractures (pp. 374-383)

  b. Home care regarding client education

      (1) Work with client to evaluate home for potential hazards

         (a) Use nonskid slippers

         (b) Remove throw rugs from floors

         (c) Install optimal lighting

(d) Place handrails in bathroom near commode and in tub or shower

(e) Use nonskid material on steps

(2) Evaluate current drug therapy for medications that may cause drowsiness or dizziness

(3) Teach client about

(a) Foods high in calcium

(b) Avoiding caffeine and alcohol

(c) Stopping tobacco use

(4) Consult with physical therapist to devise an exercise program—deep-water exercises with the use of flotation devices are excellent

(5) Encourage assistant devices if necessary, such as a walker or cane

(6) Control pain—medication if needed: narcotic or nonnarcotic, anti-inflammatory drugs, moist heat

(7) Assess fit of vertebral support—braces and neck supports

9. Evaluation protocol

a. How will I know that my client teaching has been effective?

(1) Client produces a food diary indicating foods high in calcium are being eaten

(2) Client is taking vitamin and calcium supplements

(3) Client has stopped smoking and has stopped drinking beverages with caffeine and alcohol

(4) Client has begun an exercise program of walking for 15 to 30 minutes at least once daily

(5) Client demonstrates proper use of a cane

(6) Client states that pain is controlled with an NSAID and warm, moist compresses

10. Older adult alert—osteoporosis is found predominantly in the older adult population and must be considered when treating an older adult client with new onset of skeletal pain or disability.

WEB Resources

http://www.arthritis.com
Latest news on arthritis, information and community.

http://www.nih.gov/niams
National Institute of Arthritis and Musculoskeletal and Skin Diseases.

REVIEW QUESTIONS

1. The client who has a synthetic cast applied is permitted to swim or bathe with the cast. Which of these instructions must be given?
    1. Blot the cast dry on the outside, and allow it to air-dry
    2. Flush the cast with clean water, blot the outside of the cast dry, use a hair dryer on the cool or warm setting to dry the inside padding
    3. Blot the outside of the cast dry, use a hair dryer on the cool or warm setting to dry the inside padding
    4. Flush the cast with warm to hot water, use a hair dryer on the cool or warm setting to dry the inside padding

2. A client at home calls the office nurse and states that his cast feels warm in one spot. He is asking what he should do. The best answer will depend on an understanding of what is happening. The nurse knows a hot spot is an indication of
    1. Swelling under cast
    2. Inflammation under cast
    3. Cast tightness or compartment syndrome
    4. An object stuck under the cast

3. The purpose of the abductor pillow after surgery to implant a total hip prosthesis is to
    1. Prevent mobility of the new joint until healed
    2. Prevent adduction of the lower extremities
    3. Hold the prosthesis in the acetabulum until healing can begin
    4. Hold the prosthesis in the acetabulum, and prevent slippage out of the acetabulum

4. A client with compartment syndrome will exhibit which most common assessment finding?
    1. Paresthesia in the involved extremity
    2. Increased pain in the entire limb
    3. Warm then cold skin on the involved extremity
    4. Minimal movement of the digits

5. The pain experienced by a client postoperatively after a lumbar laminectomy with spinal fusion is commonly a
    1. Sharp quality that travels down one of the legs
    2. Dull ache in the area of the buttocks
    3. Sharp incisional pain that shoots around the trunk of the client
    4. Sharp incisional pain and muscle spasms around incisional area

6. Which statement helps to distinguish between osteoarthritis and rheumatoid arthritis?
    1. Complaints of discomfort increase only in clients with osteoarthritis when there is increased humidity

    2. Pain increases with movement and use of the joints in both conditions

    3. Fever is noted in both conditions during exacerbations

    4. Pain decreases with the affected joint use in rheumatoid arthritis and increases with the affected joint use in osteoarthritis

7. A food stuff that should be restricted for a client with gouty arthritis is

    1. Chicken

    2. Eggs

    3. Legumes

    4. Cereal grains

8. An understanding of phantom pain allows the nurse to explain to a client that it is caused by

    1. Nerves stimulated at the level of the surgical incision

    2. Nerves that have been cut but are still sending impulses from the severed limb

    3. Swelling around the nerves at the surgical site

    4. Bone nerves that have been cut

9. Clients with osteoporosis must be counseled not only to include high levels of calcium in their diet but also include

    1. Vitamin C

    2. Vitamin K

    3. Vitamin D and the B vitamins

    4. Vitamins A and D

10. The initial therapy of choice for the client with rheumatoid arthritis in an acute exacerbation is

    1. Hot compresses

    2. Warm, moist compresses

    3. Cold therapy

    4. Paraffin therapy

ANSWERS, RATIONALES, AND TEST-TAKING TIPS

Rationales	Test-Taking Tips

1. Correct answer: 2

The cast must be flushed to remove traces of soap or chlorine. Blot the outside dry, and dry the inside with a warm or cool hair dryer. Clues in the stem are the words "swim" and "bath." Common sense reflects that in both of these situations the cast would need to be rinsed first, then the outside and inside padding dried.

When you compare them, similarities are found in options 2, 3, and 4 for drying the inside of the cast. Thus, eliminate option 1, because the action of air-drying is different. With air-drying, a longer time is required and the inside of the cast may not dry completely, which may cause complications. Then eliminate option 3, which omits the cleaning of chlorine or soap from the cast. Compare options 2 and 4, and note that option 2 is the most comprehensive and therefore most likely is the correct answer.

2. Correct answer: 2

The hot spot is typically caused by inflammation under the cast and should be evaluated within 24 hours by a physician. Clients complain of tingling, numbness, or loss of movement in the fingers or toes when swelling occurs under the cast. Compartment syndrome is a result of *severe* swelling under a cast. The findings for this syndrome are associated with a loss of arterial circulation and nerve function to that extremity. It is a medical emergency with the need for action within 15 minutes to 1 hour of the diagnosis. The action is typically to *bivalve* the cast, meaning to cut the cast with parallel cuts from the proximal to the distal ends of the cast. Then the cast is wrapped with an elastic

The clue in the question is the word "hot." Use common sense. Hot on the body typically indicates inflammation. Swelling would occur in more than just one spot.

Rationales	Test-Taking Tips

bandage to maintain immobility yet allow for more swelling. An object stuck under a cast usually results in pain at a specific site under the cast.

3. Correct answer: 4

Slippage of the head of the prosthesis out of the acetabulum is a very painful and dangerous complication. The abductor pillow will prevent this by holding the head of the prosthesis in the correct position. The initial part of option 1 is correct—prevent mobility of the new joint. However, the second part—until healed—is incorrect. A similar situation occurs in options 2 and 3. In option 2 the location of "lower extremities" is incorrect in a situation in which one hip is affected, and not both hips. In option 3, "until healing begins" is incorrect information.

Note that these options have two parts. If you only focused on the first part of each, you have made the question harder than it really is. To clarify the options for the purpose of eliminating wrong options, simply use the reverse reading process for each option. Read the second part first and the first part second.

4. Correct answer: 1

Loss of sensation or diminished sensation in the affected extremity is a more common finding with compartment syndrome that can occur after severe burns, trauma, or cast application. Clients' complaints result from a compression of the arteries and nerve impulse functions. Thus, deficits in these two areas occur. Pain in the entire limb may result from venous or muscle problems. Option 3 is incorrect. Option 4 might be an expected finding after trauma to any extremity.

Avoid an elimination of option 1 because you could not recall what the word paresthesia means. Go with what you know to eliminate the other options. On the other hand, if you do not know what compartment syndrome is, read the options with an open mind. The options give the clue that it involves an extremity. Then, make an educated guess and select the worst description of the options. Select option 1 in which nerve malfunction is a priority over pain, skin temperature, and minimal movement of the digits.

5. Correct answer: 4

The client feels sharp pain from the incision and muscle spasms from the procedure. Eliminate options 1 and 2 because they are in the wrong location—down one leg and in the buttocks—and there is no mention of incisional pain. Of the remaining options, option 4 is more accurate and specific to the type of surgery—in the lumbar area rather than the trunk.

Pick up on the clue in the stem about the location of the surgery, which is in the lumbar area. As you read the options, focus on the question. It is about postoperative pain, not *preoperative* pain.

6. Correct answer: 4

Pain increases with affected joint use in osteoarthritis and decreases with affected joint use in rheumatoid arthritis. Complaints of clients increase with increased humidity for both conditions. Fever only occurs in rheumatoid arthritis during exacerbations.

The clue is that osteo is an old, worn-out joint. The more these types of joints are used, the more pain increases. Remember that osteo is a short word; therefore, it is a local condition and may effect joints unilaterally. Rheumatoid is a long word; therefore it is a systemic condition that may more likely effect joints bilaterally. In systemic conditions fever may be present, as well as anemia, elevated ESR, and elevated rheumatoid factor levels.

7. Correct answer: 3

On a low purine diet, legumes such as beans and mushrooms are discouraged. Also to be avoided are organ meats, shellfish, and alcohol—including wine and beer.

The approach to correct answer selection is to "go with what you know." Eliminate chicken, which is usually not restricted. Associate a restriction from eating eggs with clients having a high serum cholesterol level. Cereal grains usually are not restricted except when glutens are a problem, as in celiac disease or gluten enteropathy. Select legumes—the only option left.

8. Correct answer: 2

Phantom pain results from impulses sent from severed nerves, and it eventually subsides. Do not confuse this

Careful reading will help you to eliminate the incorrect options. In option 1, "nerves stimulated" is not a condition of phantom limb pain.

Rationales	Test-Taking Tips

problem with phantom limb sensation, which usually is permanent. Eliminate option 4 because there is no such thing as bone nerves. Options 1 and 3 can be clustered to describe specific sites, which is too restrictive of an answer. Option 2 is the most comprehensive answer.

In option 3, "swelling around the nerves" resulting in pain is incorrect pathology. Swelling as in compartment syndrome stops nerve function, with findings of numbness and loss of feeling or movement in that area. Avoid reading too quickly and skimming over the word "bone" in option 4. You will be deciding between options 2 and 4, which are alike, except that option 2 gives more details.

9. Correct answer: 4

Vitamins A and D are required for appropriate calcium absorption. Vitamin C is important is healing and urine acidification. Vitamin K is important in the production of clotting factors in the liver. Vitamin K is absorbed from the large intestine. The B vitamins are essential mainly for nerve and RBC function and many other bodily functions, as well as being a source of energy for the body.

If you narrowed the options to 3 and 4, then think of the two categories of vitamins—the fat- and the water-soluble vitamins. Use your general knowledge that calcium needs vitamin D for absorption. Vitamin D is a fat-soluble vitamin. Select option 4, which has another fat-soluble vitamin, vitamin A. Recall that the fat-soluble vitamins are like a deck of cards without the C—— A, D, E, K—a dek.

10. Correct answer: 3

Cold therapy is used to decrease inflammation, swelling, and pain during an acute exacerbation. The other therapies are used after the acute phase.

Use common sense that in any acute inflammation, cold is used first for the initial 24 to 48 hours of the exacerbation.

12

The Integumentary System

FAST FACTS

1. The skin is frequently the first organ to show signs of illness by changes in color, texture, temperature, and hydration.
2. Normal skin turgor is when the skin returns to baseline within 3 seconds of being pinched up.
3. The usual sites to check for skin turgor are the hands, forearms, and forehead.
4. Skin elasticity decreases with age and dehydration.
5. The skin is extremely important in the development of self-esteem and self-image.
6. Skin color changes in the dark-skinned population are best observed in the sclera, conjunctiva, oral mucous membranes, tongue, lips, nail beds, palms of the hands, and soles of the feet.
7. In clients with a brown skin tone, pallor is seen as a yellow tint to the skin.
8. In clients with a dark or a very pale skin tone, cyanosis is seen as an ashen-gray color.
9. **Petechiae** indicate a low level of serum platelets, called *thrombocytopenia.*
10. *Melasma* or *chloasma* is a tan or brown pigmentation particularly on the forehead, cheeks, and nose. Also called the *mask of pregnancy,* this condition is commonly associated with pregnancy, oral contraceptive use, and hormone replacement therapy.
11. *Uremic frost* is a pale frostlike deposit of white crystals on the skin caused by kidney failure and uremia, with urea compounds and other metabolic waste products excreted through the skin.
12. The need for isolation of clients is determined by two essential criteria for skin disorders: the characteristics of the rash and the history of the skin problem.

CONTENT REVIEW

I. **The integumentary system is responsible for protecting the body from pathogen invasion, fluid loss, chemicals, and ultraviolet radiation. This system also regulates heat loss from the body, excretes wastes, and synthesizes vitamin D.**

II. **Structure and function**
   A. Largest organ of the body
   B. Two layers of the skin—the epidermis and dermis, joined together and situated above the subcutaneous layer
      1. Epidermis
         a. Comprised of the squamous epithelium, which is divided into four or five layers
         b. Has no blood supply of its own and few nerve endings in layer closest to the dermis
         c. Forms new cells in the layer closest to the dermis, which are pushed upward to the top layer of the epidermis
         d. Comprised of dead cells, the top layer is eventually rubbed off the skin surface
      2. Dermis
         a. Comprised of dense, fibrous, connective tissue
         b. Has a considerable blood supply and lymph vessels and a group of sensory receptors that supplies the dermis
      3. Accessory structures
         a. Hair—protects the scalp from heat and cold, and protects the nose and eyes from airborne particles
         b. Nails—found on tips of fingers and toes on the dorsal side; protect the digits and fingernails assist with picking up small objects
         c. Glands
            (1) Sebaceous glands—secrete **sebum** that keeps skin moist and supple
            (2) Ceruminous glands—secrete wax that lines the ear canal and prevent drying of the canal and eardrum
            (3) Sudoriferous glands—secrete sweat that assists in maintaining body temperature

III. **Targeted concerns**
   A. Pharmacology—priority drug classifications—commonly topical
      1. Antibacterial agents—alter the chemistry of the invading pathogen
         a. Expected effect—suppression of the pathogen
         b. Commonly given drugs
            (1) Bacitracin zinc (Altracin)
            (2) Polymyxin B sulfate (Polysporin ointment)

    c. Nursing considerations

       (1) Apply to skin as per physician's order

       (2) Assess skin for redness

       (3) Watch for systemic effects if there is a break in skin integrity

2. Antifungal agents—alter cell wall of fungus

    a. Expected effect—eradication of fungal infection

    b. Commonly given drugs

       (1) Nystatin (Mycostatin)

       (2) Clotrimazole (Lotrimin)

    c. Nursing considerations

       (1) Instruct client that a 2- to 3-week course, twice a day, must be completed for effective treatment

       (2) Assess skin carefully for irritation from medication

3. Antiparasitics/Pediculicides

    a. Expected effect—eradication of parasites such as lice

    b. Commonly given drugs

       (1) Lindane (Kwell)

       (2) Permethrin (Nix)

    c. Nursing considerations

       (1) Caution client to avoid getting medication into the eyes

       (2) Assess client for successful removal of parasites

       (3) Repeat treatment after 48 hours to eliminate eggs

4. **Antipruritics**—block histamine and serotonin effects

    a. Expected effect—soothes skin

    b. Commonly given drugs

       (1) Calamine lotion

       (2) Colloidal oatmeal (Aveeno Shower & Bath)

       (3) Aluminum acetate (Burow's Solution)

       (4) Boric acid wet dressing

    c. Nursing considerations

       (1) Assess for sensitivity to solution

       (2) Apply only as directed if the solution contains an anesthetic

5. Corticosteroids—reduce blood flow through their vasoconstrictive action

    a. Expected effects—decreased redness and itching

    b. Commonly given drugs

       (1) Hydrocortisone (Hytone)

       (2) Triamcinolone acetate (Kenalog)

       (3) Betamethasone dipropionate (Diprosone)

    c. Nursing considerations

       (1) Apply evenly to the skin

       (2) Assess use carefully in clients with systemic infections

       (3) Encourage short-term use only; long-term use tends to thin the skin and the client may encounter the systemic effects of corticosteroids

B. **Procedures**
   1. Skin biopsy—removal of a small piece of skin or a **lesion** to evaluate for cell composition
   2. Skin scrapings—skin is scraped for evaluation of cell composition; hair and nail scrapings also can be taken
   3. Swab samples—usually of lesions; evaluated for pathogen and effective antibiotic therapy
   4. Wood's light—high-pressure mercury light, also known as black light; used to visualize bacterial and fungal infections on the skin
   5. Allergy skin testing
      a. Patch testing—an allergen is placed on the skin and covered with a nonabsorbent patch; skin area is assessed in 48 to 72 hours for **erythema, vesicles,** and induration
      b. Intradermal skin testing—allergen is injected intradermally and a **wheal** is produced; inspected in 48 to 72 hours to evaluate for allergic reaction
      c. Scratch test—allergen is placed on an area of skin that has been scratched; if a wheal forms within 15 minutes the client is allergic to the allergen

C. **Psychosocial concerns**
   1. Anger—commonly associated with the client who has a skin disorder; a "Why me?" response
   2. Frustration—commonly seen in the client with a skin disorder as a result of many different types of treatments that may have varying degrees of success
   3. Anxiety—uncomfortable feeling associated with an unknown direct cause; common in the client with a skin disorder because of the fear of what will happen
   4. Embarrassment—common in skin disorders that are disfiguring or change the appearance, especially of the face
   5. Communication problems—written instructions for skin care medications and treatments must be given to the client because anxiety and embarrassment may prevent the client from listening to directions.

D. **Health history—question sequence**
   1. Please describe the problem you have been experiencing.
   2. When did you first notice your skin problem? How long have you had this skin problem?
   3. Have you noticed any new symptoms, such as nausea, vomiting, or diarrhea, that have begun since the skin problem started?
   4. Which symptoms are associated with the skin problem? Itching, pain, burning?
   5. Can you associate the problem with anything new you are eating, drinking, or using on your skin?
   6. Have you been using home remedies for this skin problem? Are they working? Have they made the problem worse?

7. Are you taking any prescription or over-the-counter medications for other problems?
8. Which medical problems and surgeries have you had in the past? Have you had chicken pox?
9. Do you have allergies to any foods or medications?
10. Do you have new stresses in your life?
11. Are you following a new diet?
12. Have you been traveling lately? Where?
13. Is there a family history of skin disorders?

E. **Physical examination—appropriate sequence**
   1. ABCs—vital signs
   2. Total-body skin evaluation—inspection, palpation, and olfactory evaluation
      a. Hair, scalp, and nails
      b. Mucous membranes
      c. Skin
         (1) Start at the head and work down to the feet
         (2) Evaluate for color, thickness, turgor, and temperature
         (3) Assess for **purpura** and **petechiae**
      d. General considerations
         (1) Frequently the skin is the first organ to show signs of an illness
         (2) With normal skin turgor, the skin returns to baseline within 3 seconds of being pinched up
         (3) Skin elasticity decreases with age
         (4) The skin is extremely important in the development of clients' self-esteem and self-image
         (5) Skin color changes in the dark-skinned population are best observed in the sclera, conjunctiva, oral mucous membranes, tongue, lips, nail beds, palms, and soles
         (6) In clients with a brown skin tone, pallor is seen as a yellow tint to the skin
         (7) In clients with a darker or very pale skin tone, pallor is seen as an ashen-gray color
   3. Complete assessment by evaluating the heart, lungs, and abdomen as discussed in previous chapters

IV. Pathophysiologic disorders
A. **Burn injury**
   1. Definition—dermal injury as a result of skin contact with fire, hot liquids, chemicals, radiation, or electricity
   2. Pathophysiology and etiology—burns cause destruction of the epidermis and sometimes the dermis
      a. Mechanism of injury
         (1) Thermal burns—flame or hot liquids
         (2) Chemical burns—chemicals must be diluted and removed from the skin area or burning will continue

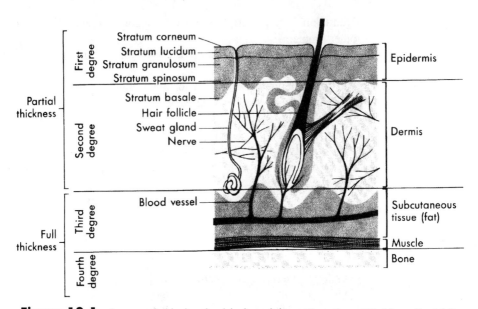

Figure 12-1 Layers of skin involved in burn injury. (From Beare PG, Myers JL: *Adult health nursing,* ed 3, St. Louis, 1998, Mosby.)

(3) Radiation burns—caused by a radioactive source, radiation therapy, and sunburn

(4) Electrical burns—create an entrance and exit wound and cause injury along the electrical path; often cause cardiac arrest. The exit wound typically has more severe damage than the entrance site.

b. Burn categorization (Figure 12-1)

(1) Superficial partial thickness (first degree)—sunburn; superficial epidermis; skin is pink, red, dry, painful, and slightly edematous

(2) Deep partial thickness (second degree)—epidermis and dermis are injured; skin is blistered and red, blanches appropriately, and is edematous and very painful

(3) Full thickness (third degree)—causes destruction of the epidermis and dermis; may include subcutaneous tissue as well. The wound is dry and leathery and may appear white or charred. The skin does not blanch. The wound itself may not be painful but the surrounding tissue is painful. Skin grafting to cover the area is required.

(4) Fourth degree—same as full thickness but also involves fat, fascia, tendons, and bones

c. Phases of burn care

(1) Emergent phase—first 48 hours after a burn; major concerns include shock, respiratory failure, and hyperkalemia

(a) Increased permeability of blood vessels allows the outpouring of plasma and colloids into the interstitial space, which accounts for the edema associated with burns

    (b) If the burn injury area is large enough, CO can be significantly decreased resulting from fluid shift into the interstitial space

  (2) Acute phase—from day 3 to several months. This phase ends when all burn wounds are covered with grafts or healed tissue. Major concerns include fluid overload, CHF with pulmonary edema, and hypokalemia.

  (3) Rehabilitation phase—from the end of the acute phase until several years later. Major concerns include an attempt to regain near normal function, scar revision, contracture control, and body-image adjustments.

  d. The pulmonary system—may be impaired if the client has inhaled noxious fumes or heat

    (1) Burn injury or inhalation injury to the airways

    (2) Airway obstruction from airway edema associated with the burn

    (3) Impaired inhalation if sufficient burn injury to the chest wall occurs such that inhalation is restricted by **eschar** or burned, noncompliant tissue

  e. The renal system—may be impaired by decreased circulating blood volume

    (1) Renal shutdown may result from decreased blood volume

    (2) Hematuria may be seen initially as a result of massive RBC destruction

  f. Burned body surface area (BBSA)

    (1) Rule of nines—rough estimate (Figure 12-2)

    (2) Lund and Browder burn assessment chart—accurate (Figure 12-3)

3. Incidence—in the United States, over 2 million persons per year seek medical assistance for burn injury; of these, over 60,000 are hospitalized. Burns are the third leading cause of accidental death.

4. Assessment

  a. Questions to ask

    (1) Are you having difficulty breathing?

    (2) Are you in pain? Can you show me where? On a scale of 0 to 10, how severe is your pain?

  b. Clinical manifestations—discussed in the section on pathophysiology

  c. Abnormal laboratory findings

    (1) Carboxyhemoglobin level—elevated, indicative of inhaled carbon monoxide and an inhalation injury

    (2) H&H—may be elevated as a result of hemoconcentration, especially in the first 24 to 48 hours

    (3) ABGs—hypoxemia and metabolic acidosis with an inhalation injury

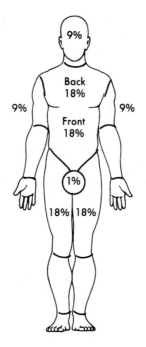

Figure 12-2 Rule of nines. (From Beare PG, Myers JL: *Adult health nursing,* ed 3, St. Louis, 1998, Mosby.)

       (4) Potassium—increased as a result of cell destruction, especially in the first 24 to 48 hours

       (5) Urinalysis—myoglobin, released from damaged muscles; damages the renal tubules

       (6) WBC—increased

       (7) Platelets—decreased

   d. Abnormal diagnostic test results

       (1) Bronchoscopy—evidence of heat injury to the airways with resultant edema

       (2) CXR—pulmonary edema as a response to an inhalation injury

5. Expected medical interventions

   a. Airway maintenance—with endotracheal tube if necessary

   b. Respiratory support—with a ventilator if necessary

   c. Fluid resuscitation—fluid administration is dictated by the percentage of burns and the client's weight; several formulas exist that establish calculations for fluid administration over the first 24 to 48 hours

   d. Treatment for burn wounds

       (1) Cleaning and debriding, removing blisters and tissue that is not adherent; hydrotherapy is most commonly used

AREA	AGE – YEARS					% 2°	% 3°	% TOTAL
	0 – 1	1 – 4	5 – 9	10 – 15	ADULT			
Head	19	17	13	10	7			
Neck	2	2	2	2	2			
Ant. Trunk	13	13	13	13	13			
Post. Trunk	13	13	13	13	13			
R. Buttock	2 1/2	2 1/2	2 1/2	2 1/2	2 1/2			
L. Buttock	2 1/2	2 1/2	2 1/2	2 1/2	2 1/2			
Genitalia	1	1	1	1	1			
R.U. Arm	4	4	4	4	4			
L.U. Arm	4	4	4	4	4			
R.L. Arm	3	3	3	3	3			
L.L. Arm	3	3	3	3	3			
R. Hand	2 1/2	2 1/2	2 1/2	2 1/2	2 1/2			
L. Hand	2 1/2	2 1/2	2 1/2	2 1/2	2 1/2			
R. Thigh	5 1/2	6 1/2	8 1/2	8 1/2	9 1/2			
L. Thigh	5 1/2	6 1/2	8 1/2	8 1/2	9 1/2			
R. Leg	5	5	5 1/2	6	7			
L. Leg	5	5	5 1/2	6	7			
R. Foot	3 1/2	3 1/2	3 1/2	3 1/2	3 1/2			
L. Foot	3 1/2	3 1/2	3 1/2	3 1/2	3 1/2			
					TOTAL			

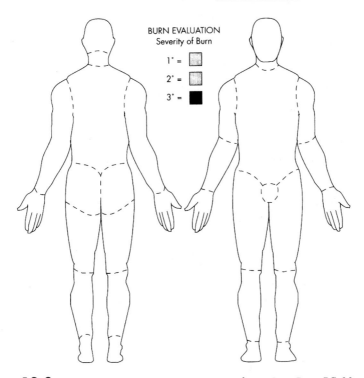

BURN EVALUATION
Severity of Burn

1° =

2° =

3° =

Figure 12-3 Lund and Browder burn assessment chart. (From Beare PG, Myers JL: *Adult health nursing,* ed 3, St. Louis, 1998, Mosby.)

(2) Applying topical antimicrobial agents such as mafenide (Sulfamylon) or silver sulfadiazine (Silvadene). Use caution because discoloration may occur to clothing or affected burned skin areas.

(3) Using a closed or open method of burn dressings, or using only antimicrobial cream and no dressing

(4) If using tape, use only paper tape because the skin in the surrounding areas is likely to tear

(5) Using biological dressings to cover wounds until grafts can be placed
   (a) Homografts come from another human
   (b) Xenografts come from an animal
   (c) Synthetic dressings also can be used

(6) Providing nutritional support—burn clients require a high calorie intake, as high as 5000 calories/day; nutritional supplements may be required

(7) Skin grafting—most common method is removing pieces of skin from unburned areas (donor sites), meshing the piece, and placing it over the burn area. Grafted tissue will grow over the cleaned burn site. Initially, the donor sites may be very painful.

6. Nursing diagnoses
   a. Fluid volume deficit related to increased capillary permeability and fluid shift into the interstitial space
   b. Risk for infection related to loss of the first line of pathogen defense, the skin
   c. Pain related to the tissue injury and exposed nerve endings
   d. Altered nutrition (less than body requirements) related to increased metabolic demands of the body

7. Client goals
   a. Client will have acceptable fluid volume as evidenced by balanced I&O and a CVP of 5 to 15 mm Hg
   b. Client will have no infection as evidenced by clean burn wounds and no exudate; client is afebrile
   c. Client will state pain has decreased from a 10 to a 2 on a scale of 0 to 10
   d. Client will maintain preburn weight or gain half a kilogram per week

8. Nursing interventions
   a. Emergent phase—first 24 to 48 hours
      (1) Airway and ventilation maintenance
      (2) Venous access for massive fluid resuscitation and pain medication
      (3) Pain management—usually morphine IV
      (4) Indwelling urinary catheter insertion to help monitor fluid volume and kidney function

      (5) Baseline and daily weights

      (6) Bathing, debriding, and dressing of wounds

      (7) Family counseling begins at this phase

  b. Acute phase—begins third day after injury until several months later

      (1) Strict aseptic technique for care of burn wounds; may require isolation if wounds are infected

      (2) Pain management by way of IV narcotics, relaxation techniques, imagery, and hypnosis

      (3) Management of severe pruritus, usually with diphenhydramine hydrochloride (Benadryl)

      (4) Splinting and positioning of the extremities to maintain function and prevent contractures

      (5) Active and passive range-of-motion exercises

      (6) Nutritional supplements to maintain high caloric needs; TPN is discouraged because of the risk of infection

      (7) Prevention of stress ulcers; check pH of stomach and administer antacids as needed

      (8) Wound care; continue cleaning and debriding wound dressings with antimicrobial agents

  c. Home care regarding client education—the rehabilitation phase

      (1) Bathe wounds daily

      (2) Clean wound three to four times daily

      (3) Dress wounds as per physician's instructions

      (4) Elevate limbs to prevent edema

      (5) Exercise the affected limbs four times daily

      (6) Resume normal activities

      (7) Keep physician appointments for follow-up

      (8) Maintain nutritional balance

9. Evaluation protocol

  a. How do I know that my interventions have been effective?

      (1) Vital signs are within 10% of baseline

      (2) Input of fluids equals output plus or minus 300 ml/day

      (3) Urine output is 30 ml/hr or over

      (4) Wounds are clean and not infected

      (5) Pain is manageable

  b. Which criteria will I use to change my interventions?

      (1) Pain is not managed

      (2) Vital signs are not within desired parameters

      (3) Urine output is under 30 ml/hr

      (4) Burn wound infection is apparent

  c. How will I know that my client teaching has been effective?

      (1) Burn wounds continue to heal without infection or severe contractures

      (2) Client reports increasing exercise daily

      (3) No evidence of edema in the extremities is seen

(4) Client is maintaining adequate nutrition

(5) Client returns to an acceptable normal daily routine

10. Older adult alert

a. The older adult client has a higher mortality rate in burn injury than in the younger adult

b. The older adult client is at a higher risk for burn injury as a result of decreased reaction time, decreased mobility, and poor peripheral sensation

c. The thinning of the older adult client's skin increases the severity of burn injury

B. Dermatitis

1. Definition—skin inflammation

2. Etiology—allergy, stress, or unknown

3. Pathophysiology—may be a response to something the skin has touched or an allergy to a known substance. The allergic response is a result of T-cell sensitivity.

4. Assessment

a. Questions to ask

(1) Which symptoms are you feeling at the site of discomfort? Pain, itching, and so forth?

(2) Are there blisters? Are they open?

(3) Is there swelling anywhere?

(4) Are you having fevers?

b. Clinical manifestations

(1) Pruritus, pain, and burning at site

(2) Reddened skin

(3) Vesicles at site

(4) Edema

(5) Fever

(6) Malaise

5. Expected medical interventions

a. Identify the cause of the disorder

b. Lubricate and hydrate the skin

c. Use topical corticosteroids

d. Administer antibiotics

e. Administer antihistamines

6. Nursing diagnoses

a. Pain related to skin response from causative agent

b. Impaired skin integrity related to the presence of an allergic agent and itching

c. Body-image disturbance related to the presence of skin lesions

7. Client goals

a. Client will state pain has decreased to a manageable level

b. Client will indicate skin is healing and lesions are decreasing in size

c. Client will state feeling comfortable with the condition of the skin

8. Nursing interventions—acute and home care
   a. Teach client to use soothing baths or solutions and how often
   b. Teach client how to use topical steroids as ordered by physician
   c. Teach client how to use systemic steroids if ordered: take with meals, do not miss a dose, and take exactly as directed
9. Evaluation protocol
   a. How will I know that my interventions have been effective?
      (1) Client exhibits stable fluid volume with a CVP of 5 to 15 cm H_2O
      (2) Client is afebrile and there is an absence of infection
      (3) Client verbalizes acceptable level of comfort
   b. Which criteria will I use to change my interventions?
      (1) Incorrect technique of time span for baths and solutions
      (2) Incorrect technique for topical steroids
      (3) Incorrect statements regarding the use of systemic corticosteroids
   c. How will I know that my client teaching has been effective?
      (1) Client reports the use of baths and solutions as per teaching
      (2) Client demonstrates how to apply topical steroids
      (3) Client states precautions associated with oral corticosteroids
10. Older adult alert
    a. There is a decrease in the number of sebaceous glands and as a result the amount of sebum. Thus, the skin of an older adult will be much drier and dermatitis will be much more difficult to control.
    b. Consider a drug interaction when observing dermatitis in the older adult taking multiple drugs
    c. The older adult client, in most instances, does not require a daily bath and should be discouraged from using hot water when bathing because of skin fragility

C. **Pressure ulcers**
   1. Definition—tissue destruction as a result of prolonged pressure on an area of the skin
   2. Etiology—commonly seen in areas of the body where bones are close to the skin. Pressure on those areas pushes the bone against the tissues underlying the skin, beginning the breakdown process.
   3. Pathophysiology—pressure on an area for a prolonged time causes decreased circulation, tissue hypoxia, and death. Shearing forces of the skin and moist skin, such as with incontinence, also contribute to ulcer formation.
   4. Assessment—see Table 12-1 for assessment factors associated with the stages of pressure ulcers
   5. Expected medical interventions
      a. Wound debridement to allow healing
      b. Skin grafting for more severe wounds
   6. Nursing diagnoses—impaired skin integrity related to prolonged pressure to an area

TABLE 13-1	Stages of Pressure Ulcers

Stage	Description	Goals of Intervention
I	A reddened area that returns to normal skin color after 15 to 20 min of pressure relief (e.g., turning to other side). The skin is intact, but the area may appear pale when pressure is initially removed.	To cover and protect
II	An area in which the top layer of skin is missing. The ulcer usually is shallow with a pinkish red base, and white or yellow eschar may be present.	To cover, protect, hydrate, insulate, and absorb
III	Deep ulcers that extend into the dermis and subcutaneous tissues. White, gray, or yellow eschar usually is present at the bottom of the ulcer, and the ulcer crater may have a lip or edge. Purulent drainage is common.	To cover, protect, hydrate, insulate, absorb, cleanse, prevent infection, and promote granulation
IV	Deep ulcers that extend into muscle and bone. These ulcers have a foul smell, and the eschar is brown or black. Purulent drainage is common.	To cover, protect, hydrate, insulate, absorb, cleanse, prevent infection, obliterate dead space, and promote granulation

From Beare PG and Myers JL: *Adult health nursing,* ed 3, St Louis, 1998, Mosby.

7. Client goal—client will have pressure ulcers with a clean base and granulation tissue at the edges
8. Nursing interventions
   a. Acute care
      (1) Wound management—follow physician's orders for wound packing with a wound cleansing agent
      (2) Stage I and II ulcers—nonabsorptive thin films and absorptive gel wafers work well
      (3) Prevention techniques
         (a) All pressure points must be visualized for breakdown at least every 2 hours
         (b) Clients who are unable to turn on their own must be turned every 2 hours
         (c) Client should be positioned in bed at a 30- to 45-degree angle, propped with pillows
         (d) Body parts should be supported with pillows
         (e) Air mattresses or air-fluidized beds are used to decrease skin pressure
         (f) Skin is cleaned immediately after incontinence or continent elimination

        (g) A turning sheet or a pad is used to pull up the client in bed and reduce skin sheering forces

        (h) Nutrition is assessed, and appropriate intake of vitamin C, zinc, and vitamin E are ensured

    b. Home care regarding client and caregiver education

      (1) Review with caregiver specific stress coping strategies used prior to hospitalization

      (2) Teach caregiver findings of healing, poor healing, and when to notify physician

9. Evaluation protocol

    a. How will I know that my interventions have been effective?

      (1) Skin will remain clean and dry, without breakdown or redness

      (2) Wounds will have a clean base and show signs of granulation tissue at the edges

      (3) Wounds will decrease in size at a slow, steady rate

    b. Which criteria will I use to change my interventions?

      (1) New skin breakdown is seen

      (2) Wound base is covered with purulent drainage or necrotic tissue

      (3) Wounds are enlarging, and no granulation tissue is seen

    c. How will I know my client and caregiver teaching has been effective?

      (1) Client and caregiver report diminished size or complete healing of pressure ulcers

      (2) Client and caregiver state complications to report to physician

10. Older adult alert—as a result of the fragile nature of their skin, older adult clients are at greater risk for pressure ulcers and must have optimal interventions to prevent them

D. Skin cancer

1. Definition—malignancy of the skin

    a. Basal cell carcinoma—most common type; originates in the basal cell layer of the epidermis

    b. Squamous cell carcinoma—fast growing; found in previously damaged skin

    c. Malignant melanoma—cancer of the melanocytes of the skin; rapidly spreading cancer

2. Etiology—most common cause is overexposure to the rays of the sun

3. Incidence—most commonly seen cancer in the United States

4. Assessment

    a. Questions to ask

      (1) How long have you had this growth?

      (2) How long has it had this appearance?

      (3) Are there other similar growths elsewhere on your body?

    b. Clinical manifestations

      (1) Basal cell carcinoma

        (a) Painless lesion

        (b) Usually found on areas of the body exposed to sun

(c) A well-defined, dome-shaped **papule** with a pearl-like appearance and raised edges

(d) Center may be ulcerated

(e) Rarely metastasizes but will invade and destroy the surrounding structures

(2) Squamous cell carcinoma

(a) Thick, rough, shallow lesions with raised edges

(b) May ulcerate in the center or have a gravel-type center

(c) Can metastasize rapidly, therefore diagnosis and treatment should be swift

(3) Malignant melanoma

(a) Superficial spreading melanoma—circle lesion with irregular borders

(b) Nodular melanoma—berrylike **nodules** with a blue-black color

(c) Lentigo melanoma—flat lesion that slowly turns black

(d) Acral-lentiginous melanoma—irregularly shaped, pigmented **macules**

  c. Abnormal diagnostic test results—incisional or total excisional biopsy positive for malignant cells

5. Expected medical interventions

  a. Excisional surgery; wide excision used for melanoma

  b. Cryosurgery—destroys tissue by freezing

  c. Mohs' chemosurgery—removes tumor layer by layer until all is gone

  d. Regional lymph node dissection—only used if nodes are involved and no metastases

  e. External beam radiation therapy—not for melanoma

  f. Topical chemotherapy

6. Nursing diagnoses

  a. Fear related to beliefs about the diagnosis of cancer and the possibility of death

  b. Anxiety related to unknown outcome and fear of disfigurement

  c. Body-image disturbance related to the possibility of disfigurement

7. Client goals

  a. Client will state fear has decreased as more information is available

  b. Client will state anxiety is decreased as more information is learned about the body changes that will occur

  c. Client will state feeling comfortable with body changes that will occur as discussed with physician

8. Nursing interventions

  a. Acute care

    (1) Help reduce anxiety before surgery by reiterating plans for surgery, grafting, or reconstruction

    (2) Care for large postoperative wounds by using drainage tubes and frequently changing large dressings

    (3) Keep the graft site immobile and clean if skin grafting is required

    (4) Provide analgesia for donor sites, which can be quite painful

  b. Home care regarding client education

    (1) Need to perform monthly skin self-assessment for new lesions and changes in existing lesions

    (2) Need for any suspicious lesions to be seen by physician as soon as possible

    (3) Need for family members to watch for skin changes

    (4) Client must use sunscreen with a sun block of over 20 when in the sun

9. Evaluation protocol

  a. How will I know that my interventions have been effective?

    (1) Does client feel less fearful after having discussed the surgical plans?

    (2) Does client feel less anxious about the changes that will occur with treatments?

  b. Which criteria will I use to change my interventions?

    (1) Increased fear

    (2) Increased anxiety or fear of changes in body image

  c. How will I know that my client teaching has been effective?

    (1) Client demonstrates appropriate technique for skin self-assessment

    (2) Client states having purchased and used appropriate sunscreen products

    (3) Client states the criteria for lesions that must be reported to the physician

10. Older adult alert

  a. Changes that occur in the skin of older adults make them especially prone to skin cancers

  b. Many skin growths in older adults are benign. Older adults should be encouraged to seek medical assistance, especially if the lesion is creating distress in relation to their appearance.

WEB Resources

http://www.ameriburn.org/home.htm
American Burn Association Home Page

REVIEW QUESTIONS

1. The client who has suffered burn injury may present with hematuria as a result of
   1. Massive tissue destruction from the burned skin
   2. Massive RBC destruction from the intensity of the heat
   3. Heat injury to the kidney
   4. Heat injury to the urinary tract

2. The dehydration seen in a client with large surface area burns is related to
   1. Large amounts of urine output
   2. Increased metabolic demands from the burns
   3. Fluid shift of plasma out of the vascular space and into the interstitial space
   4. Blood loss to the extravascular spaces

3. A client with partial-thickness burns over 30% of the body has entered the intermediate phase of care. In choosing a diet the nurse would suggest which items?
   1. Roast beef, green beans, rice, and orange juice
   2. Salad, rolls, butter, and soda
   3. Spaghetti, rolls, butter, and milk
   4. Chicken noodle soup, salad, and a milkshake

4. Burn wound coverage may take the form of only antimicrobial creams or antimicrobial creams and bulky dressings. The bulky dressings would afford the client
   1. A cleaner method for wound coverage
   2. Coverage of the wound and better pain relief
   3. Better control to minimize the bacteria
   4. Better control of fluid loss

5. An older adult client is admitted to the emergency department with second- and third-degree burns from accidentally setting the clothes on fire while making dinner. This client's burns may be more severe than a younger adult client because
   1. Older adult clients have less pain receptors so they do not pull away from fire as quickly as younger adults
   2. Older adult clients have slower reaction times. They are more prone to not move quickly from burning substances
   3. The skin of the older adult client tends to be thinner and there is less subcutaneous fat
   4. Younger adult clients wear more clothing in most cases than older adult clients

6. Teaching of clients with contact dermatitis who have been ordered a topical corticosteroid medication must include how to
   1. Apply the medication to the skin in a thick layer as needed
   2. Cover the site of ointment application with a clean dressing
   3. Apply in a thin layer only as often as ordered by the physician
   4. Have awareness that the skin does not absorb the steroid, so no systemic effects are expected

7. The best defense against decubitus ulcers is
   1. Positive pressure mattresses
   2. Airflow beds
   3. Elbow and heel protectors
   4. Identifying clients at risk with the incorporation of preventive measures for skin breakdown

8. An appropriate initial nursing diagnosis for any client with a new diagnosis of skin cancer would be
   1. Fear related to the diagnosis of cancer
   2. Anxiety related to an unknown outcome
   3. Body-image disturbance related to changes in appearance
   4. Personal identity disturbance related to the cancer therapy

9. Which of these findings is a potential problem with long-term cortisone cream use on the skin
   1. Tissue-paper-type skin
   2. Multiple superficial bruises over the area where the cream was applied
   3. Frequent colds or other upper respiratory infections
   4. Intermittent palpitations of the heart

10. A client enters the clinic with a poison ivy allergy. The prescribed medication is an antipruritic. The nurse should explain to the client that this type of medication works by which mechanism?
    1. It is a topical analgesic and numbs the skins surface
    2. The skin is soothed by the blockage of the local effects of histamine and serotonin
    3. The drug decreases redness and itching by eradication of the parasites of the ivy
    4. A suppression of the pathogen results in comfort to the client

ANSWERS, RATIONALES, AND TEST-TAKING TIPS

Rationales	Test-Taking Tips

1. Correct answer: 2

The heat from burn injuries causes lysis of body and vascular compartment cells. These lysed cells pass through the kidney, with damaging effects to the glomerular filtration or renal tubule system, and appear as hematuria or myoglobinuria. Option 1 is incorrect because of the words "from the skin." Myoglobin is found in the muscles, not the skin. For the same reason, options 3 and 4 are incorrect. Myoglobin is responsible for the red color of muscle and for its ability to store oxygen.

Think globally or in general with this question. Options 1, 3, and 4 refer to a specific site, that is, skin, kidney, and urinary tract, respectively. Option 2 is the only option that is of a general character. Select it.

2. Correct answer: 3

After burn injuries, the fluid shifts from the intravascular to the interstitial space. In burn injuries, plasma proteins are lost from destruction of the capillary membranes. Without normal levels of plasma proteins, fluid in the vascular space moves into the interstitial space. This situation also occurs with starvation—a lack of protein intake, liver failure—a lack of protein production, or the loss of protein through the kidneys such as occurs in nephrotic syndrome.

Think through each option. Option 1 is an incorrect statement. In burns with large surface areas, urine output decreases as the kidneys attempt to conserve fluid for its return into the vascular space. Option 2 is a correct statement. However, when associated with the question about dehydration and burns, it becomes incorrect. Option 4 is incorrect. In burns the blood loss is usually minimal and does not result in dehydration. The correct answer must then be option 3.

3. Correct answer: 1

A burn client needs high protein and vitamin C for the healing process. Proteins can be obtained from red meat,

This is a higher level question because the reader must think about what is needed in the healing process. Once you recall that both protein and

chicken, or pork. Of the given options, option 1 has the highest protein from roast beef and the highest vitamin C from the orange juice. All of the other meal choices have higher amounts of carbohydrates.

vitamin C are essential to healing, the options becomes easier to eliminate. If you only focused on the protein requirements for healing, you probably narrowed your choices to options 3 or 4 that have "milk" in them. At this point, the fact that both options contain "milk" should alert you that you might be missing something. Take the time to reread and rethink your answers using a more global view. Hopefully you will remember that vitamin C is also important in healing, and then select option 1.

4. Correct answer: 4

Fluid loss is controlled by pressure on the wound exerted from the dressing. The other options are incorrect statements about bulky dressings.

Use common sense in that dressings are typically used to collect drainage and minimize fluid loss. Think of the last time you used a Band-Aid or dressing for a cut or burn.

5. Correct answer: 3

As a normal course of aging the older client has less subcutaneous tissue and thin skin, which burn easily. Option 1 is a false statement about fewer pain receptors. The first part of option 2 is a correct statement. However, the second part is unrelated to the situation because the clothing caught on fire and it was not a matter of moving from the burning substance. Option 4 is false.

The question asks about the reason for a "more severe burn." The only option that most closely addresses the burn site is option 3. The others present information about reaction time or dress habits.

6. Correct answer: 3

A thin layer of corticosteroid ointment is to be applied at the ordered intervals. Option 1 is incorrect because of the word "thick." Typically, substances should be applied to the skin in a thin layer—thicker is not

If you have no idea of the correct answer, look at the options for clues. As you read think about other ointments you know about, such as nitroglycerine paste. Eliminate option 1, which contains the word "thick." Eliminate option 4 because

Rationales	Test-Taking Tips

better. A dressing would further irritate the area of the contact dermatitis. Option 4 is not true. Steroid creams may be absorbed systemically, especially if occlusive dressings are used over the site of application. Indications of systemic absorption are fever and inflammation. Therapy usually is limited to 14 days.

it its more likely that the medication in ointments or creams are absorbed systemically. To decide between options 2 and 3 select what you *know* sounds reasonable, which is option 3. If you are not sure about a clean dressing, then do not select it.

7. Correct answer: 4

Identifying the client at risk will allow the client to be treated before the decubitus begins to develop. The other options may be used to prevent or treat skin breakdown. However, the clue in the question is "best defense." This leads to selection of the most comprehensive option.

This question falls into the harder category because all of the answers are correct. You must select the priority. You can use the nursing process steps to figure out the best option. Assessment is the first step. Option 4 speaks to that. The interventions as stated in the other options are the later steps.

8. Correct answer: 1

Initially, fear is associated with a diagnosis of skin cancer. Option 2, anxiety, usually follows fear. Body-image disturbance would be a correct answer if the stem included information on the type of cancer and extensiveness of the action for removal, or if the client were in his or her teens or twenties because body image is a priority in these age groups. For option 4 to be correct more information would have to be given in the stem.

The clues in the question are "initial" and "new diagnosis." With a cancer diagnosis the first reaction of clients is fear, followed by anxiety as treatments are planned or implemented. Body image may not be of concern, especially in older clients who are more concerned about the maintenance of body functions or parts. In other words, this group says "Who cares how it looks as long as it can work."

9. Correct answer: 2

Cortisone cream applied to the skin continuously for 6 months or more interferes with platelet aggregation at the application

If you have no idea of the correct answer, categorize each option into a systemic or local effect. Option 1 is systemic in reference to the entire

site, resulting in superficial
bruises. Frequent colds and
URIs are systemic findings
with the use of oral or
injectable steroids rather than
local application. Cardiac
effects are secondary from the
retention of fluids, which is
likely with oral or injectable
but not local application of
steroids.

skin, not just at the application site.
Option 3 is systemic, with the
immune system a target of
suppression. Option 4 is systemic,
with changes in the heart function
resulting from electrical,
mechanical, hormonal, or blood
volume changes. Option 2 is the
only option specific to a problem at
the site of application.

10. Correct answer: 2

Antipruritic agents work to
minimize the effects of local
allergic skin reactions. These
agents do not numb the skin.
They may help decrease
redness and itching. Poison ivy
is not caused by parasites, as
stated in option 3. No pathogen
is associated with poison ivy
allergy.

Use the clues in the stem and the
options. The problem of an
"allergy" is a clue that histamine is
released. The clues in the options
are the terms: in option 1, "numbs";
in option 3, "parasites"; and in
option 4, "pathogen." Be aware that
the options have two parts. Careful
reading is needed to avoid selection
of an answer based on the first part
of the option, because you may
have read the second part of the
option too quickly. Option 3 is a
good example of where this may
have happened.

13

The Immune System

FAST FACTS

1. Inflammation characteristics are swelling, heat, redness, pain, and loss of function in the affected area.
2. Fever is the most commonly identified systemic indicator of inflammation: (1) temperature greater than 100.6° F, or 38.1° C; or (2) temperature greater than 99° F, or 37.2° C, in the elderly and immunocompromised clients.
3. Lymph nodes swell with infection from an increased activity to fight the infection.
4. The immune system is activated when a pathogen invades from any point of entry or when cells in the body are damaged.
5. The immune system is suppressed when the body experiences a stress response from either physical or mental stressors.
6. **Antigens** are enemies of the body
7. **Antibodies,** immunoglobulins, are friends of the body for self-defense against antigens.
8. **Complement** is a group of plasma proteins responsible for enhancement of the initial steps of the inflammatory response and mediation of the antigen-antibody response.

CONTENT REVIEW

I. Definition—the immune system is responsible for protecting the body from the invasion of organisms, for the provision of homeostasis by removing defective cells, and to monitor the body for abnormal cell growth. The immune system also is activated when cells are damaged. Extremely important to the body is the ability of the immune system to identify self and "nonself."

II. Structure and function

A. **Bone marrow—produces competent WBCs**

B. **WBCs—inadequate mature numbers are responsible for attacking any "nonself" antigen. An elevated level of WBC indicates infection, and how high the WBC count rises is an indication of the severity of the infection** (Box 13-1).

   1. WBC count over 10,000 is *leukocytosis,* which indicates an infection

   2. WBC count under 5000 is *leukopenia,* which indicates minimal defense against foreign substances

C. **Lymphoid tissue—responsible for maturation and differentiation of lymphocytes; also responsible for storing small collections of WBCs to interact with blood and lymph and quickly identify "nonself antigens"**

D. **Chemical mediators—histamine, kinins, complement, leukotrienes, prostaglandins, and interleukin-1, which is necessary to stimulate and enhance the activity of WBCs**

Box 13-1
Categories of White Blood Cells

Myeloid Stem Cells Produce
Granulocytes

Neutrophils

Mast cells (segmented or segs; mature cells)—elevated in pernicious anemia and liver disease

Basophis (immature cells)—elevated in bacterial infections, allergic reactions, and parasitic infections such as malaria

Eosinophils (mature cells)—elevated in allergic reactions and parasitic infections; do not respond to elevated levels with bacteria and viruses

Monocytes

Macrophages

Lymphoid Stem Cells Produce
T Lymphocytes

   Helper T_4 cells
   Suppressor T_8 cells
   Cytotoxic T cells

B Lymphocytes

   Plasma cells
   Memory cells

Natural killer cells

Modified from Beare PG and Myers JL: *Adult health nursing,* ed 3, St Louis, 1998, Mosby.

E. **Immunity—two types**

1. Innate (natural)—first defense; physical barriers, chemicals, and cellular defenses prevent invading pathogens from becoming rooted and multiplying

2. Acquired—action of B and **T lymphocytes** against invading pathogen using memorized reactions to known pathogens and memorizing new pathogens; can be acquired actively or passively

   a. Active acquired—introducing an antigen into the body either intentionally or through exposure to the pathogen. The initial antigen elicits a response, creating a memorized response to this antigen if it is again introduced into the body. Examples include any of the vaccinations, hepatitis B vaccine, and tetanus toxoid.

   b. Passive acquired—antibodies passed from one person to another. Transfer of antibodies from mother to fetus is a good example. Immunity is short-lived because no memory is produced. Immunity lasts only as long as the antibodies are active. Passive immunity in infants lasts 3 to 6 months. Examples of injectable forms that have antibody action for 2 to 3 weeks are the tetanus immune serum globulin given to victims of multiple trauma and Hyperab, a rabies immune serum globulin.

III. **Targeted concerns**

A. **Pharmacology—priority drug classifications**

1. Immunosuppressants—block production of WBCs by the bone marrow

   a. Expected effect—inhibition of immune response

   b. Commonly given drugs

      (1) Azathioprine (Imuran)

      (2) Cyclosporin (Sandimmune)

      (3) Lymphocyte immune globulin (Atgam)

      (4) Muromonab-CD3 (Orthoclone OKT3)

   c. Nursing considerations

      (1) Monitor client carefully for signs of infection, which will be masked by medication; temperatures of 99° F may be significant

      (2) Observe for anaphylaxis

2. Anti-inflammatory agents—block the release of leukotrienes and prostaglandins

   a. Expected effect—decreased inflammatory response

   b. Commonly given drugs

      (1) Prednisone (Deltasone)

      (2) Hydrocortisone sodium succinate (Solu-Cortef)

      (3) Methylprednisolone (Medrol)

   c. Nursing considerations

      (1) Give medication with food to prevent GI distress

      (2) Never miss a dose; missing one dose may result in adrenal crisis, especially with prolonged use

(3) Wean off medication because the risk of adrenal crisis exists if stopped abruptly

(4) Give IV push slowly to prevent decreased BP and HR

3. Drugs to treat AIDS—prevent replication of the virus

a. Expected effect—helps stop the progression of AIDS

b. Commonly given classifications and drugs (current therapy recommendations suggest a combination of these drugs)

(1) Nucleoside reverse transcriptase inhibitors (NRTIs)

(a) Zidovudine (AZT, Retrovir)

(b) Didanosine (Videx)

(2) Non-nucleoside reverse transcriptase inibitors (NNRTIs)

(a) Nevirapine (Viramune)

(b) Delavirdine (Rescriptor)

(i) Protease inhibitors (PIs)

(c) Saquinavir (Fortovase)

(d) Indinavir (Crixivan)

c. Nursing considerations

(1) Client must awaken at night to take the medication

(2) Client must avoid crowds and people with infections

(3) Client must be instructed that these medications do not eliminate the risk of transmitting HIV

(4) Liver enzyme levels must be monitored with the use of many of these preparations

B. Procedures

1. CBC—provides information about H&H as well as the specific value for various leukocytes

2. Immunodiffusion—detects antigen-antibody reactions

3. Electrophoretic assays—measure serum immunoglobulins such as IgG and IgA

4. Enzyme-linked immunosorbent assay (ELISA)—very sensitive in detecting antigens and antibodies

5. RIA—detects small amounts of antigens, antibodies, and antigen-antibody complexes

6. Lymphocyte assays—determine absolute numbers of lymphocytes

7. T-cell and B-cell surface markers—assist in diagnosing various immune disorders

8. Bone marrow aspiration and biopsy—evaluation of cellular components of blood

9. Lymph node biopsy—assesses immunologic function and evaluates for malignancy of the lymph system

C. Psychosocial concerns

1. Stresses—in relation to illness or to lifestyle. Overall stress can suppress the immune response and increase the glucose load.

2. Anxiety—uncomfortable feeling associated with an unknown cause. Clients may be unable to discuss their feelings but are aware they are uneasy about what is going to happen.

3. Fear—uncomfortable feeling associated with real danger. Clients' fear is of death.

4. Social isolation—may be a result of the illness itself or in response to fear of contracting illness as a result of immunosuppression

5. Life changes—changes in lifestyle and activities of daily living must be made in response to the illness; career changes may be needed, and the ability to work may be affected.

6. Anger—clients may be angry about suffering from these types of illnesses

D. Health history—question sequence

1. Which problems have you been experiencing?
2. Have you noticed frequent infections lately?
3. Have you ever had any surgery or trauma to your extremities?
4. Have you ever been treated for cancer? Which type?
5. Is your physician treating you for any illnesses at present?
6. Do you have any food or drug allergies?
7. Have you experienced fatigue?
8. Have you noticed that you have had an elevated temperature frequently?
9. Do you ever wake up at night covered with sweat?
10. Have you noticed pain or swelling in your neck, underarms, or groin?
11. Have you noticed a lack of appetite?

E. Physical examination—appropriate sequence

1. ABCs—vital signs
2. Inspect areas over lymph node chain—compare sides (see Figure 4-1, p. 123)
3. Inspect skin for lesions, color, rashes, temperature, and moisture
4. Inspect hair for color, texture, and distribution
5. Palpate superficial lymph nodes for size, shape, and tenderness
   a. Head and neck nodes
   b. Supraclavicular nodes
   c. Axillary nodes
   d. Upper extremity nodes
   e. Lower extremity nodes
6. Inspect breathing pattern, effort, and rate
7. Palpate chest for expansion and chest wall pain when pressure is applied
8. Auscultate breath sounds
9. Auscultate cardiac rate and rhythm for abnormal sounds
10. Inspect the abdomen for lesions, nodules, or scars
11. Auscultate for bowel sounds
12. Percuss the abdomen for abnormal dullness
13. Inspect muscle areas for swelling, and palpate for tenderness
14. Assess client for gait, muscle strength, coordination, and range of motion

IV. Pathophysiologic disorders

A. Acquired *immunodeficiency* syndrome (AIDS)

1. Definition—a disorder associated with a deficiency of cell-mediated immunity characterized by development of opportunistic infections and cancers
2. Pathophysiology
   a. HIV invades the host cell, T_4, and uses the genetic material of the cell to replicate itself
   b. The genetic code of HIV, carried on RNA instead of DNA, is transferred to the host's DNA. More DNA will then be made with the genetic code of the HIV.
   c. The HIV virus can remain dormant for an unknown period of time (Figure 13-1). HIV will be stimulated to reproduce once the host T_4 cell has been stimulated to function immunologically.
   d. More and more T_4 cells are infected, and the total number is decreased
   e. The T_8 cells, or suppressor cells, now have a higher number than the T_4, or helper cells. The suppressor cells dominate in immunologic action.
   f. The client becomes immunosuppressed
   g. Pathogens and tumors are allowed to grow in the body unchecked, allowing opportunistic infections and cancers to become prominent
   h. HIV is found in all body fluids, but only semen, blood, vaginal secretions, and breast milk have been implicated in transmission

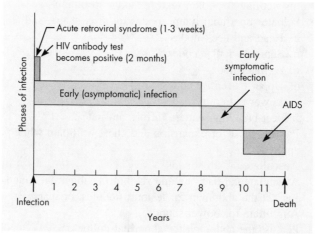

Figure 13-1 Timeline for the spectrum of HIV infection. The timeline represents the course of the illness from the time of infection to clinical manifestations of the disease. (From Lewis SM, Heitkemper MM, Dirksen SR: *Medical-surgical nursing: assessment and management of clinical problems,* ed 5, St. Louis, 2000, Mosby.)

3. Etiology—HIV, a retrovirus responsible for destruction of T and CD4 lymphocytes
4. Incidence—Most clients with HIV in the adult population are homosexual or bisexual males or clients who have abused IV drugs. The remaining population is comprised of clients who have contracted the virus through blood products, perinatally from their mother, or from infected sexual partners. The incidence in the heterosexual population is increasing.
5. Assessment
   a. Questions to ask
      (1) Have you noticed swelling in your neck or groin?
      (2) Have you noticed bruising or purple areas on your skin?
      (3) Have you noticed a white buildup on your tongue?
      (4) Do you feel tired often?
      (5) Have you been losing weight?
      (6) Do you wake up sweating at night?
      (7) Do you suffer from frequent diarrhea?
   b. Clinical manifestations
      (1) HIV disease (previously known as AIDS-related complex)
         (a) Generalized lymphadenopathy
         (b) Immune thrombocytopenia purpura
         (c) Hairy leukoplakia—raised white plaque on the tongue
      (2) AIDS
         (a) Severe fatigue
         (b) Malaise and weakness
         (c) Chronic weight loss
         (d) Chronic lymphadenopathy
         (e) Fevers
         (f) Joint pain
         (g) Night sweats
         (h) Chronic diarrhea
   c. Abnormal laboratory findings
      (1) Enzyme linked immunosorbent assay (ELISA)—positive for antibodies against AIDS; usually repeated
      (2) Western blot test—positive for antibodies against AIDS; used to confirm ELISA
      (3) P24 antigen—positive for circulating antigen
      (4) CBC and differential—WBC, lymphocytes, neutrophils, platelets, RBC, and H&H are all decreased
      (5) HIV culture—live HIV
      (6) T-cell studies—analyze numbers and functions of the specific T cells; shows decreased T_4 and increased T_8 cells
   d. Abnormal diagnostic tests—used primarily to confirm the presence of opportunistic infections or cancers
      (1) Bronchoscopy—confirms the cause of pneumonia
      (2) Pulmonary function tests (PFT)—used to assist detection of pneumonia

      (3) Electroencephalography (EEG)—shows slowed activity as a result of encephalopathy

      (4) CT and MRI scans—used to evaluate a fever of unknown origin

6. Expected medical interventions

  a. The goal of medical management is to quickly make a diagnosis and begin a treatment regimen, which is the best method known to date to assist in the repair of the immune system. It is also important to quickly diagnose and treat opportunistic infections and cancers that occur.

  b. Common opportunistic infections and treatments

      (1) *Pneumocystis carinii* pneumonia (PCP)—sulfamethoxazole (Bactrim), pentamidine isethionate 300 mg (Pentam 300)

      (2) Toxoplasmosis—sulfadoxine and pyrimethamine (Fansidar), clindamycin (Cleocin)

      (3) *Candida albicans* infection—nystatin (Mycostatin), ketoconazole (Nizoral)

      (4) Histoplasmosis—Amphotericin B, ketoconazole (Nizoral)

      (5) Tuberculosis—three-drug therapy: isoniazid (INH), ethambutol hydrochloride, and rifampin

      (6) Cytomegalovirus (CMV) infection—ganciclovir sodium (Cytovene)

      (7) Herpes simplex infection—acyclovir (Zovirax)

  c. Common opportunistic malignancies

      (1) Kaposi's sarcoma

      (2) Lymphoma

      (3) Non-Hodgkin's lymphoma

7. Nursing diagnoses

  a. Impaired gas exchange related to increased alveolar secretions secondary to pneumonia

  b. Diarrhea related to inflammation of the intestinal tract secondary to viral infection

  c. Altered nutrition (less than body requirements) related to GI inflammation secondary to viral infection

  d. Fluid volume deficit related to anorexia, nausea, and diarrhea

  e. Altered oral mucous membranes related to oral infection

  f. Fatigue related to altered nutrition and a wasting disorder

8. Client goals

  a. Client will exhibit a PaO_2 and $PaCO_2$ within normal baseline

  b. Client will exhibit decreased episodes of diarrhea (two less per day) with a more solid consistency to the stool

  c. Client will demonstrate a stable weight with no further weight loss

  d. Client will demonstrate a balanced I&O within 300 ml/day, with no further weight loss

  e. Client will state that mucosa of the mouth are less painful

  f. Client will state feeling less fatigued

9. Nursing interventions
   a. Acute care
      (1) Use standard precautions as with all clients—assume all clients are infected; follow precautions
         (a) Use barrier precautions to protect skin and mucous membranes from exposure to blood or body fluids: gloves, eyewear, gowns, and masks
         (b) Wash hands before and after caring for every client, after removing gloves, and immediately after unexpected contact with body fluids

   > ⚠️ **Warning!**
   >
   > Do not recap needles. Place all sharp items in a sharps container for disposal.

         (c) Refrain from direct client care if you have any lesions or open areas on the skin
      (2) Balance client activity and rest to decrease fatigue
      (3) Place client in position of comfort and for best respiratory effort
      (4) Monitor for symptoms of respiratory illness
      (5) Provide antidiarrheal agents as necessary to maintain appropriate fluid balance
      (6) If client is tolerating oral intake, provide diet that will improve nutritional status
      (7) If not tolerating oral intake, anticipate use of TPN
      (8) Provide viscous lidocaine or similar agent to provide oral pain relief before meals
   b. Home care regarding client education
      (1) The syndrome and which complications clients should monitor
      (2) Medications and possible side effects to report to physician
      (3) Symptoms of infection and to seek medical care immediately
      (4) Knowledge to avoid people with contagious illnesses because the client may easily contract them
      (5) Instructions on how to avoid transmission of the HIV infection
      (6) The need to avoid sharing toilet articles
      (7) Information that client must not donate blood or organs
      (8) The need to inform all appropriate health care personnel of their diseases
      (9) The need to inform sexual partners of HIV infection
      (10) Hospice intervention if necessary
10. Evaluation protocol
    a. How do I know that my interventions have been effective?
       (1) New infectious processes have been averted or decreased in intensity

      (2) Respiratory status is stable, with no increase or decrease of RR over 10% of baseline; no fluid-mucus accumulation in the lungs

      (3) Episodes of diarrhea have decreased

      (4) Weight loss has stopped, or client is gaining weight slowly

      (5) Oral mucosa are showing signs of healing

      (6) Level of fatigue has decreased

  b. Which criteria will I use to change my interventions?

      (1) New infections are apparent, or present infections are becoming more severe

      (2) Respiratory function is more impaired; client has dyspnea at rest

      (3) More episodes of diarrhea are evident

      (4) Client is still losing weight steadily, despite increased nutritional efforts

      (5) Oral pain is worse, making eating even more difficult

      (6) Client indicates fatigue is worse

  c. How will I know that my client teaching has been effective?

      (1) Client indicates having informed sexual partner of illness

      (2) Client indicates having informed physicians, dentist, and other health care workers of illness

      (3) Client states how to avoid transmission of the illness to others

      (4) Client states knowing how to take medications and for which side effects to monitor

      (5) Client states symptoms to watch for regarding new infections and how to avoid them

      (6) Client states benefits of hospice and how to obtain the help when necessary

  11. Older adult alert—this is a disorder to date found primarily in the younger adult. It is felt that if identified in the older adult client as a result of the normal changes of the aging, client illness would progress rapidly.

B. Rheumatoid arthritis

  1. Definition—chronic systemic inflammatory disorder of the connective tissue; exacerbations and remissions are characteristic

  2. Pathophysiology—synovial lining of the joint becomes inflamed, granulation tissue forms, cartilage is destroyed, and fibrous tissue is left in place of cartilage

  3. Etiology—unknown; theories suggest autoimmune disorder and infectious agents

  4. Incidence—more common in the female population

  5. Assessment

    a. Ask the following questions

      (1) When does your pain occur?

      (2) Do you have swelling of your joints?

        (3) Does the weather make your pain worse?

        (4) What else makes your pain worse?

        (5) What lessens your pain?

  b. Clinical manifestations

        (1) Joint pain, warmth, and edema

        (2) Joint motion limitation

        (3) Morning stiffness and fatigue

        (4) Proximal joints of hands and feet most commonly affected

        (5) Nodules over bony prominences

        (6) Hand deformity

        (7) Systemic findings of increased WBC and increased temperature

        (8) Anorexia and weight loss

  c. Abnormal laboratory findings

        (1) Rheumatoid factor—positive

        (2) ESR—elevated

        (3) H&H—anemia

        (4) WBC—may be elevated

  d. Abnormal diagnostic test results

        (1) Joint aspiration—increased synovial fluid volume is cloudy

        (2) Joint x-ray films—eroded joint surfaces, joint space narrowing, and unstable joint

6. Expected medical interventions

  a. Rest, especially during exacerbations; possibly splints on effected joints during severe pain

  b. Passive and active range-of-motion exercises

  c. Cold therapy during acute exacerbations, and moist heat for stiffened joints

  d. Aspirin in high doses

  e. Gold salts

  f. Corticosteroids

  g. Methotrexate

7. Nursing diagnosis

  a. Acute pain related to inflamed joint spaces

  b. Impaired physical mobility related to joint pain

  c. Fatigue related to prolonged immobility and increased metabolic demands

8. Client goals

  a. Client will state pain has decreased or has been relieved

  b. Client will demonstrate daily ability to perform active or passive range-of-motion exercise on all joints

  c. Client will state fatigue has decreased

9. Nursing interventions

  a. Acute care—postoperative joint replacement—care will be the same as for the client after hip surgery (see Chapter 11, pp. 376-379)

    b. Home care regarding client education

        (1) Instruction on when and how to take medications and the side effects to report

        (2) Maintenance of a minimal activity level without overexertion

        (3) Application of heat or cold for analgesia

        (4) Exercise of joints to the point of pain but not past the point of pain

        (5) Splint affected joints during acute exacerbations

        (6) Control weight to minimize stress on weight-bearing joints

  10. Evaluation protocol (Refer to Chapter 11, p. 382 for additional protocol)

    a. How will I know that my client teaching has been effective?

        (1) Client states performing range-of-motion exercises at least three times a day

        (2) Client demonstrates correct medication regimen and is aware of the side effects to relate to physician

        (3) Client loses weight to within 4% to 8% of ideal body weight

        (4) Client demonstrates correct procedure for moist heat application

  11. Older adult alert—this is a disorder of the older adult and should be evaluated for when assessing older adult clients

C. Lupus erythematosus

  1. Definition—a widespread connective tissue disorder

  2. Pathophysiology—widespread destruction of collagen in the body marked by exacerbations and remissions, eventually leading to organ destruction and death

  3. Etiology—unknown; theorized as an autoimmune disorder

  4. Incidence—more common in females and young adults or adolescents

  5. Assessment

    a. Questions to ask

        (1) Do you burn frequently or easily when exposed to the sun?

        (2) Have you noticed a rash across the bridge of your nose?

        (3) Have you noticed an increase in hair loss?

        (4) Have you noticed any sustained fatigue?

    b. Clinical manifestations

        (1) Symptoms that mimic arthritis

        (2) Sun sensitivity

        (3) "Butterfly rash" over the bridge of the nose

        (4) Sustained fatigue

        (5) Alopecia

        (6) Symptoms indicative of organ involvement such as renal impairment and cardiac dysrhythmias

        (7) Inflammation of skeletal muscles—polymyositis

    c. Abnormal laboratory findings

        (1) CBC—anemia

        (2) Lupus erythematosus prep—positive

        (3) Antinuclear antibody titer—positive

6. Expected medical interventions
   a. Plasmapheresis *(plasma exchange)* for exacerbations or preventive therapy
   b. High-dose steroids for exacerbations
   c. NSAID or aspirin in high doses for pain
7. Nursing diagnoses
   a. Pain related to inflammatory changes in the joint spaces
   b. Body-image disturbance related to butterfly rash
   c. Impaired mobility related to painful joints
8. Client goals
   a. Client will state pain is decreased or relieved
   b. Client will state feeling comfortable with facial or hair changes that have occurred
   c. Client will demonstrate range-of-motion exercises and less fatigue when participating in the activities of daily living
9. Nursing interventions
   a. Acute care—exacerbations
      (1) Provide support before, during, and after plasmapheresis
      (2) Treat pain
      (3) Administer steroids as per order
      (4) Teach client safe administration of steroids
   b. Home care regarding client education on remission
      (1) Teach client safe administration of high doses of NSAIDs or aspirin and findings to report to physician
      (2) Encourage client to stay out of the sun and use a sun block with a high number, >15, when in the sun
10. Evaluation protocol
    a. How will I know that my interventions have been effective?
       (1) Client states pain has decreased
       (2) Client states desired effects from medication or plasmapheresis
    b. Which criteria will I use to change my interventions?
       (1) Client states pain is increased or unrelieved
       (2) Client states plans to take steroids before or between meals
       (3) Client reports severe fatigue that interferes with activities of daily living or work
    c. How will I know that my client teaching has been effective?
       (1) Client indicates that an NSAID or aspirin will be taken with food or milk
       (2) Client states plan to avoid being in sun or to wear a sun block >15 when in the sun
11. Older adult alert—this disorder is uncommon in older adults

WEB Resources

http://hivinsite.ucsf.edu/
   HIV

REVIEW QUESTIONS

1. Maintenance of the nutritional status of a client with AIDS is best accomplished by
   1. Providing for pain relief of mouth lesions, a diet high in calories and protein, and appealing food
   2. Starting TPN when clients are unable to take in oral substances
   3. Initiating enteral feedings with high-calorie, high-protein feedings
   4. Offering foods that the client finds appealing and small frequent meals

2. Client teaching about AZT must include that
   1. The medication will arrest the HIV virus
   2. The client must wake up at night to take the medication
   3. Medication dosages can be spread across the time the client is awake
   4. The medication kills the HIV virus

3. A common manifestation the nurse would expect to see in the client with AIDS is
   1. Constipation
   2. High fevers
   3. Night sweats
   4. Painful lymph nodes

4. During meals a nursing assistant must help a client who has HIV infection. Universal precautions that the nurse instructs the nursing assistant to take would consist of
   1. No protective devices needed
   2. Gloves
   3. Gown
   4. Mask

5. To plan care for a client with an acute exacerbation of lupus erythematosus, the nurse begins teaching the client about the appropriate administration of prednisone. The teaching must include that this medication
   1. Must be taken on an empty stomach for appropriate absorption
   2. Should be taken for only 10 days and then stopped
   3. Must be taken with food or antacids
   4. Must be taken with large amounts of water

6. The client with an acute exacerbation of rheumatoid arthritis must have which of these interventions placed on the plan of care?
   1. Application of warm moist compresses to the inflamed joints
   2. Institute range-of-motion exercises at least four times a day
   3. Splint affected joints after range-of-motion exercises done at least once a day
   4. After a PRN medication is given, exercise affected joints to just past the point of pain

7. A client who slobbers, has inadequate chewing from poor dentition, and who has HIV infection requires assistance during meals. Universal precautions that the nurse should observe the nursing assistant using at meal times with this client would consist of

1. No precautions needed
2. Gloves
3. Gown
4. Mask

8. Which laboratory test result is expected if the client has suspected rheumatoid arthritis?

1. Antibody titers are negative
2. Elevated ESR
3. Severely elevated WBC
4. An abnormal hemoglobin, with a normal hematocrit

9. A client has been given an IV dose of hydrocortisone (Solu-Cortef) and exhibits a significant decrease in BP and increase in HR. These findings indicate which of these items?

1. An allergic reaction to the medication
2. An expected untoward effect when the drug is given too quickly by the IV route
3. An expected untoward effect when the drug is given too slowly by the IV route
4. An indication that the dosage was too high for the client

10. A client is brought to the emergency center with suspected bites from a rabid raccoon. After confirmation that the raccoon was indeed rabid, the nurse anticipates administration of the drug Hyperab. To teach this client, the nurse must have an understanding that

1. The use of this medication falls into the category of active acquired immunity
2. The drug is an immune serum globulin, which has an antibody action for a few weeks
3. The intent is to establish passive acquired immunity with a half-life of 72 hours
4. Repeat injections are required bimonthly for at least 1 year

ANSWERS, RATIONALES, AND TEST-TAKING TIPS

Rationales	Test-Taking Tips

1. Correct answer: 1

Mouth ulcer pain must be attended to before clients can ingest foods with comfort. Diet should be high in protein and calories, and should include foods the client likes. Options 2 and 3 are correct statements but do not best answer the question about maintenance of nutritional status. Both options introduce the assumption that the client cannot take food by mouth, which is new information. The stem gives no information to even consider that enteral or parenteral routes are needed. Option 4 is correct information. When you narrow the options to 1 and 4, recognize that option 4 is included in option 1. Therefore, option 1 is the best answer.

Note that each option is lengthy. To clarify the information as you read, write down a few notes on paper for each option.
Option 1—mouth care, high prot. & cal., foods liked.
Option 2—IV nutrition if not PO.
Option 3—food via tubes, high prot. & cal.
Option 4—foods liked, sm. freq.
Doing so makes it clearer and easier to make a decision when you see the information with fewer words.

2. Correct answer: 2

The client must awaken at night to take the required dose of AZT. Options 1 and 4 are incorrect information. In bacterial and viral infections around-the-clock medication results in better effects. Thus, even though option 3 sounds good, it is not the best choice.

If you narrowed the options to 2 or 3, you have done well. Then associate the fact that antiviral agents are ideally given around the clock. Giving this medication only when the client is awake may allow for 8 to 10 hours without the medication.

3. Correct answer: 3

Night sweats are a common manifestation in AIDS. Note that night sweats also are associated with four other conditions: TB, Hodgkin's disease, hypoglycemic

Keep in mind the problem, an immune deficiency. Eliminate option 1, constipation, which has little to do with the immune system. Eliminate options 2 and 4 because high fevers and painful lymph nodes are

episodes, and menopause. The
other options are incorrect.
Typically diarrhea, *low-grade*
fevers, and *painless* enlarged
lymph nodes are seen.

unlikely in immune deficiency. The
immune system must be functioning
normally to see these findings.

4. Correct answer: 1

Unless contact with bodily fluids is
a concern, protective devices are
not necessary. When one feeds a
client and no extenuating
condition exists, there usually is
no contact with body fluids. If
the option had included that the
client has excessive drooling or
a condition exists in which the
spitting of food occurs, then a
mask, gown, and gloves may be
required. Be sure to read
carefully if the question is in
general or if a specific condition
exists.

Be cautious when you think you know
that the first option is the correct
answer because then you may not
bother to read the other options, or
read them too quickly. This bad
habit often results in wrong
answers, and you may fail the test.
To correct this problem, read the
answers in reverse order, that is, by
starting with option 4.

5. Correct answer: 3

Corticosteroids cause increased
stomach acid. They must be
taken with food or antacids, are
not to be stopped abruptly, and
have no association with water
intake. In fact, water intake
may be monitored because
steroids cause water and
sodium retention.

Approach medication questions with
the thought that all medications
need to be taken with food except
tetracycline, Carafate, and some
sulfonamides. Sulfonamides require
a full glass of water with each dose
to prevent the formation of sulfate
crystals in the urinary tract.

6. Correct answer: 3

Affected joints in the acute
exacerbation phase should be
splinted to prevent
contractures. Range-of-motion
exercises for all joints must be
done at least once a day to
keep them flexible. Applying
cold to acute inflammation
decreases swelling and has an
anesthetic effect. Application of
heat is usually withheld for 48

Careful reading is needed to make this
question easy. If you missed the
"acute exacerbation" period in the
question, all of the options will
seem to be correct. Also, if you
read option 4 quickly you may have
missed "just past the point of pain"
and thought it sounded reasonable.
But it is an incorrect action.

Rationales	**Test-Taking Tips**

to 72 hours after the initial event, and heat usually is applied as dry rather than moist compresses. Moist compresses are more often used for pulled or strained muscles. In the acute phase, completing range-of-motion exercises four times a day would irritate the affected joint. These actions are appropriate after the inflammation has resolved. For client comfort and to prevent further damage, exercise the arthritic joint only to the point of pain, not beyond.

7. Correct answer: 2

The nurse would expect the nursing assistant to use gloves for protection when the mouth area requires wiping. Note that the client slobbers and has poor chewing. Therefore, it is likely that food will fall out of the oral cavity as the client chews. A gown and mask might be needed if the client spits out food and fluids during meals.

Careful reading is required to make this the easy question that it is. Remember when specific information is given in the stem, it can lead you to the right answer by giving you a clue.

8. Correct answer: 2

Of the given answers, option 2, an elevated ESR, indicates an abnormal process present in the body. If you selected option 1, you may have ready only the initial part of the option "antibody titers," which is an appropriate test for this problem. Antinuclear antibodies, ANA, are positive in rheumatoid arthritis and many other autoimmune diseases. Option 3 typically

Avoid reading too quickly only for test identification without the given direction of change in the test. This action leads you to select option 1. Then you may be tempted to skip reading the other options because you know titers are important in rheumatoid arthritis. When this happens, go to option 4 and read the options in reverse order to force yourself to read all of the options and to increase your thinking skills.

indicates a severe infection or
leukemia if immature WBCs
are prevalent. Option 4 is
incorrect because the
hematocrit is usually three
times the hemoglobin if the
RBCs are within normal
structure and function.

9. Correct answer: 1

Significant decreases in the BP
and increases in the HR are
indications of a reaction to any
substance. No information is
given in the stem for options 2,
3, or 4 to be considered
correct. More details would
need to be provided such as the
dose, administration rate, or
frequency.

If you have no idea of a correct
answer, take an educated guess.
Significant changes in BP and HR
indicate sudden change in bodily
functions. An IV medication is
more likely to result in significant
changes in vital signs than
medications given by other routes.
Select the option with an allergic
reaction.

10. Correct answer: 2

The client has been exposed to
rabid agents and needs
immediate protection, which
immune serum globulins
provide. This is similar to
being exposed to hepatitis B,
with the need for hepatitis
immune globulin. Option 1 is
an incorrect statement.
Vaccines provide active
acquired immunity, which
usually takes from 4 to 8
weeks before clients are
protected. Option 3 is incorrect
because the half-life has
nothing to do with the
medication, and the
terminology "passive acquired
immunity" is not usually used.
Also, passive immunity does
not occur in only 72 hours.
Option 4 is incorrect. In
injections for rabies exposure
the immune globulin is given

In the terms vaccine and immune
globulin, an "A," for Active
immunity, is found only in the word
vAccine. Thus, associate the fact
that vAccines provide Active
immunity, which means the body
Actively produces substances to
protect the client. This Action
usually takes a minimum of a few
weeks before the client is protected
from an antigen. In passive
immunity such as the injection of
immune globulins, the protective
substances are injected into the
body and provide immediate
protection against the antigen.

at same time as the first rabies
vaccine. The method is to
infiltrate the wound with a
half-dose of the immune
globulin, then administer the
rest IM. Then, a 1-ml dose of
vaccine is given on days 3, 7,
14, and 28.

14

Essential Odds and Ends

FAST FACTS

This chapter offers information about disease processes that may not commonly be seen in the acute clinical setting. The diagnosis will be briefly discussed, and then you may be directed to another area in the book for discussion of the client's nursing care with the particular problem.

I. Bell's palsy
A. **Definition—a disorder of the seventh cranial nerve; may be related to a reactivation of the herpes simplex virus, usually from chicken pox**
B. **Common symptoms**
   1. Initial onset may be preceded by an outbreak of herpes vesicle around the ear
   2. Fever
   3. Tinnitus
   4. Hearing deficit
   5. Flaccidity on one side of the face
   6. Drooping of the mouth and drooling on the affected side
   7. Inability to close the affected eye which has excessive tearing
   8. Muscle weakness on the affected side
C. **Diagnostic studies—EMG**
D. **Treatment**
   1. Corticosteroids
   2. Analgesics
   3. Acyclovir (Zovirax)
   4. Alternative therapies

E. **Nursing Interventions**
1. Provide pain relief
2. Teach to chew on unaffected side
3. Teach client to wear dark glasses for eye protection
4. Provide supportive care for weeks up to months

II. Diabetes insipidus

A. **Definition—a syndrome distinguished by the inability of the kidneys to concentrate urine. The syndrome is due to a relative or an absolute deficiency in antidiuretic hormone (ADH) or to a lack of renal responsiveness to the circulatory ADH. The most common cause is injury to the posterior lobe of the pituitary gland (neurohypophysis) by surgery or trauma. Other causes are idiopathic or familial/congenital.**

B. **Common findings**
1. Thirst with excessive water intake (polydipsia)
2. Urine output of 5 to 15 L/day (polyuria)
3. Low specific gravity
4. High serum sodium
5. Note that if fluid volumes are not maintained the client will suffer from hypovolemic shock from severe dehydration

C. **Diagnostic studies**
1. Attempt to find the source to diagnose the type: neurogenic, nephrogenic, dipsogenic, or gestagenic
2. Urine—low specific gravity
3. Water-deprivation test

D. **Treatment**
1. IV fluid replacement
2. Hormone replacement of ADH (vasopressin) subcutaneous (SC), IM, or IV
3. Desmopressin acetate (DDAVP) nasally for long-term therapy

E. **Nursing interventions**
1. Monitor fluid volume balance carefully
2. Teach proper administration of long-term medication

III. Disseminated intravascular coagulation (DIC)

A. **Definition—a serious bleeding disorder caused by excess clotting initiated by another condition (shock, septicemia, tissue disruptions such as burns, transfusion reactions). DIC is always a secondary diagnosis and not a primary problem.**

B. **Common symptoms—caused by consumption of clotting factors and platelets in the microcirculation with a lack of platelets and clotting factors in the microcirculation**
1. Bleeding with no overt cause
2. Weakness
3. Fever

    4. Pallor

    5. Petechiae

    6. Tachycardia with hypotension

C. Diagnostic studies

    1. PT

    2. APTT

    3. Fibrin split product (FSP) assay, also called fibrin degradation product (FDP) assay—increased owing to breakdown of excessive fibrin

    4. D-dimer—assesses both thrombin and plasmin activity. D-dimer is a fibrin degradation fragment that is made through fibrinolysis. As plasmin acts on the fibrin polymer clot, FDPs and D-dimer are produced.

        a. Provides a highly specific measurement for the amount of fibrin degradation. Normal plasma does not have detectable amounts of fragment D-dimer.

        b. Provides a simple and confirmatory test for DIC. Positive results of the D-dimer assay correlate with those of the FDP assay. The D-dimer assay is more specific but less sensitive than the FDP assay. Therefore, combining the FDP and D-dimer assays provides highly sensitive and specific tests for recognizing DIC in a client.

D. Treatment—controversial

    1. Supportive therapy as needed

    2. Treatment of the underlying cause if possible

    3. Platelets

    4. Cryoprecipitate

    5. Fresh frozen plasma

    6. Heparin—to replace antithrombin III, a cofactor of heparin

E. Nursing Intervention would be very much like the care of the client with anemia found in Chapter 6, pp. 125-126.

IV. Guillain-Barré syndrome

A. Definition—postinfection ascending polyneuropathic paralysis, loss of myelin, edema and inflammation of the affected nerves, and cell-mediated immunologic reaction. This syndrome frequently follows a viral infection or trauma. Some clients recover fully and others only partially.

B. Common symptoms

    1. Occur 1 to 3 weeks after a viral syndrome

    2. Weakness to paralysis of lower extremities that has an ascending pattern of movement

    3. Numbness and tingling in extremities

    4. Autonomic nervous system dysfunction (orthostatic hypotension, bradycardia, bowel and bladder dysfunction)

    5. Pain—paresthesias and muscle aches and cramps, which are worse at night

6. Complication—respiratory failure from ascending muscular paralysis
C. **Diagnostic studies**
   1. Spinal tap with CSF evaluation
   2. EMG
D. **Treatment**
   1. Plasmapheresis
   2. Supportive care—ventilation as necessary from weeks to months
   3. Treatment with high-dose immunoglobulins
E. **Nursing Interventions would be much like the care of the client with degenerative neurologic disorders as discussed in Chapter 1, pp. 26-27**

V. Meniere's disease
A. **Definition—idiopathic disease of the inner ear. The hallmark manifestations are an attack of prostrating vertigo with nausea and vomiting, worsening tinnitus, and sensory hearing loss with a feeling of fullness or pressure in the affected ear.**
B. **Common recurrent findings**
   1. Vertigo
   2. Tinnitus
   3. Hearing loss
   4. Feeling of fullness in the ear
   5. May affect both ears
   6. Begins between 30 and 60 years of age
   7. May last from a few hours to a day and then gradually subside
   8. Between acute attacks the person suffers progressive hearing loss and a persistent background humming and has an intolerance to loud noises
C. **Diagnostic studies**
   1. Audiometric studies (hearing tests)
   2. Vestibular tests
   3. Glycerol test
D. **Treatment**
   1. Sedatives—diazepam (Valium)
   2. Anticholinergics (atropine)
   3. Antihistamines—diphenhydramine hydrochloride (Benadryl)
   4. Diuretics during the acute attack
   5. Reduced caffeine, nicotine, and alcohol
   6. Low-sodium diet to minimize fluid retention
E. **Nursing Interventions can be found in Chapter 1 (Hearing Loss), pp. 34-35**

VI. Obstructive sleep apnea
A. **Definition—cessation of inhalation during sleep, usually related to the soft palate or the tongue obstructing the pharynx. Severe hypoxemia occurs during the obstruction and may occur as many as 600 times during a night's sleep.**

   B. **Common symptoms**
   1. Frequent awakening during sleep
   2. Insomnia
   3. Excessive sleepiness during the day
   4. Loud snoring
   5. Morning headaches
   6. Irritability
   C. **Diagnostic studies**
   1. Polysomnography
      a. Chest and abdominal air movement
      b. Oral and nasal airflow
      c. SaO_2
      d. Ocular movements
      e. HR and heart rhythms
      f. All of these are evaluated during a sleep-stage test, which includes all stages of sleep
   D. **Treatment**
   1. No alcohol or sedatives before bed
   2. Weight loss
   3. Nasal continuous positive airway pressure (n-CPAP)—to keep airway open
   4. Surgical excision of pharyngeal and palate tissue
   E. **Nursing interventions**
   1. Teaching needs
      a. Use of n-CPAP
      b. Weight loss and diet control
      c. Avoid alcohol and sedatives 3 to 4 hours before bed
   2. Support groups for clients with sleep apnea
   3. Assessment for depression and encouragement for client to obtain medical evaluation

VII. Paget's disease

   A. **Definition—skeletal bone disorder characterized by replacement of normal marrow by fibrous connective tissue. The bone is then weaker, resulting in deformities. Abnormalities are seen in the pelvis, long bones, spine, ribs, sternum, and cranium.**
   1. Beware—do not get this confused with the "Paget's disease of the nipple," which is nipple cancer. If the question is about *"Paget's disease,"* then think of the skeletal bone problem.
   B. **Common symptoms**
   1. May be asymptomatic for years
   2. Skeletal pain
   3. Fatigue
   4. Waddling gait
   5. Pathologic fractures

C. **Diagnostic studies**
1. X-ray films—abnormal bone contour with thickened bone cortex
2. Serum alkaline phosphatase levels—elevated

D. **Treatment**
1. Supportive care
2. Surgery to correct bone deformities
3. Calcitonin to decrease bone changes
4. Alendronate sodium (Fosamax) and tiludronate disodium (Skelid) to help reduce bone resorption of calcium

E. **Nursing interventions**
1. Teaching needs
   a. Firm mattress for sleeping
   b. Instructions on how to wear braces
   c. Instructions on activities not to engage in such as contact sports
   d. Analgesics and muscle relaxants
   e. Balanced nutrition high in vitamin D, calcium, and protein

VIII. Syndrome of inappropriate secretion of antidiuretic hormone (SIADH); Schwartz-Bartter syndrome

A. **Definition—antidiuretic hormone is released in excess levels, resulting in decreased urine output. This syndrome is caused by malignancies, various drugs, hypothyroidism, and head trauma resulting in increased ICP.**

B. **Common symptoms**
1. Hyponatremia—low sodium
2. Muscle cramps and weakness
3. Low urinary output
4. Mental confusion from cerebral edema and low serum sodium

C. **Diagnostic studies**
1. Simultaneous urine and serum osmolality
2. Serum sodium decreased below 130
3. Decreased BUN
4. Decreased creatinine clearance

D. **Treatment**
1. Fluid restrictions
2. Hypertonic saline solution
3. Diuretics

E. **Nursing Interventions**
1. Accurate hourly intake and output
2. Daily weights
3. Careful neurologic assessment
4. Fluid restrictions
5. Elevated head of bed
6. Seizure precautions

IX. Systemic inflammatory response syndrome (SIRS) and multiple organ dysfunction syndrome (MODS)

A. **Definitions**—SIRS is an abnormal response to several bodily insults characterized by widespread inflammation in organs not in close proximity to the original insults. MODS is progressive failure of more than one organ as a result of SIRS, and may also be a consequence of trauma or sepsis.

B. **Common symptoms**
1. HR under 60 beats per minute
2. Systolic BP under 60 mm Hg
3. Respiratory distress or arrest—symptoms of ARDS
4. Decreased urine output
5. CNS depression

C. **Diagnostic studies**
1. ABGs—abnormal
2. BUN and creatinine—elevated
3. Clotting studies—abnormal
4. Serum bilirubin—elevated

D. **Treatment—prognosis is poor, with a mortality rate of 95%**
1. Maintain ventilatory support and attempt normalization of ABGs
2. Prevent infection
3. Provide nutritional support
4. Support failing organs with renal dialysis, and so forth

E. **Nursing interventions will be very much like the care of the client with ARDS discussed in Chapter 5, pp. 158-159**

X. Trigeminal neuralgia (tic douloureux)

A. **Definition—disorder of the fifth cranial nerve**

B. **Common symptoms**
1. Severe pain in the lip, upper or lower gums, cheek, forehead, or side of the nose
2. Twitching, grimacing, blinking, or tearing of the eye occurs during an acute attack
3. Episodes may have a triggering mechanism and may last for 2 to 3 minutes

C. **Diagnostic studies**
1. CT scan of the head
2. Arteriography
3. Spinal tap with CSF evaluation

D. **Treatment**
1. Phenytoin (Dilantin), carbamazepine (Tegretol), or valproic acid (Depakene)
2. Nerve blocking
3. Glycerol injection into the trigeminal nerve
4. Several intracranial surgical approaches

E. **Nursing interventions—care of the client is similar to the client having intracranial surgery (Chapter 1, pp. 15-16)**

Glossary

Abduction   Moving a part of the body away from the midline of the body. (Think of abduction: moving people away from their home.)

Absorption   Small particles of digested food cross the membranes of the intestines and enter the bloodstream.

Adduction   Moving a part of the body toward the midline of the body. (Use the first three letters "add" to think of "adding" to the body.)

Afterload   Resistance to ventricular emptying from forces that oppose ventricular ejection of blood, that is, aortic size, blood pressure, and blood viscosity.

Amenorrhea   Absence of menstruation.

Antibodies   Also known as immunoglobulins. They are responsible for the control or destruction of nonself antigens.

Antigens   Protein markers on cells that identify a cell as self or nonself.

Ataxia   An unsteady or staggering gait, postural imbalance, or both; impaired ability to coordinate movement.

Azotemia   Toxic condition in which there exists an excess of nitrogenous waste (urea nitrogen) in the blood.

B lymphocytes   Lymphocytes that do not mature in the thymus of two varieties: memory cells, which are responsible for storing information about nonself antigens and the appropriate response, and (2) plasma cells, which produce the immunoglobulins also known as antibodies.

Cardiac output (CO)   The amount of blood ejected from the ventricles; CO = Heart rate × Stroke volume.

Circumscribed   A specified area limited by a border.

Client education   Process of meeting the client's needs for the acquisition of skills, knowledge, or attitudes to deal with a pathologic condition in the arenas of primary, secondary, or tertiary health promotion as based on the prior skills, knowledge, and attitudes of the client.

Complement   A group of plasma proteins responsible for enhancing the initial steps of the inflammatory response and mediating the antigen-antibody response; also acts as an opsonin for phagocytosis.

Conduction   The movement of formed electrical impulses through the heart; these impulses stimulate the chambers of the heart to contract.

Contractility The force of myocardial contraction.

Core temperature Temperature of the body in the chest, abdomen, and head.

Diastole Relaxation of the chambers of the heart results in filling of the chambers; the desired diastolic blood pressure is under 90 mm Hg.

Diffusion The movement of solutes across a semipermeable membrane from an area of higher concentration to an area of lower concentration until an equal distribution is established between the two areas.

Digestion Breaking down of proteins, polysaccharides, and fat through the action of acids and enzymes secreted into the gastrointestinal tract.

Diurnal A pattern of the rise and fall of hormone levels in the blood within a 24-hour time period.

Dysmenorrhea Painful menstruation.

Dysphagia Difficulty swallowing.

Dysuria Painful urination.

Ecchymosis Discoloration of the skin as a result of blood extravasating into the area; a bruise. The initial color is purplish blue. After about 3 to 5 days the color changes to yellowish green.

Efflux Movement of urine from the kidneys through the ureter to the bladder.

Endocrine glands These glands secrete their hormones directly into the bloodstream or lymph system.

Epididymitis Acute or chronic inflammation of the epididymis from venereal disease, urinary tract infection, prostatitis, or after a prostatectomy.

Equilibrium The body's orientation in space.

Erythema Redness.

Eschar Scab or dried crust resulting from burns, infection, or excoriation of the skin.

Exhalation The second phase of ventilation; air exiting the lungs is a passive maneuver.

Exocrine glands These glands secrete hormones through a duct into the gastrointestinal tract.

Frequency The feeling of a need to void often.

Glomerular filtration rate (GFR) The amount of fluid that is passed through all of the nephrons in one minute.

Hemostasis Termination of bleeding by chemical or mechanical means.

Homeostasis A balance or constancy in the internal functioning of the body.

Hormone A chemical agent secreted by the endocrine glands into the blood; it is responsible for eliciting a response from a target organ or structure.

Hypoxemia Oxygen pressure (PO_2) is less than 80 mm Hg in arterial blood.

Hypoxia Cellular deprivation of oxygen.

Immunocompetence Appropriate or intact functioning of the immune system.

Immunodeficiency Incompetence of the immune system; inability to destroy or control invading organisms.

Incontinence Uncontrolled leakage of urine from the bladder; refer to Ch. 8, pp. 276, 277 for specific definitions of incontinence.

Indurated Hardened, raised tissue.

Inspiration The first phase of ventilation; air entering the lungs is an active maneuver.

Lesion Change in the normal skin structure.

Leukocytes   White blood cells (WBCs), the active components of inflammatory and the immune response (Box 13-1).

Macule   A small, flat, discoloration of the skin such as a freckle or rash.

Menorrhagia   Abnormally heavy menstruation.

Metrorrhagia   Uterine bleeding not associated with menstruation.

Micturition   Urination, voiding; the process of emptying the bladder.

Mobility   The ability to move or have motion.

Motility   The action of peristalsis of the bowel or the urinary tract.

Negative feedback   A method the body uses to bring the hormone to an appropriate level, but not to allow it to increase to an unacceptable level.

Nerve impulse   Depolarization and repolarization of a neuron generated by a chemical or physical stimulus.

Neurotransmitter   Chemical secreted by the neuron axon terminals that is responsible for transmission of nerve impulses across synapses or spaces between either the neurons, neurons and muscle fibers, or neurons and glandular cells.

Nocturia   The urge to urinate in the middle of the night, usually several times during the night.

Nodule   A small, rounded mass.

Nonspecific immune response   Immediate response to invading organisms with neutrophils and macrophages; the result is inflammation.

Nursing process   The process used as the basis of nursing practice, which includes five steps: (1) assessment, (2) selection of a nursing diagnosis, (3) planning, (4) intervention, and (5) evaluation.

Opsonins   Substances that coat nonself antigens making them more susceptible to phagocytosis.

Osmosis   The movement of a pure solvent, such as water, across a semipermeable membrane from an area with a lower solute content to one with a higher solute content.

Papule   A solid, raised lesion less than one centimeter in size.

Paresthesias   A feeling of pins and needles or numbness in the extremities.

Perfusion   The flow of blood through blood vessels.

Peripheral vascular resistance (PVR)   Also called afterload. An impedance to blood flow from the ventricles; it involves three factors: (1) aortic pressure, (2) vessel size, and (3) blood viscosity.

Peristalsis   Rhythmic contraction of the smooth muscles of the gastrointestinal tract responsible for movement of solid matter through the tract.

Petechiae   Flat, tiny, red or purple spots that appear on the skin, usually the upper anterior chest wall or under the upper arms, as a result of tiny hemorrhages in the dermal or mucosal layer.

Phagocytosis   Cells engulf microorganisms for destruction and cellular debris for removal.

Plasma   Liquid portion of the blood.

Preload   Volume of blood returning to the atria; also referred to as the end-diastolic volume of the ventricles--stretching of the chamber wall by chamber volume increases resistance in the wall muscle and subsequently the contractile force.

Proprioception An individual's ability to sense body position and movement.

Pruritus Itching.

Purpura A bleeding disorder that results in bleeding under the skin or mucous membranes; produces ecchymosis or petechiae.

Range of motion Degree of movement in a joint.

Reflex Protective, learned response to a change in the pattern or frequency of sensory impulses that reach the spinal cord, such as pain.

Reflux Movement of urine in a backward motion from the bladder into the ureters and possibly to the kidneys.

Respiration The exchange of oxygen and carbon dioxide at the alveolar and cellular levels.

Retention Inability to empty the bladder completely.

Sebum Oil produced by the sebaceous glands.

Secretion Release of a chemical substance from gland cells of the gastrointestinal system.

Serum Plasma that has had some substances removed.

Specific immune response Also known as cell-mediated immunity. Response by lymphocytes programmed to respond to nonself antigens.

Stem cells Also called parent cells in bone marrow. They are responsible for producing leukocytes.

Systole Contractions of the chambers of the heart result in emptying of the chambers; desired systolic blood pressure is under 140 mm Hg.

T lymphocytes Lymphocytes that mature and establish various roles in the thymus; the varieties of T lymphocytes are helper cells, suppressor cells, natural killer cells, and cytotoxic cells.

Target gland Glands affected by the action of a hormone from another gland.

Tidal volume The volume of air inspired and then exhaled during one ventilation; approximately 600 to 800 ml.

Uremia Presence of excess urea and other waste in the blood.

Urgency The feeling of a need to void immediately.

Urticaria Hives.

Vasoconstriction Contraction or squeezing of the walls of the blood vessels causing a decrease in diameter of the vessel lumen.

Vasoconstrictor Any agent that will cause contraction of the walls of blood vessels.

Vasodilation Expansion of the size of a blood vessel, causing an increase in the diameter of the lumen of the vessel.

Vasodilator Any agent that will cause an increase in the diameter of the lumen of a blood vessel.

Ventilation Air moving in and out of the lungs and includes the alveolar sacs.

Vesicle Small, thin-walled, fluid-filled, raised lesion, such as a blister.

Wheal A raised, reddened, solid lesion of the skin, usually caused by an allergen.

Work of breathing The amount of energy expended to accomplish ventilation; the respiratory effort.

Bibliography

Banks PA: Acute and chronic pancreatitis. In Feldman M, Sleisenger MH, Scharschmidt BF, eds. *Sleisenger and Fordtrans Gastrointestinal and Liver Disease,* ed 6, Philadelphia, 1998, WB Saunders Co., 809-838.

Beare PG, Myers JL: *Adult Health Nursing,* ed 3, St Louis, 1998, Mosby.

Belcher A: *Blood Disorders,* St Louis, 1993, Mosby.

Belcher A: *Cancer Nursing,* St Louis, 1992, Mosby.

Black JM, Matassarin-Jacobs E: *Luckman & Sorensen's Medical-Surgical Nursing: A Psychophysiologic Approach,* ed 5, Philadelphia, 1997, WB Saunders.

Brundage DJ: *Renal Disorders,* St Louis, 1994, Mosby.

Chipp E, Clanin N, Campbell V: *Neurologic Disorders,* St Louis, 1992, Mosby.

Clark J, Queener S, Karb V: *Pharmocological Basis of Nursing Practice,* ed 6, St Louis, 2000, Mosby.

Deglin JH, Valler and AH: *Davis's Drug Guide for Nurses,* ed 6, Philadelphia, 1999, FA Davis.

Dennison R: *PASS CCRN,* ed 2, St Louis, 2000, Mosby.

Des Jardins T, Burton GC: *Clinical Manifestations and Assessment of Respiratory Disease,* ed 3, St Louis, 1995, Mosby.

Doughty DB: *Gastrointestinal Disorders,* St Louis, 1993, Mosby.

Eliopoulous D: *Gerontological Nursing,* ed 4, Philadelphia, 1997, JB Lippincott.

Gahart B, Nazareno A: *2000 Intravenous Medications,* ed 6, St Louis, 2000, Mosby.

Gray M: *Genitourinary Disorders,* St Louis, 1992, Mosby.

Josephson DL: *Intravenous Infusion Therapy for Nurses,* Albany, 1999, Delmar.

Lewis SM, Heitkemper MM, Dirksen SR: *Medical-Surgical Nursing: Assessment and Management of Clinical Problems,* ed 5, St. Louis, 2000, Mosby.

Mosby's Nursing Drug Reference, St Louis, 2000, Mosby.

Mosby's Medical, Nursing, & Allied Health Dictionary, ed 5, St Louis, 1998, Mosby.

Mudge-Grout CL: *Immunologic Disorders,* St Louis, 1992, Mosby.

Nickolaus M: Diabetes Insipidus: a current perspective. *Critical Care Nurse* (19)6, pp. 18-30.

Pagana KD, Pagana TJ: *Mosby's Manual of Diagnostic and Laboratory Tests,* ed 4, St Louis, 1999, Mosby.

Phipps WJ, Sands JK, Marek JF: *Medical-Surgical Nursing: Concepts and Clinical Practice,* ed 6, St Louis, 1999, Mosby.

Rollant PD: Acing multiple choice exams, American Journal of Nursing Career Guide for 1994, *AJN* 36 (January 1994):18-21.

Rollant PD: *Soar to Success: Do Your Best on Nursing Tests,* St Louis, 1999, Mosby.

Swearingen P: *Manual of Medical-Surgical Nursing Care,* ed 4, St Louis, 1997, Mosby.

Index